DIETARY SUPPLEMENTS

A FRAMEWORK FOR EVALUATING SAFETY

Committee on the Framework for Evaluating the
Safety of Dietary Supplements
Food and Nutrition Board
Board on Life Sciences

INSTITUTE OF MEDICINE *AND*
NATIONAL RESEARCH COUNCIL
OF THE NATIONAL ACADEMIES

THE NATIONAL ACADEMIES PRESS
Washington, D.C.
www.nap.edu

THE NATIONAL ACADEMIES PRESS 500 Fifth STREET, N.W. Washington, DC 20001

NOTICE: The project that is the subject of this report was approved by the Governing Board of the National Research Council, whose members are drawn from the councils of the National Academy of Sciences, the National Academy of Engineering, and the Institute of Medicine. The members of the committee responsible for the report were chosen for their special competences and with regard for appropriate balance.

This study was supported by Contract Number 223-00-2458 between the National Academy of Sciences and the Food and Drug Administration. Additional support came from Institute of Medicine internal funds. Any opinions, findings, conclusions, or recommendations expressed in this publication are those of the author(s) and do not necessarily reflect the views of the organizations or agencies that provided support for the project.

Library of Congress Cataloging-in-Publication Data

Dietary supplements : a framework for evaluating safety / Committee on the Framework for Evaluating the Safety of Dietary Supplements, Food and Nutrition Board [and] Board on Life Sciences.
p. ; cm.
Includes bibliographical references and index.
ISBN 0-309-09110-1 (hardcover)
1. Dietary supplements—Evaluation. 2. Dietary supplements—Toxicology.
[DNLM: 1. United States. Food and Drug Administration. 2. Dietary Supplements—standards—United States. 3. Safety—United States. 4. Government Regulation—United States. 5. Product Surveillance, Postmarketing—methods—United States. QU 145.5 D5639 2004] I. Committee on the Framework for Evaluating the Safety of Dietary Supplements.
RM258.5.D543 2004
613.2′8—dc22
2004022339

Additional copies of this report are available from the National Academies Press, 500 Fifth Street, N.W., Lockbox 285, Washington, DC 20055; (800) 624-6242 or (202) 334-3313 (in the Washington metropolitan area); Internet, http://www.nap.edu.

For more information about the Institute of Medicine, visit the IOM home page at: **www.iom.edu.**

Printed in the United States of America.

Cover photo of red ginger taken by Dr. Aniko Solyom, University of Arizona.

THE NATIONAL ACADEMIES

Advisers to the Nation on Science, Engineering, and Medicine

The **National Academy of Sciences** is a private, nonprofit, self-perpetuating society of distinguished scholars engaged in scientific and engineering research, dedicated to the furtherance of science and technology and to their use for the general welfare. Upon the authority of the charter granted to it by the Congress in 1863, the Academy has a mandate that requires it to advise the federal government on scientific and technical matters. Dr. Bruce M. Alberts is president of the National Academy of Sciences.

The **National Academy of Engineering** was established in 1964, under the charter of the National Academy of Sciences, as a parallel organization of outstanding engineers. It is autonomous in its administration and in the selection of its members, sharing with the National Academy of Sciences the responsibility for advising the federal government. The National Academy of Engineering also sponsors engineering programs aimed at meeting national needs, encourages education and research, and recognizes the superior achievements of engineers. Dr. Wm. A. Wulf is president of the National Academy of Engineering.

The **Institute of Medicine** was established in 1970 by the National Academy of Sciences to secure the services of eminent members of appropriate professions in the examination of policy matters pertaining to the health of the public. The Institute acts under the responsibility given to the National Academy of Sciences by its congressional charter to be an adviser to the federal government and, upon its own initiative, to identify issues of medical care, research, and education. Dr. Harvey V. Fineberg is president of the Institute of Medicine.

The **National Research Council** was organized by the National Academy of Sciences in 1916 to associate the broad community of science and technology with the Academy's purposes of furthering knowledge and advising the federal government. Functioning in accordance with general policies determined by the Academy, the Council has become the principal operating agency of both the National Academy of Sciences and the National Academy of Engineering in providing services to the government, the public, and the scientific and engineering communities. The Council is administered jointly by both Academies and the Institute of Medicine. Dr. Bruce M. Alberts and Dr. Wm. A. Wulf are chair and vice chair, respectively, of the National Research Council.

www.national-academies.org

COMMITTEE ON THE FRAMEWORK FOR EVALUATING THE SAFETY OF DIETARY SUPPLEMENTS

BARBARA O. SCHNEEMAN (*Chair*), Departments of Nutrition and Food Science, Division of Clinical Nutrition and Metabolism, and Office of University Outreach, University of California, Davis

DANIEL L. AZARNOFF, D.L. Azarnoff Associates and Clinical/Regulatory Affairs, Cellegy Pharmaceuticals, South San Francisco, California

CINDY LYNN CHRISTIANSEN, Center for Health Quality, Outcomes, and Economic Research, Bedford V.A. Hospital, and Boston University School of Public Health, Massachusetts

ALICE M. CLARK, Office of Research and Sponsored Programs, University of Mississippi, Oxford

NORMAN R. FARNSWORTH, Department of Medicinal Chemistry and Pharmacognosy, University of Illinois at Chicago

TED GANSLER, Medical Information Strategy, American Cancer Society, Atlanta, Georgia

JAMES E. GIBSON, Department of Pharmacology and Toxicology, The Brody School of Medicine at East Carolina University, North Carolina

STEPHEN A. GOLDMAN, Stephen A. Goldman Consulting Services, LLC, Morris Plains, New Jersey

PHILIP S. GUZELIAN, Department of Medicine, University of Colorado Health Sciences Center, Denver

ELIZABETH JEFFERY, Department of Food Science and Human Nutrition, University of Illinois at Urbana-Champaign

LOREN D. KOLLER, Loren Koller and Associates, LLC, Corvallis, Oregon

JOSEPH LAU, Institute for Clinical Research and Health Policy Studies, Tufts New England Medical Center, Boston, Massachusetts

RUSSELL J. MOLYNEUX, USDA Western Regional Research Center, Albany, California

SUSAN S. PERCIVAL, Department of Food Science and Human Nutrition, University of Florida, Gainesville

CHERYL L. ROCK, Department of Family and Preventive Medicine, University of California, San Diego, La Jolla

JERROLD M. WARD, Division of Intramural Research, National Institute of Allergy and Infectious Diseases, National Institutes of Health, Bethesda, Maryland

Consultants

LEWIS A. GROSSMAN, Washington College of Law, American University, Washington, D.C.
JOSEPH RODRICKS, ENVIRON International, Arlington, Virginia

Staff

ALLISON A. YATES, Study Director
MARILEE SHELTON-DAVENPORT, Program Officer
JANICE OKITA, Program Officer
CRYSTAL RASNAKE, Research Assistant
SANAIT TESFAGIORGIS, Senior Project Assistant

PROTOTYPE MONOGRAPHS

Chaparral Consultants

CYNTHIA K. ARON, University of Massachusetts Memorial Medical Center, Worcester

MARILYN BARRET, Pharmacognosy Consulting Services, San Carlos, California

CARL K. WINTER, Department of Food Science and Technology, University of California, Davis

Chromium Picolinate Consultants

AARON BARCHOWSKY, Department of Pharmacology and Toxicology, Dartmouth Medical School, Hanover, New Hampshire

MAX COSTA, Department of Environmental Medicine, New York University Medical School, New York City

JIM K. LIU, College of Pharmacy, University of New Mexico, Albuquerque

STEVEN R. PATIERNO, Department of Pharmacology, George Washington University School of Medicine, Washington, D.C.

STEVEN R. SMITH, Pennington Biomedical Research Center, Louisiana State University, Baton Rouge

BARBARA STOECKER, Department of Nutritional Sciences, Oklahoma State University, Stillwater

Glucosamine Consultants

H.B. "SKIP" MATTHEWS, Consultant, Hertford, North Carolina

TIMOTHY EDWARD McALINDON, Boston University School of Medicine, Massachusetts

DONALD ALLAN McCLAIN, Division of Endocrinology and Metabolism, University of Utah School of Medicine, Salt Lake City

Melatonin Consultants

ANITA CAVALLO, Cincinnati Children's Hospital Medical Center, Cincinnati, Ohio

STANLEY T. OMAYE, Department of Nutrition, University of Nevada, Reno

PHYLLIS C. ZEE, Neurobiology and Physiology, Northwestern University Institute for Neuroscience, Chicago, Illinois

Saw Palmetto Consultants

SHUTSUNG LIAO, Ben May Institute, University of Chicago, Chicago, Illinois
LEONARD S. MARKS, Urological Sciences Research Foundation, Culver City, California
STEPHEN H. SAFE, Department of Veterinary Physiology and Pharmacology, Texas A&M University, College Station

Shark Cartilage Consultants

SAMUEL M. COHEN, Department of Pathology and Microbiology, University of Nebraska Medical Center, Omaha
SUSAN E. CRAWFORD, Department of Pathology, Northwestern University Medical School, Chicago, Illinois
JOSEPH A. SCIMECA, General Mills, Inc., St. Louis Park, Minnesota
KIN-PING WONG, College of Science and Mathematics, California State University, Fresno

FOOD AND NUTRITION BOARD

Preface

The Committee on the Framework for Evaluating the Safety of Dietary Supplements was asked to develop a framework for use by the Food and Drug Administration (FDA) to evaluate the safety of dietary supplement ingredients (see Appendix B for scope of work). It was to include, from a science-based perspective, a system for prioritizing review of dietary supplement ingredients that could be extended to new ingredients as notifications regarding intent to market are submitted by manufacturers. Although evaluation of data regarding the efficacy of such ingredients to maintain health is of interest to many, a review of these data was specifically not included in the charge to the committee.

Once a proposed framework was constructed, FDA requested that it be made available to the dietary supplement industry and other stakeholders for review and comment. In addition, it requested that six prototype safety monographs be developed using the proposed framework. In July 2002, the proposed framework was released for comment, along with the list and a brief rationale for which six dietary supplement ingredients were to undergo a safety review and development of a prototype safety monograph. The committee valued the input received regarding the workability and utility of the proposed framework (see summary in Appendix B). Subsequently, new members with expertise in toxicology, natural product chemistry, pharmacokinetics, and pharmacoepidemiology were added to the committee and several aspects of the proposed framework were revised.

Included in the proposed framework released in July 2002 was a requirement that, prior to the completion of a monograph, there would be a sharing of information obtained to date on the dietary supplement ingredient under review and a request for additional information regarding its safety. Thus during the fall and early spring of 2002–2003, comments were received on the six prototype monographs as well as on the framework itself.

What follows in this report is a framework for prioritizing and evaluating the safety of dietary supplements based on existing information available to FDA and others. This framework, the primary work of the committee, was developed in the context of the current law regulating dietary supplements, the Dietary Supplement Health and Education Act of 1994 (DSHEA). It has been nearly 10 years since Congress passed DSHEA, and considerable experience has been gained in attempting to protect public health under its provisions. Consequently, in the process of completing our task, the committee identified several ways that the law could be more effective in meeting the goal of protecting public health, and these findings and recommendations are included in this report. Although some might consider such recommendations to be outside the scope of the task, the committee felt it had gained valuable insight into this challenging task through its work on the framework and felt it was important to convey this information to policy-makers.

Although this study is under the primary management of the staff of the Food and Nutrition Board (FNB) of the Institute of Medicine (IOM), it has been conducted as a collaborative project within the National Academies by the FNB and the Board on Life Sciences (BLS) of the Division of Earth and Life Studies of the National Research Council (NRC).

The committee was assisted in its task by the invaluable contributions of a number of individuals. Christine Lewis Taylor, Ph.D., Director of FDA's Office of Nutritional Products, Dietary Supplements, and Labeling and the FDA's Project Officer for this project; Susan Walker, M.D., Director of the Division of Dietary Supplement Programs; and Elizabeth Yetley, Ph.D., Lead Scientist for Nutrition, all from the Center for Food Safety and Applied Nutrition of FDA, met with the committee in open session at almost every meeting to respond to questions and provide insight into what would be useful to the agency in developing the framework. We appreciated their clear presentations about the committee's task.

The committee also recognizes the significant contributions made by two former members of the committee, Lars Noah of the University of Florida and Adriane Fugh-Berman of George Washington University, who resigned during the development of the initial report released for comment in 2002; their insights were very valuable to the initial thinking of the proposed process. We also gratefully acknowledge the significant assistance of the four consultants: Dr. Kenneth Fisher, now with the Office of Dietary Supplements at the National Institutes of Health, who assisted in the early development of the proposed framework report; Dr. Edward Bortnichak,

Sanofi-Synthelabo, who was also involved in the early phases; Mr. Lewis Grossman, American University, who came into the project to assist after Mr. Noah resigned and guided us through the areas of food and drug law; and Dr. Joseph Rodricks of Environ International, who provided significant assistance in how risk assessment and toxicology are applied to chemicals and other substances. We also gratefully appreciate the assistance of Stephen F. McNamara of Hyman, Phelps, and McNamara, for his early technical review of Chapter 1.

During the development of the prototype monographs, we were fortunate to have outstanding experts as consultants who participated in the working groups on the ingredients reviewed. Their input was invaluable for the monograph development which also helped the committee rethink aspects of the framework. These experts are listed in the front of this report, and we do appreciate their assistance.

The committee was greatly assisted by the very able work of Dr. Marilee Shelton-Davenport, program officer for BLS, who has provided major and critical assistance in the management and conceptual development of the framework; her efforts to move the project forward have been key to the process. Dr. Janice Rice Okita, who served as the monographer for the project, provided the resources, knowledge, and organizational skills to help the working groups complete their tasks in a timely manner. Throughout all aspects of the project Dr. Allison A. Yates, Study Director, has provided valuable insight and input for accomplishing the task of the committee. We also greatly appreciate the able and dedicated assistance of FNB research associates Alice Vorosmarti and Vivica Kraak, as well as senior project assistant Sybil Boggis, who assisted in the early phases with the proposed framework, and most recently the significant dedication and assistance of Crystal Rasnake, research assistant for the second phase of the study and for the monograph documentation. Thanks also go to Sanait Tesfagiorgis, senior project assistant, who assisted with the completion of this final report; Gail Spears for her editorial assistance; Gary Walker and Elisabeth Rimaud for financial management; and members of IOM's Office of Reports and Communication for assistance in the production and dissemination of the report.

This report has been reviewed in draft form by individuals chosen for their diverse perspectives and technical expertise, in accordance with procedures approved by the NRC's Report Review Committee. The purpose of this independent review is to provide candid and critical comments that will assist the institution in making its published report as sound as possible and to ensure that the report meets institutional standards for objectivity, evidence, and responsiveness to the study charge. The review comments and draft manuscript remain confidential to protect the integrity of the deliberative process. We wish to thank the following individuals for their review of this report:

Neal L. Benowitz, University of California, San Francisco; Joseph M. Betz, National Institutes of Health; Steven Dentali, Dentali Associates; John Edgar, Honorary Fellow, CSIRO Livestock Industries; Kenneth D. Fisher, KD Consultants; Freddie Ann Hoffman, HeteroGeneity, LLC; Marvin M. Lipman, Consumers Union of U.S., Inc.; Richard A. Merrill, The University of Virginia and Covington & Burling; Robert M. Russell, Tufts University; Meir Stampfer, Harvard University; Brian L. Strom, University of Pennsylvania; and Roy Upton, American Herbal Pharmacopoeia.

Although the reviewers listed above have provided many constructive comments and suggestions, they were not asked to endorse the conclusions or recommendations nor did they see the final draft of the report before its release. The review of this report was overseen by Sanford A. Miller, Virginia Polytechnic Institute and State University, coordinator, appointed by the IOM, and Ronald Estabrook, The University of Texas Southwestern Medical Center at Dallas, monitor, appointed by the NRC's Report Review Committee. The coordinator and monitor were responsible for making certain that an independent examination of this report was carried out in accordance with institutional procedures and that all review comments were carefully considered. Responsibility for the final content of this report rests entirely with the authoring committee and the institution.

As a final note, I extend the appreciation and respect of the committee to our Study Director, Dr. Allison Yates, as she completes her position of director of the Food and Nutrition Board and wish her the best in future endeavors. I personally am grateful to my fellow committee members for their commitment to the work of the committee under a rather demanding time schedule. Their quick and constructive responses to the many drafts of the report, their respect for each other's opinion and willingness to find common ground, has made the task possible. It has been a pleasure to work with this entire group.

Barbara O. Schneeman
Committee Chair

Contents

APPENDIXES

DIETARY SUPPLEMENTS

A FRAMEWORK FOR EVALUATING SAFETY

Executive Summary

Consumer interest in health and self-care has expanded the market for a wide range of products, including dietary supplements. Total sales of dietary supplements have grown to over $18 billion per year. As with conventional foods, when used as recommended, many dietary supplements are probably safe. However, increased use of supplements and the broad spectrum of products that qualify as dietary supplements as defined by the Dietary Supplement Health and Education Act of 1994 (DSHEA) make the determination of risk to the health of the consumer, a sizeable task. In addition, the limitations imposed by DSHEA—that the Food and Drug Administration (FDA) determine what is unsafe without requiring that specific information on safety be presented by manufacturers prior to marketing or that manufacturers submit to the FDA any reports they have received on serious adverse events associated with dietary supplement use—serve to make the safety regulation of dietary supplements a sizeable challenge.

THE COMMITTEE'S TASK

FDA must approach evaluating the safety of dietary supplement ingredients in a manner that is cost effective and science based within this regulatory environment. In order to assist in developing such an approach, FDA turned to the Institute of Medicine and the National Research Council of the National Academies to provide a framework for evaluating the safety of dietary supplement ingredients. FDA requested that a committee of experts (1) develop a proposed framework for categorizing and prioritizing dietary supplement ingredients sold in the United States based on safety issues, (2) describe a process for developing a system of scientific reviews, (3) utilize the proposed framework to develop at least six scientific reviews or monographs as prototypes, and (4) revise the framework based on comments received.

The final Framework described in this report is the result of the committee's deliberations over the last 30 months and comments received on the proposed framework issued in July 2002. This Framework includes guidance on considering the various categories of data, taking into consideration methods other expert bodies have used to categorize and review supplement safety issues.

REGULATORY BACKGROUND

Current regulatory approaches to the safety evaluation of dietary supplements in the United States are a product of several key pieces of legislation that span the twentieth century, culminating in the passage of DSHEA in 1994. Since the passage of the 1938 Federal Food, Drug, and Cosmetic Act (FDCA), FDA has wrestled with the most appropriate approach to regulating dietary supplements and several attempts have been met with resistance by industry as well as by segments of the public.

In 1958, the Food Additives Amendment to the FDCA defined food additives and provided that they must undergo a premarket approval process unless they were considered to be generally recognized as safe (GRAS) (Table ES-1). FDA subsequently attempted to regulate the botanical industry by alleging that individual botanical products were unapproved food additives; this approach was subsequently struck down by the courts, recognizing that the applicability of the provisions of the FDCA to products containing a vitamin, mineral, or botanical ingredient (whether it was considered a drug or a food, for example) depended on the product's *intended use*, as determined usually by the labeling and advertising claims for the product.

Congress acted further to delineate FDA's authority by passing DSHEA in 1994. DSHEA established the first comprehensive definition of dietary supplements as legally equivalent to foods (Box ES-1). Most importantly, DSHEA established a regulatory framework for dietary supplements that defined FDA's authority over these products. FDA bears the burden of proof in determining that a dietary supplement ingredient presents a "significant or unreasonable risk of illness or injury" (see Box ES-2) rather than being authorized by statute to require the manufacturer to provide data supporting its safety, as is authorized for substances added to foods[1] or for drugs.

[1]Food ingredients not declared or listed as GRAS.

For new dietary ingredients (those not marketed in the United States prior to passage of DSHEA in 1994), manufacturers or distributors must notify FDA at least 75 days before introducing a dietary supplement ingredient and must provide FDA with the information that is the basis upon which the manufacturer[2] has concluded that dietary supplement or ingredient will reasonably be expected to be safe.

THE SAFETY FRAMEWORK FOR DIETARY SUPPLEMENTS

The definition developed for a "framework" was based on review of other existing frameworks. The Framework consists of two components: (1) a process for prioritizing, evaluating, and describing available information to establish risk of harm, and (2) a set of science-based principles that serve as guidelines for evaluating risk to human health.

For the Framework to be useful, FDA must have adequate resources for implementation. To be credible, it must be scientifically based and include guidelines for obtaining and integrating the totality of the information from many areas of science. Adequate staff with appropriate expertise must be available within FDA to administer the process and evaluate the information.

The Framework described here (see Figure ES-1) characterizes the nature of the scientific evidence that FDA is likely to encounter and describes a process for organizing this evidence to assess where a dietary supplement ingredient[3] lies on a spectrum of concern.[4] As the level of concern increases, so does the potential for a "significant or unreasonable risk," the standard warranting regulation under the FDCA, as amended by DSHEA.

I. The Process

Three major components comprise the process:

- Signal detection
- Initial review of available information
- Integrative evaluation

---

[2]The term manufacturer is used for simplicity, but the statutes related to dietary supplements refer to both manufacturers and distributors, which may or may not be the same for a given dietary supplement ingredient or product.

[3]In order to be consistent with the FDA's regulatory role, the definition of "dietary supplements" used is that of DSHEA (Box ES-1).

[4]The use of the term "concern" denotes a need for further investigation and inquiry by FDA based on a relative level of interest arising from initial information.

TABLE ES-1 Current Status of Foods, Food Additives, Drugs, and Dietary Supplements under the Food and Drug Administration (FDA) Regulations

Status	Dietary Supplements: Containing Ingredients in Use prior to DSHEA[a]	Dietary Supplements: Containing "New" Ingredients Introduced after DSHEA (10/15/94)	Conventional Foods[b]
Premarket approval required	No	No; FDA notification 75 days prior to sale required; FDA has 3 options: (1) respond with objection, (2) respond with no objection, (3) not respond	No[e]
Postmarket reporting or surveillance by industry required	No	No	No
Burden of proof of safety	FDA must demonstrate significant or unreasonable risk of harm to remove product from market	FDA must demonstrate significant or unreasonable risk of harm to prevent product from being marketed	FDA must demonstrate that food is injurious to health to remove product from market

[a] DSHEA = Dietary Supplement and Health Education Act of 1994.

[b] Here "conventional foods" refers to whole agricultural commodities.

[c] This description applies to "new" drugs. Many over-the-counter drugs are regulated under FDA's Over-the-Counter Drug Review procedures, which do not provide for post-marketing surveillance.

[d] GRAS = generally recognized as safe (as defined by the 1958 Food Additives Amendment to Food, Drug, and Cosmetic Act).

	Substances Added to Foods		
New Drugs[c]	GRAS[d] Pre-1958	GRAS Notice (previously, "Affirmation" Petition)	Food Additive Petition
Yes	No	No; manufacturer voluntarily may notify FDA of basis of self-declaration as GRAS[f]; FDA will respond with letter of objection or no objection within 90 days	Yes; with FDA approval becomes an approved food additive
Yes	No	No	Rarely
Manufacturer provides risk/ benefit analysis acceptable to FDA	FDA conducts risk assessment to determine if GRAS recognition should be withdrawn	Manufacturer must demonstrate reasonable certainty of no harm for intended use through scientific procedure or history of use	Manufacturer must present adequate risk assessment to demonstrate reasonable certainty of no harm for intended use

[e] In 2001 FDA proposed in the *Federal Register* (66:4706) a rule requiring marketers of food developed through biotechnology to notify the agency at least 120 days before commercial distribution and to provide information to demonstrate that the product is as safe as its conventional counterpart.

[f] While the final regulations for the notification procedure are not yet published, the interim policy outlined by FDA in the proposed regulations invites interested persons who determine that a substance is GRAS to notify FDA of such GRAS determinations as described in the proposed regulation 21 C.F.R. § 170.36 (b) and (c).

BOX ES-1
Legal Definition of a Dietary Supplement as Defined by the Dietary Supplement Health and Education Act of 1994

The term dietary supplement:

(1) means a product (other than tobacco) intended to supplement the diet that bears or contains one or more of the following dietary ingredients:
   (A) a vitamin;
   (B) a mineral;
   (C) an herb or other botanical;
   (D) an amino acid;
   (E) a dietary substance for use by man to supplement the diet by increasing the total dietary intake; or
   (F) a concentrate, metabolite, constituent, extract, or combination of any ingredient described in clause (A), (B), (C), (D), or (E).

Dietary supplements are further defined as products that are labeled as dietary supplements and are not represented for use as a conventional food or as a sole item of a meal or the diet. Supplements can be marketed for ingestion in a variety of dosage forms including capsule, powder, softgel, gelcap, tablet, liquid, or, indeed, any other form so long as they are not represented as conventional foods or as sole items of a meal or of the diet (FDCA, as amended, § 402).

Signal Detection

Given the large number of dietary supplement ingredients and that dietary supplements are assumed to be safe in general, it is unlikely that FDA will have the resources or need to evaluate each ingredient uniformly. Thus it is assumed that some "signal" will indicate that an ingredient's safety may need to be reviewed. When a signal is detected and the credibility of the signal and its relationship to a serious adverse effect in humans is evaluated, it is up to FDA to decide to take the next step.

Given the significant number of dietary supplement ingredients, **FDA's attention should focus on signals that indicate that a *serious*[5] health problem may result due to ingestion of a dietary supplement ingredient.**

[5]Serious—any experience resulting in any of the following outcomes: death, a life-threatening adverse experience, inpatient hospitalization or prolongation of existing hospitalization, a persistent or significant disability/incapacity, or a congenital anomaly/birth defect. Important medical events that may not result in death, be life-threatening, or require hospitalization may be considered serious when, based upon appropriate medical judgment, they may jeopardize the individual and may require medical or surgical intervention to prevent one of the outcomes previously listed (in accordance with 21 C.F.R. § 600.80 [2002] and 21 C.F.R. § 314.80 [2002]).

BOX ES-2
Safety Standards for Dietary Supplements as Established by DSHEA

Section 4. Safety of Dietary Supplements and Burden of Proof on FDA.

DSHEA amends § 402 (21 U.S.C. 342) by adding the following:

(f) (1) If it is a dietary supplement or contains a dietary ingredient that—

- (A) presents a significant or unreasonable risk of illness or injury under –
  - (i) conditions of use recommended or suggested in labeling, or
  - (ii) if no conditions of use are suggested or recommended in the labeling, under ordinary conditions of use;
- (B) is a new dietary ingredient for which there is inadequate information to provide reasonable assurance that such ingredient does not present a significant or unreasonable risk of illness or injury;
- (C) the Secretary declares to pose an imminent hazard to public health or safety, except that the authority to make such declaration shall not be delegated and the Secretary shall promptly after such a declaration initiate a proceeding in accordance with sections 554 and 556 of title 5, United States Code to affirm or withdraw the declaration; or
- (D) is or contains a dietary ingredient that renders it adulterated under paragraph [402](a)(1) under the conditions of use recommended or suggested in the labeling of such dietary supplement.

In any proceeding under this paragraph, the United States shall bear the burden of proof on each element to show that a dietary supplement is adulterated. The court shall decide any issue under this paragraph on a de novo basis.

(2) Before the Secretary may report to a United States attorney a violation of the paragraph (1)(A) for a civil proceeding, the person against whom such proceeding would be initiated shall be given appropriate notice and the opportunity to present views, orally and in writing, at least 10 days before such notice, with regard to such proceeding.

SOURCE: FDCA, P.L. 75-717 § 402, as amended 21 U.S.C. § 342(f) (2001).

In contrast to reacting based on detecting a signal, FDA may decide to proactively initiate a review of a dietary supplement ingredient due to high prevalence of use in the general population, high level of use by a particularly vulnerable population, or other factors.

One of the requirements of the study was to develop a framework that would include criteria for how the review of safety of dietary supplements

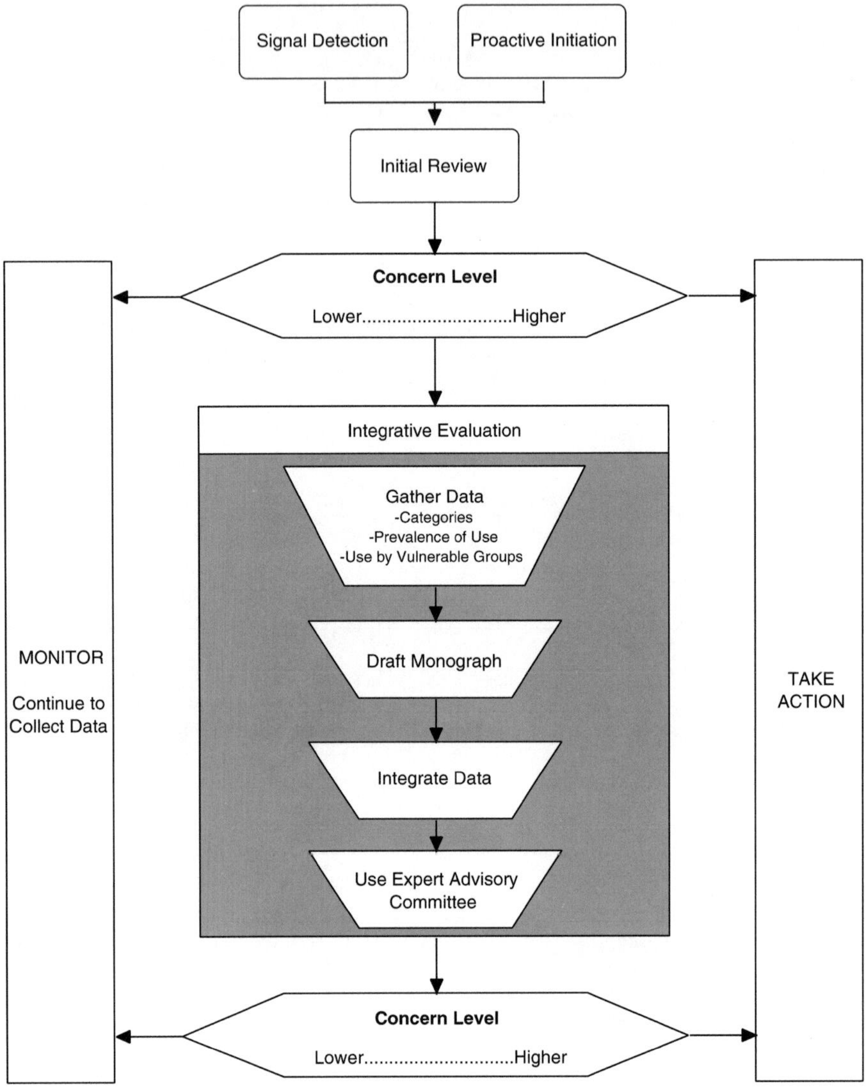

FIGURE ES-1 Diagram of the three components of the Safety Framework: signal detection, identification of level of concern in an initial review, and integrative evaluation, as well as how these components feed into FDA's decision to take action.

and ingredients should be prioritized. However, given the wide variety of dietary supplement ingredients available, the multiple forms of an ingredient for sale (e.g., pills, concentrates, extracts), the voluntary and thus varying nature of the data available on an ingredient, and the wide variety of adverse effects that are possible for dietary supplements and the dependence of such effects on exposure levels, a simple scheme for priority setting is not feasible nor scientifically defensible.

Initial Review of Available Information

The second component of the Framework is to conduct an initial review of available information. First, the nature of the information generating the signal is examined to determine the appropriate level of concern regarding a risk to human health. This component is not envisioned as a detailed analysis of data, but rather as an assessment of the concern level warranted by the nature of the evidence (e.g., quality of the report, applicability to humans, route of exposure) and whether the information raises questions that require further examination.

Second, some effort may be made to gather easily available data to place the detected signal in context; such additional information may come from many sources, including other categories of data. Thus this initial review of the signal information need not be limited to reviewing only the information associated with the signal. If reviewing the signal results in a moderate level of concern, data from other categories should be considered as well.

Since it is assumed by DSHEA that dietary supplements are safe, there should be relatively few dietary supplement ingredients that will be categorized as of higher concern after the initial review and thus warrant further examination. This allows FDA to focus its efforts on the few dietary supplement ingredients that are strong candidates for regulation.

Integrative Evaluation

The third step of the Framework is conducting an integrative evaluation for those dietary supplement ingredients that are deemed to warrant further investigation based on the preliminary data reviewed in the second step. There are four aspects to the Integrative Evaluation component (see Figure ES-1): in-depth literature searching and reviewing, drafting of a safety monograph based on this information, integrating the available data into an analysis to complete the monograph, and possibly referring the draft monograph and accompanying information to an expert advisory committee for additional input prior to FDA determining whether to take regulatory action.

Focused Versus Broad-Based Evaluation. An integrative evaluation may be reactive to the signal and focused in nature in that it is being conducted to examine a specific moderate or high-level concern about an ingredient, or it may be more proactive and broad-based in that it looks for any risk associated with use of the dietary supplement ingredient. For example, a proactive integrative evaluation might be initiated simply because a large percentage of the population is using the ingredient, rather than as a reaction to a particular safety concern.

Drafting a Safety Monograph. In most cases, the integrative evaluation will be documented in a monograph that summarizes the categories of data available and their use in drawing conclusions about the potential risk associated with use of the ingredient; it should include the conclusions of the expert committee and/or FDA. The science-based guiding principles described in the following section of this summary, and explained in detail in Chapters 4 through 10, should be used to reach a decision regarding whether there is an unreasonable risk of illness or injury.

Integrating the Data to Determine Risk. When evidence on a dietary supplement ingredient presents a moderate or higher level of concern relative to this risk, biological plausibility and consistency should be evaluated, especially when independently convincing data are not available. Such an analysis can be represented by creating a causal model diagram—a tool to visualize how the different types of available data link together to establish risk (described in Chapter 10).

The principles described for considering the various categories of data (Chapters 4 through 8), as well as the principles describing how to integrate among and within categories of data (Chapter 10), are applied in the integrative evaluation.

It is expected that FDA may want further input from an advisory committee on many of the dietary supplement ingredients undergoing an integrative evaluation because only ingredients with significant potential for concern are likely to reach this stage.

Decision to Take Action. The results of the integrative evaluation should play a pivotal role in establishing that a supplement ingredient is unsafe. If an advisory committee is used, its findings and rationale should be posted with the monograph on FDA's website. One of the important components of DSHEA was that the public should be educated about dietary supplements. FDA thus has a responsibility to educate consumers about the safety of supplement ingredients, and the public availability of the completed monographs can be an important aspect of the educational process.

Decision to Continue to Monitor. When review of information, either at the initial review step or as a result of an integrative evaluation, indicates a lower level of concern, FDA should continue to monitor information it receives relative to the dietary supplement ingredient. Monitoring consists of either passively watching for new signals of other concerns about the ingredient, as well as maintaining search strategies to routinely search the scientific literature for new data to address specific existing concerns or to identify new concerns. FDA relies on the industry to perform this function in the case of drugs as part of the required postmarketing surveillance; since there is no required postmarketing surveillance for dietary ingredients, ongoing assessment of relevant literature is thus FDA's responsibility.

II. Applying Science-Based Principles to Establish Risk

Given the variety of types of information that are likely to be available, the Framework classifies scientific information into four broad *categories* for use in determining the potential for serious harm for a specific dietary supplement ingredient (see Box ES-3):

- human data,
- animal studies,
- information on related substances, and
- *in vitro* experiments.

Individual chapters describe the types of information that may be available in each of these data categories and considerations for using the different categories of data in evaluating the potential of a dietary supplement ingredient to cause harm (Chapters 4 through 7). Also described are how to consider the potential for dietary supplement interactions with drugs and other xenobiotics[6] (Chapter 8), important considerations that should be factored into evaluations when vulnerable populations consume dietary supplements (Chapter 9), and considerations for integrating the available data from various sources to weave together the information to determine an overall level of concern (Chapter 10) using a causal model diagram.

Spectra of Concern

The Framework also includes a qualitative method to evaluate the nature of the evidence for a specific piece of information within a particular

[6] A chemical substance or compound that is foreign to the human body or to other living organisms.

BOX ES-3
Guiding Principles for Evaluating Data to Determine Unreasonable Risk

- General principles

— Absence of evidence of risk does not indicate that there is no risk.

— Proof of causality or proof of harm is not necessary to determine unreasonable or significant risk.

— Integration of data across different categories of information and types of study design can enhance biological plausibility and identify consistencies, leading to conclusions regarding levels of concern for an adverse event that may be associated with use of a dietary supplement.

- Human data

— A credible report or study finding of a serious adverse event in humans raises concern about the ingredient's safety and requires further information gathering and evaluation; final judgment, however, will require consideration of the totality of the evidence.

— Historical use should not be used as *prima facie* evidence that the ingredient does not cause harm.

— Considerable weight can be given to a lack of adverse events in large, high-quality, randomized clinical trials or epidemiological studies that are adequately powered and designed to detect adverse effects.

- Animal data

— Even in the absence of information on adverse events in humans, evidence of harm from animal studies is often indicative of potential harm to humans.

- Related substances

— Scientific evidence for risk can be obtained by considering if the plant constituents are compounds with established toxicity, are closely related in structure to compounds with established toxicity, or the plant source of the botanical dietary supplement itself is a toxic plant or is taxonomically related to a known toxic plant.

— Supplement ingredients that are endogenous substances or that may be related to endogenous substances should be evaluated to determine if their activities are likely to lead to serious effects. Considerations should include the substance's ability to raise the steady-state concentration of biologically active metabolites in tissues and whether the effect of such increases would be linked to a serious health effect.

- *In vitro* data

— Validated[a] *in vitro* studies can stand alone as independent indicators of risk to human health if a comparable exposure is attained in humans and the *in vitro* effects correlate with a specific adverse health effect in humans or animals.

---

[a] In this report, *in vitro* assays are considered validated when their results have been proven to predict a specific effect in animals and/or humans with reasonable certainty (not necessarily universally accepted or without detractors).

data category (i.e., human, animal, *in vitro*, or information about related substances). Distinguishing characteristics determine where a piece of information falls on the continuum or spectrum of lower level to higher level of concern. This is summarized in diagrams (see the figures in Chapters 4 through 8) referred to as *spectra of concern.*

Evidence that results in a higher level of concern indicates a more immediate priority for investigating further to determine if an unreasonable risk to public health exists. In contrast, a single piece of information resulting in a lower level of concern may suggest continued routine monitoring for new evidence is warranted—monitoring for new evidence that might elevate the level of concern and thus its priority for increased scrutiny.

It is important to recognize that for most dietary supplement ingredients it will be difficult, if not impossible, to find optimal information from all data categories.

General Principles and Concepts When Considering Data

Concentration of Substances at the Sites of Action. A critical factor in determining toxicity of an ingredient is not necessarily the ingested amount, but the concentration of a dietary supplement's active constituents at its sites of action.

Absence of Evidence. Absence of evidence of risk does not indicate that there is no risk. Even if a study showing lack of adverse effects is reported, if the study is not adequately designed to identify risk (e.g., not sufficiently powered, incompletely reported, does not include positive controls, or otherwise has inadequate mechanisms for detecting adverse events), it is not scientifically valid to use such information to mitigate suggested risk from other sources.

Consistency and Biological Plausibility. Data will frequently need to be collated within the same category or across several categories to determine the appropriate overall level of concern. In integrating observations across categories of data, consistency and evidence of biological plausibility should raise the level of concern. This weaving together of available information can be facilitated, and conceptually illustrated, by the use of causal evidence models.

APPLICATION OF THE FRAMEWORK

In order to evaluate the initial framework proposed, prototype monographs were developed for a variety of dietary supplement ingredients.

Significant changes made to the initial framework resulted from this opportunity to test it, as well as from comments received after its initial release for comment (see Appendix B). Summaries of the six prototype[7] monographs are included in Appendixes D through I. The full prototype monographs are available for viewing at www.iom.edu/fnb. Appendixes J and K contain examples of two focused prototype monographs to show how the FDA could focus on determining a level of concern related to one specific adverse effect.

FACTORS INFLUENCING USE OF THE FRAMEWORK

By definition, this Framework cannot be used to consider the possible benefits of consuming dietary supplements. The Framework also focuses on ingredients rather than products available in the marketplace. Another limitation is that, as with any evaluation of dietary supplement ingredients under the current regulatory scheme, the determination of what is unsafe depends on publicly available data or data made available voluntarily by industry.

FINDINGS

Ability to Determine Unreasonable Risk

Because of the limited and variable amount and types of data available, definitive statements judging safety may be difficult to completely substantiate scientifically. However, the principles used by the scientific community to determine the risk associated with the consumption or use of various substances, some of which are medical products, should also apply to dietary supplement ingredients, bearing in mind that dietary supplements, by virtue of DSHEA, have been *assumed* to be safe, but have not been required to be *proven* safe. Thus, **the appropriate scientific standard to be used to overturn this basic assumption of safety is to demonstrate significant or unreasonable risk, not *prove* that an ingredient is unsafe.**

[7]The monographs were developed as a test of the processes and framework and are thus considered prototypes because it was not possible to duplicate the access and information available to FDA within the committee process, and because of time constraints (discussed in Chapter 11). The monographs should not be considered as representing authoritative findings related to these six dietary supplement ingredients.

What Constitutes a Scientific Assessment of Unreasonable Risk?

Approaches taken by diverse organizations and governmental bodies, both within and outside the United States, which evaluate the safety and, at times, efficacy of dietary supplement ingredients vary in their relevance to the protection of the American public from risks associated with consumption of dietary supplement ingredients.

A number of these resources were reviewed to identify criteria for evaluating the relevance of other approaches. The purpose of such efforts varies substantially from organization to organization, focusing on quality, efficacy, safety, or a combination of these. Criteria outlined in Chapter 2 include importance of reliance on scientific data, consideration of all categories of such data (including animal data, *in vitro* data, data about the safety of related substances, and data on human use), use of appropriate expertise, and objectivity. Often the approaches were not sufficiently detailed or transparent to give a complete picture of the data considered, how sparse data were weighed and considered, the rationale behind the conclusions, or other questions regarding safety.

RECOMMENDATIONS

The following recommendations, while not part of the Framework itself, are designed to enhance the utility of the Framework and enhance the ability of FDA to protect consumers from unreasonable risk of illness or injury resulting from use of dietary supplements.

- **A prospective, systematic monitoring and tracking mechanism for dietary supplement ingredients should be maintained and refined.**

A prospective, systematic method for recording and monitoring the history of safety issues of specific dietary supplements is necessary to implement the Framework so that FDA can evaluate the safety of dietary supplement ingredients. During the period of this study, FDA developed a new method of monitoring and tracking dietary supplement adverse event reports. However, a prospective system is required that enables tracking of information leading to all levels of concern.

The system should be open, transparent, and useful for establishing varying levels of concern related to dietary supplements as outlined in the Framework. Resources to support these activities should be provided to FDA.

- **Adequate resources to protect the consumer under DSHEA must be provided.**

While the committee did not conduct an analysis of the cost of implementing this Framework, implementation of any framework for comprehensive safety evaluation will generate an additional workload for the responsible staff at FDA. For the Framework to be effective, adequate resources must be available to FDA to collect and analyze available information.

- Adverse Event Reporting:

— DSHEA should be amended to require that a manufacturer or distributor report to the FDA, in a timely manner, any serious adverse event associated with use of its marketed product of which the manufacturer or distributor is aware.

— FDA should continue to work with the Poison Control Centers as a source of adverse event reports, and sufficient resources to support this activity should be provided.

— FDA should increase efforts to inform health care professionals and consumers that they should use the MedWatch adverse event reporting program to report adverse events associated with the use of dietary supplement ingredients.

— FDA MedWatch toll-free telephone number should be provided on product labels to facilitate reporting of adverse events.

Reports of adverse events are an important source of information by which FDA becomes aware of potential risks to public health from exposure to dietary supplement ingredients. It has been estimated that FDA receives reports of less than 1 percent of all adverse events associated with dietary supplements. While spontaneous adverse event reports have recognized limitations, they have considerable strength as potential warning signals of problems requiring attention, making monitoring by FDA crucial.

- **To initiate the 75-day premarketing review period, both the distributor and manufacturer should be required to provide FDA with all available data, both favorable and unfavorable, regarding the safety of the product.**

- **When the formulation or processing of a dietary supplement ingredient is changed, it should be considered a new dietary ingredient and subject to regulatory oversight as such.**

Many dietary supplement ingredients on the market today have new formulations and are produced through very different processes than related dietary supplement ingredients in traditional usage, or even other dietary supplement ingredients bearing the same name. This may result in markedly different bioactive substances of potential harm and very different kinetics (e.g., absorption, distribution in the body, metabolism, and excretion).

- **The FDA initiative to establish current Good Manufacturing Practices for dietary supplement ingredients is supported and additional efforts to develop standards for content uniformity should be undertaken. Sufficient resources to support these efforts should be provided by Congress.**

While the focus of this report is on developing a framework and not on safety issues related to good manufacturing practices, these are inseparable because variability in content hampers the evaluation of safety.

- **Adoption of the labeling changes recommended in the report *Inspector General Report: Dietary Supplement Labels: Key Elements* is urged.**

Required labeling information that would be of use to the consumer in making informed decisions about safety is limited. Current regulations related to source of a product only require the name and place of business of the manufacturer, packer, or distributor to be on the label. There are usually few manufacturers of a product, but many distributors or packers. Thus both sources need to be on the label.

- **Additional Research on the Potential to Cause Harm:**

— The continued development of effective working relationships and partnerships between FDA and the National Institutes of Health is encouraged.

— FDA should ensure that its own National Center for Toxicological Research and the overall Department of Health and Human Services National Toxicology Program are optimally utilized when research is needed to further evaluate concerns.

— All federally supported research on dietary supplements conducted to assess efficacy should be required to include the collection and reporting of all data related to safety of the ingredient under study.

There is no legal or regulatory requirement that dietary supplement ingredient manufacturers conduct toxicology or safety pharmacology studies on their products or ingredients. Thus experiments and studies to address safety issues will, in most cases, be initiated by FDA or other federal agencies.

BARRIERS TO EVALUATING THE SAFETY OF DIETARY SUPPLEMENTS

Through the process of developing the Framework to evaluate the safety of dietary supplement ingredients, a number of legal and regulatory barriers were identified that hamper FDA's ability to protect the public health. New drugs are subject to premarket approval, yet DSHEA excludes all dietary supplements from this requirement despite the fact that they may possess biological activities similar to those found in medications, and survey data demonstrate that dietary supplements are used by consumers for medicinal purposes. Further, under the provisions of DSHEA, FDA has no authority to require the collection or reporting of specific safety data from dietary supplement manufacturers or distributors after their products are made available for sale to the public.

It is very challenging to carry out the mandate of DSHEA given the limitations it imposes on the quantity and quality of the currently available scientific data related to the safety of dietary supplement ingredients. One of the key premises of DSHEA is that history of use is evidence of safety when applied to dietary supplements; as indicated in Chapters 4 and 6, there are significant scientific problems with this assumption.

In line with these findings, members of the scientific and medical community have strongly advised that the regulatory mechanisms for monitoring the safety of dietary supplements, as currently defined by DSHEA, be revised. The constraints imposed on FDA with regard to ensuring the absence of unreasonable risk associated with the use of dietary supplements make it difficult for the health of the American public to be adequately protected.

1

Introduction and Background

A significant number of new dietary supplement products have appeared in the marketplace since the U.S. Congress passed the Dietary Supplement and Health Education Act (DSHEA) of 1994 (P.L. 103-417). At the time DSHEA was enacted, an estimated 600 U.S. dietary supplement manufacturers marketed about 4,000 products (CDSL, 1997). The Food and Drug Administration (FDA) estimates that more than 29,000 different dietary supplements are now available to consumers, and an average of 1,000 new products are introduced annually (Sarubin, 2000).

Consumer interest in health and self-care has been identified as providing the impetus for the expanded market of a wide range of products that includes dietary supplements (Prevention Magazine, 2001). In 2002, sales of dietary supplements increased to an estimated $18.7 billion per year, with herbs/botanical supplements accounting for an estimated $4.3 billion in sales (NBJ's Annual, 2003). Vitamin and mineral supplement use by the U.S. population has been a growing trend since the 1970s (Bender et al., 1992; Subar and Block, 1990), suggesting that Americans are becoming more receptive to alternatives to conventional food sources for nutritional health benefits (ADA, 2000). This is despite research-based dietary recommendations supporting the position that the best nutrition strategy for optimal health and reducing the risk of chronic disease is to obtain adequate nutrients from a wide variety of foods (Hunt, 1996; Hunt and Dwyer, 2001).

Many of the substances currently marketed as dietary supplements fall into the following categories: vitamins, minerals, herbs or other botanicals, amino acids, animal-derived products, hormones and hormone analogs,

BOX 1-1
Legal Definition of a Dietary Supplement as Defined by the Dietary Supplement Health and Education Act of 1994

The term dietary supplement:

(1) means a product (other than tobacco) intended to supplement the diet that bears or contains one or more of the following dietary ingredients:
- (A) a vitamin;
- (B) a mineral;
- (C) an herb or other botanical;
- (D) an amino acid;
- (E) a dietary substance for use by man to supplement the diet by increasing the total dietary intake; or
- (F) a concentrate, metabolite, constituent, extract, or combination of any ingredient described in clause (A), (B), (C), (D), or (E).

Dietary supplements are further defined as products that are labeled as dietary supplements and are not represented for use as a conventional food or as a sole item of a meal or the diet. Supplements can be marketed for ingestion in a variety of dosage forms including capsule, powder, softgel, gelcap, tablet, liquid, or, indeed, any other form so long as they are not represented as conventional foods or as sole items of a meal or of the diet (FDCA, as amended, § 402).

and enzymes, as well as concentrates, metabolites, constituents, or extracts of these.[1] Within each of these categories, products may be pure single entities of known or unknown chemical constituents, mixtures in which all or some components are known, or mixtures of unknown chemical components.

Within its definition of dietary supplements (Box 1-1), DSHEA included ingredients that have not traditionally been recognized as nutrients or as having nutritional functions, such as botanicals and hormones (Nesheim, 1999). It clarified that these substances could be considered supplement ingredients, not drug ingredients, when labeled appropriately. As with conventional foods, dietary supplements are to be presumed safe—that is, it is assumed that they do not present a significant[2] or unreasonable risk of injury or illness when consumed as recommended.

---

[1]While these are not dietary supplement categories specified by DSHEA, they illustrate the diversity of products currently marketed as dietary supplements.

[2]The origin of the use of the standard "significant or unreasonable risk" relative to dietary supplements is the DSHEA legislation; thus "significant" is used qualitatively and does not imply a statistical determination.

However, questions have been raised about the safety of some dietary supplements. When these questions are raised, FDA needs a methodology to rapidly review and further evaluate the safety of ingredients about which it has concerns. This has created a sizeable regulatory challenge for FDA because of the increased availability and use of supplements, as well as the broad spectrum of ingredients that qualify as dietary supplements under the DSHEA legislation.

COMMITTEE CHARGE

To expeditiously and efficiently monitor the continually evolving and growing patterns of dietary supplement use, as well as their potential interactions with other consumed substances, FDA needs a cost-effective and scientifically sound approach to consider the safety of dietary supplement ingredients. For these reasons, FDA turned to the Institute of Medicine and the National Research Council of the National Academies to propose a framework for evaluating the safety of dietary supplement ingredients marketed in the United States. Specifically, FDA requested that a committee develop a proposed framework for categorizing and prioritizing dietary supplement ingredients based on safety issues, describe a process for developing a system of scientific reviews with specifications for evaluating the safety of dietary supplement ingredients, and develop at least six scientific reviews as prototypes for the system. The proposed framework was to include a methodology to review data with regard to the safety of dietary supplement ingredients, taking into consideration methods other expert bodies have used to categorize and review supplement safety and efficacy issues. FDA, in its request, asked that a framework for setting priorities and evaluating the safety of dietary supplement ingredients be proposed and released for comment, followed by the development of six prototype monograph reviews using the procedures outlined in the proposed framework. After development of the prototype monograph reviews and based on comments received on the initial framework released for comment, the framework was to be revised (see Appendix B for the detailed scope of work and the comments received).

The committee held a total of seven meetings while preparing the initial framework, reviewing comments on it, and revising the framework. Six of these meetings included open sessions so the committee could hear from the sponsor and a number of individuals and organizations regarding aspects of evaluating the safety of dietary supplement ingredients. In addition, representatives of a number of agencies and organizations that currently evaluate chemical substances for safety or efficacy were invited to discuss their methodologies and frameworks for conducting their reviews. (See Appendix L for a list of those who contributed comments or made presentations to the committee at the open sessions.)

GENERAL BACKGROUND INFORMATION ABOUT DIETARY SUPPLEMENTS

National surveys, such as the Third National Health and Nutrition Examination Survey (1988–1994) and the 1987 and 1992 National Health Interview Surveys, indicate that 40 to 46 percent of Americans reported taking at least one vitamin or mineral supplement at some time within the month surveyed (Balluz et al., 2000; Slesinski et al., 1995). However, data from national surveys collected before the enactment of DSHEA in 1994 may not reflect current supplement consumption patterns (Costello and Grumpstrup-Scott, 2000), and there are limitations to interpreting user characteristics from sales data (Radimer et al., 2000). Several studies have also explored the prevalence of *nutrient supplement* (thought to be primarily vitamin and mineral formulations) use and trends in the United States (Balluz et al., 2000; Bender et al., 1992; Kim et al., 1993; Koplan et al., 1986; Slesinski et al., 1995; Subar and Block, 1990), as well as users' motivation for taking vitamin and mineral supplements (Neuhouser et al., 1999) and characteristics of users versus nonusers (Dwyer et al., 2001; Ford, 2001; Hartz et al., 1988; Lyle et al., 1998; Nayga and Reed, 1999; Pelletier and Kendall, 1997; Subar and Block, 1990). However, knowledge about the use prevalence and trends of *dietary supplements* (which include nonvitamin, nonmineral supplements) is limited (Radimer et al., 2000).

Results from a more recent national survey of 2,000 adults indicated that 85 percent of respondents had used one or more dietary supplements in the previous 12 months (Prevention Magazine, 2001). If this sample of U.S. consumers was representative of the total population, it would translate into more than 44 million consumers using botanical remedies and an estimated 24 million using specialty supplements (e.g., bee pollen, dehydroepiandrosterone, chondroitin sulfate, kava kava, shark cartilage, and S-adenosylmethionine) (Prevention Magazine, 2001; Radimer et al., 2000; Ramos, 2000).

Existing studies of reported dietary supplement use suggest an association between increased use of dietary supplements by older individuals and those who report having more healthful lifestyles (Radimer et al., 2000). The most frequent reason given for dietary supplement use in one national survey was desire for self-care (Prevention Magazine, 2001). Some consumers report using supplements because of a belief that these products will ensure good health. Generally, labeling for a dietary supplement may not claim to "diagnose, mitigate, treat, cure, or prevent a specific disease or class of diseases" (DSHEA, P.L. 103-417, § 6 [1994]; (FDCA), 21 U.S.C. § 343(r)(6)(C) [2001]). Nonetheless, consumers have reported using supplements for purposes such as to treat and prevent illnesses, colds, and flu and to alleviate depression (Prevention Magazine, 2001). There is also a reported link of more frequent dietary supplement use among Americans with one or more health problems (Bender et al., 1992), with specific diseases such as breast cancer (Newman et al., 1998), with higher alcohol consumption (Radimer et al., 2000), and with obesity (Radimer et al., 2000). Evidence suggests that supplement use may not be associated with better food intake in all populations and may differ by ethnicity and across income strata (Kraak et al., 2002; Pelletier and Kendall, 1997).

Consumer Expectations About Dietary Supplement Safety

Surveys have suggested that many Americans may assume dietary supplements are subject to existing government regulations similar to those required for over-the-counter (OTC) drugs sold without a prescription (Blendon et al., 2001). When consumers purchase OTC drugs, such drugs have typically undergone an FDA review that has deemed them to be safe and effective as labeled. Most OTC drugs have been through FDA's OTC Drug Review, in which the agency assesses the safety and effectiveness of the active ingredients of OTC drugs and then issues detailed monographs restricting the labeling and formulation of products containing these ingredients. Other OTC drugs have been specifically approved by FDA under its rigorous new drug application (NDA) process and then have been reviewed by the agency again before being changed from prescription to OTC status.

Only a few national surveys exploring the views and perceptions of Americans regarding the safety of dietary supplements have been conducted. One compilation was based on four national opinion surveys conducted from 1996 to 1999 by the Roper Center for Public Opinion; however, supplement users were not differentiated from nonusers, thereby limiting the usefulness of the findings (Blendon et al., 2001). The Sloan Survey explored general patterns of medication use in the ambulatory adult population from 1998 to 1999 and examined use of vitamins, minerals, botanicals, and other dietary supplements, in addition to drugs. Conducted among 2,590 U.S. consumers, it reported that 16 percent of prescription drug users also took one or more "herbal or other natural supplements" (Kaufman et al., 2002). A more recent telephone survey, conducted by the Princeton Survey Research Associates for Prevention Magazine, used a nationally representative sample of 2,000 U.S. adults. The results suggested a high degree of consumer confidence in supplements based on the finding that nearly two-thirds of respondents believed that herbal supplements were either safe or completely safe (Prevention Magazine, 2001).

Another analysis was based on two separate data sources that compared the views of dietary supplement users with those who were nonusers (Blendon et al., 2001). In the first survey reviewed, which was designed collaboratively by researchers at National Public Radio, the Kaiser Family

Foundation, and the John F. Kennedy School of Government and conducted by the Princeton Survey Research Associates in 1999, 1,200 randomly selected adults participated in telephone interviews. A second survey was conducted with 1,013 randomly selected adults. Results from the analysis of these two surveys revealed that regular users of dietary supplements reported not discussing use of dietary supplements with their physicians because they believed that the physicians knew little or nothing about these products and might be biased against them (Blendon et al., 2001). In addition, many users felt so strongly about the potential health benefits of some of the products used that they would continue to take them even if the products were shown to be ineffective in scientifically conducted clinical studies (Blendon et al., 2001).

Because dietary supplements are regulated as foods, they are subject to different regulatory requirements in comparison with OTC medications or other drugs. With the passage of DSHEA, the burden of proof concerning the safety of dietary supplements was placed on FDA by requiring FDA to determine that a dietary supplement ingredient presents a "significant or unreasonable risk of illness or injury" (see Box 1-2), rather than requiring a manufacturer[3] to provide data supporting its safety, as is done with food additives[4] (21 C.F.R. § 170) and new drugs (21 C.F.R. § 314). Manufacturers of dietary supplements that contain new dietary ingredients (those ingredients not in use prior to the passage of DSHEA) must notify FDA at least 75 days before introducing the dietary supplement into interstate commerce and provide FDA with information that is the basis upon which the manufacturer has concluded that the dietary supplement will reasonably be expected to be safe (DSHEA, P.L. 103-417, § 8 [1994]). This submission is not a premarket approval process, as further described below.

History of the Federal Regulation of Dietary Supplements

A framework for the evaluation of safety of dietary supplement ingredients must be carried out within the regulatory environment under which the ingredients are to be evaluated; thus the regulatory history of dietary supplements is received here. Many herbals and other botanicals have been used much longer than other types of dietary supplements, as ancient cultures employed them medicinally. People have long used plants and other substances to supplement their diets in an attempt to prevent or ameliorate

[3]The term "manufacturer" is used for simplicity, but the statutes refer to both manufacturers and distributors, which may not be the same for a dietary supplement ingredient or product.

[4]Food ingredients not declared or listed as generally recognized as safe (GRAS).

BOX 1-2
Safety Standards for Dietary Supplements as Established by DSHEA

Section 4. Safety of Dietary Supplements and Burden of Proof on FDA.

DSHEA amends § 402 (21 U.S.C. 342) by adding the following:

(f) (1) If it is a dietary supplement or contains a dietary ingredient that—

(A) presents a significant or unreasonable risk of illness or injury under –
(i) conditions of use recommended or suggested in labeling, or
(ii) if no conditions of use are suggested or recommended in the labeling, under ordinary conditions of use;
(B) is a new dietary ingredient for which there is inadequate information to provide reasonable assurance that such ingredient does not present a significant or unreasonable risk of illness or injury;
(C) the Secretary declares to pose an imminent hazard to public health or safety, except that the authority to make such declaration shall not be delegated and the Secretary shall promptly after such a declaration initiate a proceeding in accordance with sections 554 and 556 of title 5, United States Code to affirm or withdraw the declaration; or
(D) is or contains a dietary ingredient that renders it adulterated under paragraph [402](a)(1) under the conditions of use recommended or suggested in the labeling of such dietary supplement.

In any proceeding under this paragraph, the United States shall bear the burden of proof on each element to show that a dietary supplement is adulterated. The court shall decide any issue under this paragraph on a de novo basis.

(2) Before the Secretary may report to a United States attorney a violation of the paragraph (1)(A) for a civil proceeding, the person against whom such proceeding would be initiated shall be given appropriate notice and the opportunity to present views, orally and in writing, at least 10 days before such notice, with regard to such proceeding.

SOURCE: FDCA, P.L. 75-717 § 402, as amended 21 U.S.C. § 342(f) (2001).

specific symptoms. Patent medicines became popular in the 1800s as advertising increased, and the lack of trained medical personnel and the inability of conventional medicines to adequately treat many diseases drove consumers to look elsewhere for help. Patent medicines were often secret formulations and were directly marketed to consumers (CDER, 2002).

In the early years of development, the growing pharmaceutical industry marketed its medicines directly to health professionals. There were few regulations for these or patent medicines to assist the consumer or health professional in distinguishing between valid and false assertions made by purveyors of the different products. While some efforts were made by states, federal regulation of these substances and products in the 1800s was essentially nonexistent (Millikan, 1999).

Food and Drugs Act of 1906

The Federal Food and Drugs Act (also known as the Pure Food and Drug Act) of 1906 (21 U.S.C. 1 et seq.), and its companion bill, the Federal Meat Inspection Act of 1906 (21 U.S.C. 601 et seq.), were the earliest comprehensive efforts by the U.S. government to bring greater emphasis both to the safety of marketed products and to the accurate characterization of the benefits derived from their use. The 1906 acts resulted from a convergence of public, industry, and scientific support that was partially motivated by concerns about the safety of food and patent medicines, as well as about widespread fraud in the growing food and drug industry (Barkan, 1985; FDA, 2002). The triggering event was the exposure of unsafe conditions in the meat packing industry (Sinclair, 1906). The passage of the 1906 acts has also been attributed to industry's desire to restore competitiveness to their products in weak foreign and domestic markets (Barkan, 1985).

The 1906 acts established the broad authority of the federal government to protect the public from adulterated or misbranded foods and drugs, and thus imposed new regulations on these industries (Barkan, 1985; FDA, 2002). Specifically, the laws introduced accountability by requiring that regulated products be labeled accurately and that they be safe. With the passage of the Food and Drugs Act in 1906, FDA[5] was placed in a "policing" role (rules of conduct specified; agency has authority to punish violators). Also, FDA bore the burden of establishing that a food or drug was adulterated or misbranded before it could take action against the product.

Federal Food, Drug, and Cosmetic Act of 1938

A movement for increased regulation of ingested substances came about in the 1930s, eventually culminating in Congress passing the Federal Food,

[5]For clarity, FDA and its predecessors are referred to in this text simply as "FDA." The actual name Food and Drug Administration was established in 1930. Predecessors were the Bureau of Chemistry, which began in 1862, and the Food, Drug, and Insecticide Administration, which was created in 1927 when regulatory functions of the Bureau of Chemistry were separated from nonregulatory research (FDA, 2002).

Drug, and Cosmetic Act in 1938 (FDCA, P.L. 75-717, 52 Stat. 1040 [1938]). The FDCA replaced the 1906 law that had become obsolete due to the technological changes in the production and marketing of food and drugs (FDA, 1981). This new act created a complex system of federal regulations for foods, drugs, cosmetics, and medical devices. Some of the more important changes implemented by the FDCA were further introduction of food standards[6] and a refocus of FDA from that of a policing agency that had been concerned primarily with challenging adulterated drugs to that of a regulatory agency involved with oversight for evaluating new drugs (but not foods) (Wax, 1995).

The FDCA transferred the responsibility of proving the safety of new drugs to the drug manufacturer and required manufacturers to submit NDAs to FDA that establish safety before marketing.[7] While FDA no longer had the burden of establishing that an unapproved new drug was unsafe before taking action against it, FDA continued to bear the burden of establishing that a conventional food product was adulterated, as the agency does to this day[8] (CDSL, 1997).

The FDCA contained provisions that applied to foods, drugs, and cosmetics. The applicability of these provisions to products containing a vitamin, mineral, or botanical ingredient (e.g., whether the product was considered a drug or a food) depended on the product's *intended* use, as determined usually by the labeling and advertising claims for the product.

The 1938 act, as originally enacted, contains a number of definitions that continue to guide FDA actions according to the regulations derived from it. One definition of a drug is an article "intended for use in the diagnosis, cure, mitigation, treatment, or prevention of disease in man or other animals . . ."; a second definition is "articles (other than food) intended to affect the structure or any function of the body of man or other animals . . ."; and a third definition states that a product is a drug if it is "recognized in the official U.S. Pharmacopeia (USP), official Homeopathic Pharmacopoeia of the United States, or official National Formulary, or any supplement to any of them" (FDCA, P.L. 75-717, 52 Stat. 1040 [1938], as amended 21 U.S.C. § 321(g) [2001]).

---

[6]Food standards were required to promote honesty and fair dealing in the interest of consumers (FDA, 1981). The standards consist of definitions of what constitutes a food (e.g., mayonnaise must contain a certain percentage of egg and oil, etc.).

[7]In 1962, the FDCA was amended to require NDAs to establish the efficacy, as well as the safety, of new drugs.

[8]However, food colors and food additives must be approved by FDA via the food additive petition process; other substances added to food that are not approved via this process must be declared or affirmed to be GRAS based on intended use before they may be sold in a food product. Dietary ingredients marketed in dietary supplements are exempt from this requirement.

The original 1938 act contains no specific provisions for vitamin, mineral, or botanical products, except in Section 403(j), which indicates that a food is misbranded if it is claimed to be "for special dietary uses" but its label does not bear FDA-prescribed statements about its "vitamin, mineral, and other dietary properties" sufficient to inform the consumer about its value for such uses (FDCA, P.L. 75-717 § 403(j) [1938], as amended 21 U.S.C. § 343(j) [2001]).

Congress intended in 1938 that Section 403(j) would allow FDA to regulate claims for vitamins, minerals, and botanical foods more closely than for conventional foods (Pendergast, 1997). However, in enacting Section 403(j), it has been asserted that FDA was most concerned with the problems of nutritional deficiency and inadequacy of the diet and thus did not address either acceptable claims for vitamins, minerals, and botanical products or when these products should be regulated as drugs as opposed to foods (Pendergast, 1997).

Early Attempts to Regulate the Industry

Eventually FDA did focus attention on claims for vitamins, minerals, and especially botanical products. FDA began to use extensive litigation directed at claims to regulate the botanical industry in the 1940s. Botanical products were treated as unapproved drugs not only if they made claims concerning the treatment or prevention of disease, but also if they made claims concerning the products' effects on the structure and function of the body—a type of claim foods were allowed to make without being considered drugs. FDA also took action against manufacturers that made therapeutic claims for vitamins and minerals (FDA, 1941).

FDA did not, however, rigorously apply the FDCA's third definition of drugs, the definition that categorizes as drugs all products listed in the USP, the offical Homeopathic Pharmacopoeia of the United States, or the National Formulary. This definition would have included most vitamins and minerals and many botanical preparations. In 1944, when FDA charged that certain vitamin B capsules were misbranded as food and as drugs, the courts dismissed the food counts, holding that the capsules were drugs by definition because vitamin B was listed in the USP (Pendergast, 1997). FDA did not fully exploit this reasoning in future cases, however, and appeared to abandon this legal premise after several court cases in the 1960s (Pendergast 1997), declaring that a USP listing was insufficient to confer drug status on a product (FDA, 1966).

FDA's focus on regulation of labeling claims it deemed unapproved and indicative of drug status was closely followed by increased use of publications such as self-help books and magazine articles that explained claims and intended uses. This approach was a "possible way [for supplement manufacturers] to avoid FDA [enforcement]" (Pendergast, 1997). Debate about what constituted "labeling" ensued as FDA attempted to broaden labeling to include books and other materials. Some characterized this approach as restricting the First Amendment right to free speech, resulting in a number of court cases between the 1940s and 1960s.[9] The resulting debate about First Amendment rights and labeling restrictions has been considered by some to be a significant factor that eventually led to DSHEA as an attempt to resolve the situation (McNamara, 1995).

Food Additives Amendment of 1958

FDA's attempt at applying the Food Additives Amendment of 1958 (P.L. 85-929, 72 Stat. 1784 [1958]) to botanical products has also been described as a factor leading to the passage of DSHEA (Pendergast, 1997). A food additive is defined by statute as "any substance the intended use of which results, or may reasonably be expected to result, directly or indirectly, in its becoming a component or otherwise affecting the characteristics of any food . . . if such substance is not generally recognized . . . to be safe under the conditions of its intended use" (FDCA, 21 U.S.C. § 321(s) [2001]). Unless the substance at issue could be considered as "generally recognized as safe" (GRAS) by the manufacturer for its intended use or had been sanctioned or approved by FDA or the U.S. Department of Agriculture prior to 1958, manufacturers were required to obtain premarket approval from FDA for the substance. In general, the result of the Food Additives Amendment was to shift the burden of proof of safety for new substances added to food away from FDA and to the manufacturers (FDA, 2002).

While the Food Additives Amendment provides a petition process by which FDA can approve a food additive that has not been determined to be GRAS, manufacturers also have the option of determining for themselves that a substance is GRAS. The GRAS determination of a substance by a manufacturer must be based on "generally available and accepted scientific data, information, methods, or principles, which ordinarily are published . . ." and there must be a "consensus among qualified experts about the safety of the substance for its intended use" (FDA, 1997). If these conditions are met, manufacturers can "self-affirm" the GRAS status of a substance. Alternatively, they may either petition FDA to affirm their determination (21 C.F.R. § 170.35) or voluntarily notify FDA that the manufacturer has determined the substance to be GRAS, pursuant to the interim

---

[9]*See United States v Detroit Vital Foods*, 218 F Supp 208 (ED Mich 1963); *United States v Articles of Drug . . . Honey*, 344 F2d 288 (6th Cir 1965); *United States v Kordel*, 164 F2d 913 (7th Cir 1947), aff'd, 335 U.S. 345 (1948); and *United States v "Sterling Vinegar and Honey" . . . Balanced Foods*, 338 F2d 157 (2d Cir 1964).

policy delineated in the proposed rule regarding the notification procedure (FDA, 1997).

In notifying FDA that it has determined a substance to be GRAS for its intended use, the manufacturer voluntarily provides FDA with a summary of the basis upon which it has made the determination. FDA can respond with a letter of no objection to its determination of GRAS or can identify a problem with the notice. The manufacturer can also determine the food substance to be GRAS and market a product containing it without prior notification of FDA. If it does so, and then FDA determines that it is not GRAS, FDA can take action by declaring the product adulterated, seizing the product, and removing it from commerce.

Shortly after the Food Additives Amendment was passed, FDA clarified the regulatory status of many food substances that were in use prior to 1958, listing them as GRAS when used for the purposes indicated and in accordance with good manufacturing practice (GMP). Moreover, over the years, FDA has affirmed GRAS status for other substances upon petition from manufacturers and others. Substances not so listed or affirmed, or those that are to be used for purposes other than those indicated on the GRAS listing, are required to either be evaluated via the food additive petition process or to be subjected to the GRAS self-determination mechanisms described above.

Some have pointed to parallels between the processes for regulating GRAS substances and food additives and the system of regulating older (before October 15, 1994) versus newer dietary ingredients as delineated by DSHEA. The presumption that for both substances added to foods prior to 1958 and dietary ingredients in use prior to October 15, 1994 are to be considered safe based on prior common use is similar. However, there is a major difference in the evaluation of new ingredients to be used in food versus new dietary ingredients to be used in dietary supplements (Table 1-1). The underlying principle of law is different. The starting assumption is one of safety for dietary supplements because FDA bears the burden of determining that a "significant and unreasonable risk of harm" exists in order to prevent a new dietary ingredient from being marketed in a dietary supplement (DSHEA, P.L. 75-717; see Box 1-2). By contrast, the starting assumption is one of a *lack* of safety for new food ingredients because, before FDA approves a food additive or affirms or determines that it is GRAS, the manufacturer must demonstrate to FDA a reasonable certainty of no harm for the substance when added to food (21 C.F.R. § 170.3 (i); FDA, 1997). The difference in the underlying assumption has a major impact in determining what is allowed to be sold in interstate commerce, as is illustrated with the botanical *stevia* (see Box 1-3).

Prior to the passage of DSHEA, FDA instituted action in the early 1990s against many popular dietary supplement ingredients, applying food additive regulations and contending that they were unapproved food additives. FDA interpreted the definition of "food additive" as applying to single ingredient supplements in capsule form. For example, FDA argued, unsuccessfully, that black currant seed oil in a capsule was a food additive (*United States v Two Plastic Drums . . . Black Currant Oil*, 984 F2d 814 [7th Cir 1993]). The courts eventually struck down FDA's efforts to broadly interpret the food additive definition (*United States v Two Plastic Drums . . . Black Currant Oil*, 984 F2d 814, 819 [7th Cir 1993]; *United States v An Article of Food*, 792 F Supp. 139 [D Mass 1992]).

1976 "Proxmire Amendments"

Prior to the overturn by the court in 1993 of FDA's attempts to apply the food additive provisions to dietary supplements, the regulation of botanical, vitamin, and mineral supplements had been inconsistent and was based on a combination of enforcement and judicial decisions. Court actions required long periods of time and considerable resources; thus in the 1970s FDA attempted to have a broader impact on dietary supplement use by implementing tighter regulations of vitamin and mineral supplements, consistent with the U.S. Supreme Court's endorsement in 1973 of FDA action to control entire product classes with regulations rather than relying only on litigation (FDA, 2002).

In 1973 FDA issued regulations that prohibited certain representations on vitamin and mineral supplement labels, established standards of identity for vitamin and mineral supplements, and established that preparations containing more than 150 percent of the U.S. Recommended Daily Allowance (U.S. RDA) per serving were drugs (FDA, 1973). Both industry and consumers protested the attempts by FDA to set maximum levels (Hutt and Merrill, 1991; Khatcheressian, 1999; Pendergast, 1997), eventually leading Congress to enact the Health Research and Health Services Amendments in 1976. Also known as the "Proxmire Amendments," these amendments prohibited FDA from ". . . establishing standards limiting potency of vitamins and minerals in food supplements or regulating them as drugs based solely on potency" (FDA, 2002). FDA revised its vitamin–mineral regulations in response to this legislation and, after a subsequent successful court challenge (*National Foods Associations v Matthews,* 557 F2d 325 [2d Cir 1977]), ultimately revoked its 1973 regulations about maximum potency and drug status in 1979 (FDA, 1979).

The Nutrition Labeling and Education Act of 1990 and Health Claims

With the suppression of FDA's attempts at more restrictive rulemaking, the realm of products sold as dietary supplements continued to expand and

TABLE 1-1 Current Status of Foods, Food Additives, Drugs, and Dietary Supplements Under the FDA Regulations

	Dietary Supplements		
Status	Containing Ingredients in Use prior to DSHEA[a]	Containing "New" Ingredients Introduced After DSHEA (10/15/94)	Conventional Foods[b]
Premarket approval required	No	No; FDA notification 75 days prior to sale required; FDA has 3 options: (1) respond with objection, (2) respond with no objection, (3) not respond	No[e]
Postmarket reporting or surveillance by industry required	No	No	No
Burden of proof of safety	FDA must demonstrate significant or unreasonable risk of harm to remove product from market	FDA must demonstrate significant or unreasonable risk of harm to prevent product from being marketed	FDA must demonstrate that food is injurious to health to remove product from market

[a] DSHEA = Dietary Supplement and Health Education Act of 1994.

[b] Here "conventional foods" refers to whole agricultural commodities.

[c] This description applies to "new" drugs. Many over-the-counter drugs are regulated under FDA's Over-the-Counter Drug Review procedures, which do not provide for post-marketing surveillance.

[d] GRAS = generally recognized as safe (as defined by the 1958 Food Additives Amendment to Food, Drug, and Cosmetic Act).

	Substances Added to Foods		
New Drugs[c]	GRAS[d] Pre-1958	GRAS Notice (previously, "Affirmation" Petition)	Food Additive Petition
Yes	No	No; manufacturer voluntarily may notify FDA of basis of self-declaration as GRAS[f]; FDA will respond with letter of objection or no objection within 90 days	Yes; with FDA approval becomes an approved food additive
Yes	No	No	Rarely
Manufacturer provides risk/benefit analysis acceptable to FDA	FDA conducts risk assessment to determine if GRAS recognition should be withdrawn	Manufacturer must demonstrate reasonable certainty of no harm for intended use through scientific procedure or history of use	Manufacturer must present adequate risk assessment to demonstrate reasonable certainty of no harm for intended use

[e] In 2001 FDA proposed in the *Federal Register* (66:4706) a rule requiring marketers of food developed through biotechnology to notify the agency at least 120 days before commercial distribution and to provide information to demonstrate that the product is as safe as its conventional counterpart.

[f] While the final regulations for the notification procedure are not yet published, the interim policy outlined by FDA in the proposed regulations invites interested persons who determine that a substance is GRAS to notify FDA of such GRAS determinations as described in the proposed regulation 21 C.F.R. § 170.36 (b) and (c).

BOX 1-3
Regulation of Stevia Under the Dietary Supplement and Health Education Act (DSHEA) Versus as a Food Additive

The status of the botanical stevia illustrates how the different starting assumptions for dietary supplements and for food additives, based on the FDCA and its amendments, result in different regulatory decisions. Stevia leaves are a product of Brazil and Paraguay, and stevia, or its extract, stevioside, has been in use in other countries, such as Japan, but not in the United States. It is described as a "natural" noncaloric sweetener and is discussed as an alternative to other non-nutritive sweeteners, such as saccharin and aspartame. Studies relevant to the safety of stevia include those that found reduced sperm production and testicular cell proliferation in rodents when high levels of stevia were ingested. Other experiments suggested that offspring were smaller and fewer in number when pregnant rodents ingested large amounts of steviol (a stevioside derivative). *In vitro* experiments indicated that steviol could be metabolized into a mutagenic compound. The FDA concluded that toxicological data on stevia was inadequate to determine safety as a food additive or to affirm its status as GRAS and, as a result, rejected food additive petitions to approve stevia (as have the European Community regulatory authorities).

However, when considered as a new dietary supplement ingredient, FDA has not found the same safety-related information on stevia to be sufficient to determine that stevia presents a significant or unreasonable risk, the standard required in order for the agency to take action to remove supplements containing it from the marketplace.

That the same information can simultaneously be insufficient to demonstrate safety when intended to be used as a food additive, while also insufficient to conclude that it presents a significant or unreasonable risk of illness or injury when used in a dietary supplement, presents an interesting dichotomy.

The result is an FDA policy to seize, as adulterated, foods for sale to which stevia leaves or stevioside have been added, unless the items are labeled as dietary supplements. That is, the starting assumption of DSHEA, that dietary supplement ingredients, like conventional foods, are safe unless proven otherwise, results in substantial differences in how the data are interpreted and applied.

SOURCE: Cardello et al., 1999; FDA, 1995; Pezzuto et al., 1985; Scientific Committee on Food, 1999; Wasuntarawat et al., 1998; Yamada et al., 1985.

included botanicals and amino acids, as well as vitamin and mineral products. This expansion during the late 1970s and the 1980s was accompanied by some reports of serious illnesses attributed to a few of the dietary supplements available at that time. In 1978, for example, an infant with colic was reportedly given a fatal dose of a potassium chloride supplement based on erroneous advice in a parenting book, despite medical knowledge that use of such doses of the supplement would induce cardiac arrest (Wetli and

Davis, 1978). In 1989 there were widespread reports that some L-tryptophan supplements were associated with eosinophilia-myalgia syndrome.[10]

Both the L-tryptophan incidents and FDA's concerns about unsubstantiated claims appearing on the label led to new attempts by FDA to regulate the industry in the 1980s. By this time, mounting scientific evidence had led several food companies to start promoting their conventional foods based on the potential of some of their ingredients or substances to reduce the risk of specific diseases. While not endorsed by FDA, some have purported that when similar claims were made in reference to dietary supplements, FDA responded more harshly, contending that by virtue of claims made regarding the supplement they were unapproved drugs (Pendergast, 1997). This unequal approach toward regulating supplements versus foods became more evident when in 1987 FDA proposed criteria for what it would consider as an acceptable health claim (FDA, 1987). These proposed rules indicated that it might be more difficult for dietary supplement claims to meet FDA's criteria, which could be interpreted as acknowledging that foods and dietary supplements were not the same (Pendergast, 1997).

The Nutrition Labeling and Education Act (NLEA), which Congress passed in 1990 (P.L. 101-535), explicitly authorized "health claims,"[11] but did not silence the controversies surrounding the different treatment of supplements and foods (Pendergast, 1997). The NLEA provided that health claims describing the relationship of a nutrient to a disease or health-related condition were allowed for both traditional foods and dietary supplements if the claims complied with FDA regulations. FDA was charged with proposing the criteria needed for foods or supplements to make health claims (NLEA, P.L. 101-535, § 3(b) 104 Stat 2353, 2361 [1990]). Concerns that FDA would treat supplements too harshly may have contributed to the subsequent passage of DSHEA (Pendergast, 1997). Food industry advocacy efforts first resulted in a 1-year moratorium on NLEA provisions being applied to supplements (*Prescription Drug User Fee Act,* P.L. 102-571, 106 Stat. 4491 [1990]); such advocacy efforts continued until DSHEA was passed (Khatcheressian, 1999).

[10]Evidence suggesting that the problem might have been associated with the manufacturing process eventually surfaced, but the issue has not been definitely resolved (FDA, 2001a).

[11]A health claim is defined as a claim that "characterizes the relationship" between a substance in a food and damage, disease, or dysfunction of the human body (NLEA, P.L. 101-535). In effect, the NLEA allowed claims that previously would have been regarded as illegal drug claims if made for a food.

The Dietary Supplement and Health Education Act of 1994

In 1993, following the passage of the NLEA, FDA issued an advance notice of proposed rulemaking regarding dietary supplements, which was accompanied by the suggestion that some products marketed as dietary supplements might be more appropriately considered under other regulatory categories (FDA, 1993). Amino acids, for example, might be considered unapproved food additives, and some botanicals might be more appropriately considered as drugs (FDA, 1993). Vitamins and minerals were also considered a potential target of regulation, as FDA suggested that their strength should be limited to levels that approximated the U.S. RDA (FDA, 1993).

The dietary supplement industry and consumers reacted strongly to these potential regulatory restrictions (Khatcheressian, 1999). Extensive public debate ensued over the importance of dietary supplements in health, consumers' freedom to access information about supplements, and the controversy over FDA's regulatory approach. Subsequently, Congress passed DSHEA, signed into law October 15, 1994, which limited and proscribed the regulation of dietary supplements by FDA (DSHEA, P.L. 103-417, § 2 [1994]).

DSHEA can be characterized as the most important dietary supplement legislation enacted to date. In its findings, Congress recognized the wide use of dietary supplements and stated in the legislation that currently available dietary supplements are generally safe. Passage of DSHEA was based on the concept that ". . . legislative action that protects the right of access of consumers to safe dietary supplements is necessary to promote wellness" (DSHEA, P.L. 103-417, § 2 [1994]; OIG, 2001). DSHEA established the first comprehensive definition of dietary supplements (see Box 1-1), resulting in botanicals and amino acids being considered as foods based on intended use, as were vitamins and minerals, which were already classified as food based on intended use. Importantly, DSHEA established a new regulatory framework for dietary supplements that limited FDA's authority over these products to that of conventional foods, as compared with its authority over food additives or new drugs (see Table 1-1 for comparison and Box 1-3 for discussion of an example).

DSHEA specifically exempted dietary ingredients in dietary supplement products from being regulated under the category of food additives (DSHEA, P.L. 103-417 [1994]). Because FDA does not have the authority to consider dietary supplement ingredients as food additives unless they are added to a conventional food and marketed as a food, there is no requirement for a manufacturer to obtain premarket approval (Khatcheressian, 1999) or establish GRAS status (McNamara, 1995; Pendergast, 1997). Thus DSHEA eliminated one of the key approaches FDA had taken to restrict the availability of some dietary supplements (e.g., black currant oil and especially multi-ingredient products).

DSHEA and Dietary Supplement Safety. DSHEA also established safety standards for dietary supplements. It states that a dietary supplement will be considered adulterated (i.e., illegal) if it "presents a significant or unreasonable risk of illness or injury under conditions of use recommended or suggested in labeling" (DSHEA, P.L. 103-417, § 4 [1994], as codified in FDCA 21 U.S.C. § 342 [2001]). Most importantly, FDA now bears the burden of proof if it decides to assert that a supplement is adulterated (Khatcheressian, 1999; McNamara, 1995). In summary, while a manufacturer is charged with ensuring the safety of its products, the manufacturer is not required to reveal the basis of its safety determination unless the Secretary of the Department of Health and Human Services declares that the product poses an imminent hazard or FDA brings an action in court alleging the product is adulterated (see Box 1-2).

DSHEA and New Dietary Ingredients Marketed After 1994. DSHEA provided additional requirements for supplements containing "new dietary ingredients" that were not marketed in the United States before October 15, 1994. Products containing them are deemed adulterated under DSHEA unless the new ingredient has been present in the conventional food supply in a form in which the food has not been chemically altered, or unless there is a "history of use or other evidence of safety establishing that the dietary ingredient when used under the conditions recommended or suggested in the labeling . . . will reasonably be expected to be safe" (DSHEA, P.L. 103-417, § 8 [1994]). In addition, the law required that to avoid adulteration in the latter instance, the manufacturer must provide FDA with the information that is the ". . . basis on which [it] has concluded that the dietary supplement containing [the new] ingredient will reasonably be expected to be safe" at least 75 days prior to marketing the ingredient (DSHEA, P.L. 103-417, § 8 [1994]). FDA may examine the submission and indicate to the manufacturer that the submission does not provide sufficient evidence to demonstrate that the ingredient is safe. However, FDA approval is not required before sale (Young and Bass, 1995). If a manufacturer receives such an FDA response and nonetheless chooses to market the product, FDA may decide to take legal action against the product. However, as with the case of pre-1994 ingredients, in any such proceeding the government bears the burden of proof (21 U.S.C. § 342 (f)(1); Young and Bass, 1995).

The manufacturer is responsible initially for determining whether or not an ingredient is new (i.e.,". . . present in the food supply as an article used for food in a form in which the food has not been chemically altered . . ." [DSHEA, P.L. 103-417, § 8, 108 Stat. 4331-4332 {1994}]; Young and

Bass, 1995). If the ingredient is "new," the manufacturer must notify FDA 75 days in advance of introducing it or a dietary supplement containing it into commerce (DSHEA, P.L. 103–417, § 8, 108 Stat. 4331 (1994)]. If FDA disagrees with a manufacturer's determination of new when a manufacturer sells an ingredient without giving the 75-day notification to the agency, the government bears the burden of proof to show that the substance is a new dietary ingredient requiring such a submission and that the product containing it is therefore adulterated.

It is important to note that the 75-day notification period applies to new dietary ingredients, but not new products. A product that is a new combination of ingredients marketed prior to October 1994 does not require submission of a 75-day notification.

DSHEA and Marketing and Labeling

Although less relevant to this report, DSHEA also provided for a government commission to consider the marketing and labeling of dietary supplements. The findings of this commission are described in the *Report of the Commission on Dietary Supplement Labels* (CDSL, 1997), which addressed health claims, nutritional support statements, substantiation files for claims and safety, and publications used in conjunction with sales.

FDA Actions Following DSHEA

Since a dietary supplement manufacturer is generally not required to share its basis for safety determinations with FDA before marketing, FDA determines possible safety issues from publicly available information it collects and from data that it generates in its own laboratories. In some cases, FDA may not be able to gather enough data to be confident about the safety of a particular product; without demonstrating that a substance does not meet the standard of safety—representing a reasonable certainty of no harm—FDA has no authority to remove it from the marketplace. FDA has acted when aware of possible harmful effects with various levels of response: it may warn consumers as it did in 2001 with comfrey and lipokinetix; it may warn health care practitioners that a supplement may be a serious health risk and ask them to review and report cases of adverse effects as it did with lipokinetix and with kava in 2001; or it may request a voluntary recall by manufacturers and distributors as it did with aristolochic acid in 2001. In the case of ephedrine alkaloids in 2003, for the first time FDA issued a warning letter to the manufacturer or distributor of a dietary supplement ingredient indicating that it intended to take action to remove a product; this was incorporated into a final rule in 2004 (21 C.F.R. § 119). Recently, manufacturers of androstenedione were notified by FDA that their products were considered adulterated as the agency had determined that their ingredients were new dietary ingredients about which FDA had not been notified 75 days in advance of sale, and that failure to cease distribution of the product could result in enforcement action (CFSAN, 2004).

Consumer and health care advisory letters from FDA cautioning use have occasionally led to voluntary product recalls by manufacturers (East Earth Herb, 2000; FDA, 2000; Vital Nutrients, 2001). In addition, warnings about specific dietary supplement ingredients issued in response to a variety of potential health problems identified by FDA as possible concerns have been posted on FDA MedWatch website (FDA, 2004).

Good Manufacturing Practices

As dietary supplements, like foods, can be contaminated with foreign toxic substances, FDA must consider more than the "inherent" safety of specific dietary supplement ingredients to adequately evaluate the potential for public health concerns. Supplement products vary in their quality and composition, which impacts the safety of specific products. Dietary supplement products tainted by improper raw materials, heavy metals, pesticides, or microorganisms, for example, can be unsafe due to these contaminants. DSHEA provides that FDA may define current GMPs for dietary supplement production. Proposed GMPs for the dietary supplement industry were published in early 2003 (FDA, 2003). While GMPs are designed to enhance safety, they are focused on purity and consistency rather than whether a dietary supplement ingredient itself is safe. As requested by FDA, this report focuses on evaluating the inherent safety of a dietary supplement ingredient in the absence of such contamination.

REFERENCES

ADA (American Dietetic Association). 2000. Nutrition and you: Trends 2000. What do Americans think, need, expect? *J Am Diet Assoc* 100:626–627.

Balluz LS, Kieszak SM, Philen RM, Mulinare J. 2000. Vitamin and mineral supplement use in the United States: Results from the Third National Health and Nutrition Examination Survey. *Arch Fam Med* 9:258–262.

Barkan ID. 1985. Industry invites regulation: The passage of the Pure Food and Drug Act of 1906. *Am J Public Health* 75:18–26.

Bender MM, Levy AS, Schucker RE, Yetley EA. 1992. Trends in prevalence and magnitude of vitamin and mineral supplement usage and correlation with health status. *J Am Diet Assoc* 92:1096–1101.

Blendon RJ, Earaches CM, Benson JM, Brodie M, Altman DE. 2001. Americans' views on the use and regulation of dietary supplements. *Arch Intern Med* 161:805–810.

Cardello HMAB, Da Silva MAPA, Damasio MH. 1999. Measurement of the relative sweetness of stevia extract, aspartame and cyclamate/saccharin blend as compared to sucrose at different concentrations. *Plant Foods Human Nutr* 54:119–130.

CDER (Center for Drug Evaluation and Research). 2002. *The Patent Medicine Menace*. Online. Food and Drug Administration. Available at http://www.fda.gov/cder/about/history/gallery/galleryintro.htm. Accessed March 4, 2002.

CDSL (Commission on Dietary Supplement Labels). 1997. *Report of the Commission on Dietary Supplement Labels*. Washington, DC: U.S. Government Printing Office.

CFSAN. 2004. *Androstenedione Warning Letters*. Online. Food and Drug Administration. Available at http://www.cfsan.fda.gov/~dms/andrlist.html. Accessed March 15, 2004.

Costello RB, Grumpstrup-Scott J. 2000. Zinc: What role might supplements play? *J Am Diet Assoc* 100:371–376.

Dwyer JT, Garceau AO, Evans M, Li D, Lytle L, Hoelscher D, Nickas TA, Zive M. 2001. Do adolescent vitamin-mineral supplement users have better nutrient intakes than nonusers? Observations from the CATCH tracking study. *J Am Diet Assoc* 101:1340–1346.

East Earth Herb. 2000. *East Earth Herb Recalls Jade Pharmacy Brand Meridian Circulation and Quell Fire Because of Possible Health Risk*. Online. November 21. News release. Available at http://www.fda.gov/oc/po/firmrecalls/eastearth11_00.html. Accessed March 3, 2002.

FDA (Food and Drug Administration). 1941. Regulations for the enforcement of the Federal Food, Drug, and Cosmetic Act. *Fed Regis* 6:5921–5926.

FDA. 1966. Dietary supplements and vitamin and mineral-fortified foods. *Fed Regis* 31: 15730–15736.

FDA. 1973. Definitions and standards of identity for food for special dietary use. Dietary supplements of vitamins and minerals. *Fed Regis* 38:20730.

FDA. 1979. Vitamin and mineral drug products for over-the-counter human use. *Fed Regis* 44:16125–16200.

FDA. 1981. The story of the laws behind the labels part II: 1938—The Federal Food, Drug, and Cosmetic Act. *FDA Consumer*. Online. Available at http://vm.cfsan.fda.gov/~lrd/histor1a.html. Accessed June 6, 2002.

FDA. 1987. Food labeling; Public health messages and label statements. Proposed rules. *Fed Regis* 52:28843–28849.

FDA. 1993. Regulation of dietary supplements. Advanced Notice of Proposed Rulemaking 21, CFR Chapter 1. *Fed Regis* 58:33690.

FDA. 1995. *75-Day Notification for Stevia from Sunrider Corporation, Docket 95S-0316*. Online. Available at http://www.fda.gov/ohrms/dockets/dockets/95s0316/m000002.pdf. Accessed March 24, 2004.

FDA. 1997. Substances generally recognized as safe, Proposed rule. *Fed Regis* 62:18937–18964.

FDA. 2000. *FDA Warns Against Consuming Dietary Supplements Containing Tiratricol*. Online. FDA Talk Paper. November 21. Available at http://www.fda.gov/bbs/topics/ANSWERS/ANS0105.html. Accessed March 8, 2002.

FDA. 2001a. *Information Paper on L-Tryptophan and 5-Hydroxy-L-tryptophan*. Online. Available at http://vm.cfsan.fda.gov/~dms/ds-tryp1.html. Accessed March 26, 2004.

FDA. 2001b. Premarket notice concerning bioengineered foods. *Fed Regis* 66:4706–4738.

FDA. 2002. *FDA Backgrounder. Milestones in U.S. Food and Drug Law History*. Online. Available at http://www.fda.gov/opacom/backgrounders/miles.html. Accessed March 13, 2004.

FDA. 2003. Current good manufacturing practices in manufacturing, packing, or holding dietary ingredients and dietary supplements. Proposed rule. *Fed Regis* 68:12157–12263.

FDA. 2004. *Medical Product Safety Information. MedWatch Safety Information.* Available at http://www.fda.gov/medwatch/safety.htm. Accessed March 14, 2004.

Ford ES. 2001. Vitamin supplement use and diabetes mellitus incidence among adults in the United States. *Am J Epidemiol* 153:892–897.

Hartz SC, Otradovec CL, McGandy RB, Russell RM, Jacob RA, Sahyoun N, Peters H, Abrams D, Scura LA, Whinston-Perry RA. 1988. Nutrient supplement use by healthy elderly. *J Am Coll Nutr* 7:119–128.

Hunt JR. 1996. Position of the American Dietetic Association: Vitamin and mineral supplementation. *J Am Diet Assoc* 96:73–77.

Hunt JR, Dwyer J. 2001. Position of the American Dietetic Association: Food fortification and dietary supplements. *J Am Diet Assoc* 101:115–132.

Hutt PB, Merrill RA. 1991. Regulation of vitamin-mineral supplements. In: *Food and Drug Law. Cases and Materials*. 2nd ed. Westbury, NY: The Foundation Press. Pp. 204–228.

Kaufman DW, Kelly JP, Rosenberg L, Anderson TE, Mitchell AA. 2002. Recent patterns of medication use in the ambulatory adult population of the United States. The Sloan Survey. *J Am Med Assoc* 287:337–344.

Khatcheressian LAW. 1999. Regulation of dietary supplements: Five years of DSHEA. *Food Drug Law J* 54:623–644.

Kim I, Williamson DF, Byers T, Koplan JP. 1993. Vitamin and mineral supplement use and mortality in a U.S. cohort. *Am J Public Health* 83:546–550.

Koplan JP, Annest JL, Layde PM, Rubin GL. 1986. Nutrient intake and supplementation in the United States (NHANES II). *Am J Public Health* 76:287–289.

Kraak V, Pelletier DL, Dohhahite J. 2002. Food, health, and nutrient supplements: Beliefs among food stamp-eligible women and implications for food stamp policy. *Fam Econ Nutr Rev* 14:21–35.

Lyle BJ, Mares-Perlman JA, Klein BEK, Klein R, Greger JL. 1998. Supplement users differ from nonusers in demographic, lifestyle, dietary and health characteristics. *J Nutr* 128:2355–2362.

McNamara SH. 1995. Dietary supplements of botanicals and other substances: A new era of regulation. *Food Drug Law J* 50:341–348.

Millikan LE. 1999. Anecdotal therapies. *Adv Exp Med Biol* 455:407–411.

Nayga RM, Reed DB. 1999. Factors associated with the intake of dietary supplements. *Fam Econ Nutr Rev* 12:43–48.

NBJ's Annual Industry Overview VIII. 2003. *Nutr Bus J* 8:1–9.

Nesheim MC. 1999. What is the research base for the use of dietary supplements? *Public Health Nutr* 2:35–38.

Neuhouser ML, Patterson RE, Levy L. 1999. Motivations for using vitamin and mineral supplements. *J Am Diet Assoc* 101:1340–1346.

Newman V, Rock CL, Faerber S, Flatt SW, Wright FA, Pierce JP. 1998. Dietary supplement use by women at risk for breast cancer recurrence. *J Am Diet Assoc* 98:285–292.

OIG (Office of Inspector General). 2001. *Adverse Event Reporting for Dietary Supplements. An Inadequate Safety Valve*. OEI-01-00-00180. Boston, MA: OIG, Department of Health and Human Services.

Pelletier DL, Kendall A. 1997. Supplement use may not be associated with better food intake in all population groups. *Fam Econ Nutr Rev* 10:32–44.

Pendergast WR. 1997. Dietary supplements. In: Brady RP, Cooper RM, Silverman RS, eds. *Fundamentals of Law and Regulation. An In-Depth Look at Foods, Veterinary Medicines, and Cosmetics*. Washington, DC: Food and Drug Law Institute. Pp. 257–283.

Pezzuto JM, Compadre CM, Swanson SM, Nanayakkara NPD, Kinghorn AD. 1985. Metabolically activated steviol, the aglycone of stevioside, is mutagenic. *Proc Natl Acad Sci* 82:2478–2482.

Prevention Magazine. 2001. *Consumer Use of Dietary Supplements*. Emmaus, PA: Rodale. Pp. 1–79.

Radimer KL, Subar AF, Thompson FE. 2000. Nonvitamin, nonmineral dietary supplements: Issues and findings from NHANES III. *J Am Diet Assoc* 100:447–454.

Ramos L. 2000. SAMe as a supplement: Can it really help treat depression and arthritis? *J Am Diet Assoc* 100:414.

Sarubin A. 2000. *The Health Professional's Guide to Popular Dietary Supplements*. Chicago, IL: American Dietetic Association.

Scientific Committee on Food. 1999. *Opinion on Stevioside as a Sweetener*. European Commission. CS/ADD/EDUL/167 final. Brussels: European Commission. Available at http://europa.eu.int/comm/food/fs/sc/scf/out34_en.pdf. Accessed March 25, 2004.

Sinclair U. 1906. *The Jungle*. New York: Doubleday.

Slesinski MJ, Subar AF, Kahle LL. 1995. Trends in use of vitamin and mineral supplements in the United States: The 1987 and 1992 National Health Interview Surveys. *J Am Diet Assoc* 95:921–923.

Subar AF, Block G. 1990. Use of vitamin and mineral supplements: Demographics and amounts of nutrients consumed. The 1987 Health Interview Survey. *Am J Epidemiol* 132:1091–1101.

Vital Nutrients. 2001. *Vital Nutrients Recalls Joint Ease and Verified Quality Brand Joint Comfort Complex Because of Adverse Health Risk Associated with Aristolochic Acid*. Online. May 21. News release. Available at http://www.fda.gov/oc/po/firmrecalls/vital5_01.html. Accessed March 8, 2002.

Wasuntarawat C, Temcharoen P, Toskulkao C, Mungkornkarn P, Suttajit M, Glinsukon T. 1998. Developmental toxicity of steviol, a metabolite of stevioside, in the hamster. *Drug Chem Toxicol* 21:207–222.

Wax PM. 1995. Elixirs, diluents, and the passage of the 1938 Federal Food, Drug and Cosmetic Act. *Ann Intern Med* 122:456–461.

Wetli CV, Davis JH. 1978. Fatal hyperkalemia from accidental overdose of potassium chloride. *J Am Med Assoc* 240:1339.

Yamada A, Ohgaki S, Noda T, Shimizu M. 1985. Chronic toxicity study of dietary *stevia* extracts in F344 rats. *J Food Hyg Soc Japan* 26:169–183.

Young AL, Bass IS. 1995. The Dietary Supplement Health and Education Act. *Food Drug Law J* 50:285–292.

2

Approaches Used by Others and Existing Safety Frameworks

In its charge, the committee was specifically asked to consider methods other expert bodies have used to categorize and review supplement safety and efficacy issues. Considering the strengths and weaknesses of other organizations' approaches was an initial step in developing the framework described in this report. Assessing the relevance of other organizations' efforts to safety evaluation by the Food and Drug Administration (FDA) was also important because these resources may be referred to by some as authoritative sources on the safety of dietary supplements. A list of considerations was developed for evaluating the usefulness to FDA of existing and future resources of dietary supplement information. These considerations, which are not part of the proposed framework, are summarized in the first part of this chapter.

Frameworks developed for reviewing the safety of other substances (i.e., in foods, in pharmaceuticals, and in the environment) were also considered to prepare the committee to undertake its charge. The objective was to identify aspects applicable to developing a framework for evaluating dietary supplement ingredient safety. Brief descriptions of the frameworks the committee reviewed are provided in Appendix A.

The knowledge gained from reviewing existing dietary supplement resources and frameworks for other substances, as well as discussions in open sessions with many individuals, informed the development of a list of attributes of a framework for setting priorities and evaluating the safety of dietary supplement ingredients. These attributes are summarized in the second part of the chapter.

RESOURCES ON DIETARY SUPPLEMENTS

Several organizations have compiled resources that review the safety, efficacy, and/or quality of dietary supplements. A list of considerations was developed for assessing the relevance of different resources to a safety review, and samples of these resources were reviewed. The considerations are described below, followed by a table indicating how each resource met these considerations and a narrative description of each resource. This discussion focuses on resources that appeared to be the product of organization or government-sponsored committees or a peer-reviewed process. Inclusion does not constitute endorsement of resources, nor should this review be considered inclusive of all efforts to consider safety, efficacy, and/or quality of dietary supplements. Additional publications, although not reviewed here, may also be informative (Ernst, 2000; Foster and Tyler, 1999; Grieve, 1996).

Considerations for Evaluating Resources

Eighteen considerations were developed to assess the relevance of various resources to safety/risk evaluation. They address the objectives and focus of the resource, the authors and review process, the literature procurement and type of information considered, and the limitations of product-specific evaluations.

1. Was review of safety/risk a primary goal of the document? Does the review have a clear focus on safety, rather than a focus on quality or potential therapeutic uses? For example, some resources focus mainly on efficacy, with safety issues seemingly an afterthought. Also, some reviews focus on objectives, such as verifying that the label is accurate and determining whether the substance is contaminated. These are useful approaches because quality and purity issues are important and can impact the safety of dietary supplements to a significant degree, but they are product focused, rather than focused on a particular dietary supplement ingredient's inherent safety.

2. Does the review rely on primary sources of information rather than secondary sources? Primary sources are original research articles that generate data, while secondary sources are compilations that may include statements of opinion in addition to facts. A review that summarizes data from primary sources is a more appropriate resource for assessing safety. If a resource's conclusion about safety is based on scientific evidence from the primary literature, then it is more likely to be factual and less likely to be an opinion. Use of primary literature to support statements is a daunting task, but when it is possible, it minimizes the risk of carrying forward anecdotal statements that are not possible to document. Use of primary literature also increases credibility of resources when persons or organizations involved in producing them might be perceived to have a bias or conflict of interest.

3. Does the review consider all types of information available, including data from *in vitro* studies and animal studies, as well as information about the safety of closely related plants or substances? A review that attempts to integrate a variety of data types, especially in the absence of good quality human data, will be a more appropriate resource for assessing safety. Because it is scientifically appropriate to consider concerns raised by animal data, *in vitro* studies, or information about related substances (see Chapters 4–7), reviews that conclude a substance is *safe* by focusing exclusively on human data should not be considered as adequate sources of safety conclusions. The converse is not true. That is, reviews that conclude a *risk* exists by exclusively focusing on human data are acceptable.

4. Has appropriate scientific expertise and objectivity been used in weighing different types of information? Good reviews will explain why some information is considered more important than other information in reaching overall conclusions. Clearly stating the logic that underpins the data interpretation enables other experts to understand the basis for the evaluative judgment and determine whether appropriate objectivity and scientific expertise were used.

5. What are the limitations to the safety review? Does the review explain why it may be difficult to make a conclusion about the safety of an ingredient? Does the review describe where insufficient, inconsistent, or inadequate data preclude an accurate assessment of safety? Discussion of limitations in data, such as how much is known and how definitively it is known, is useful in understanding safety. Also, an appropriate discussion about the limitations in interpreting the available data lends credibility to the review. Limitations may be of two types. First is the individual study's limitations, such as limitations in interpreting the data or in experimental design, sometimes described by the study authors themselves. Another type is derived from developing the review itself, such as difficulty in interpreting data from foreign language sources or inconsistent data from different sources.

6. Were the strategies used to search the literature adequately described? A good review will describe how the search for pertinent data was performed. Ideally, this description will include a list of databases searched, when they were searched, what search terms were used, and if there was a strategy for selecting information to review. This allows the user of the information to determine if the breadth and depth of the search was appropriate.

7. How current is the information? A good review includes relevant current information, in addition to older information published in reputable journals and historic information. Of course, all published reviews cannot claim to be current after they are published, but some will be updated with new information, if available. Evaluations that use resources that do not consider recent data should be supplemented with information available after publication of the review to determine if new data might have affected safety conclusions.

8. **Are the primary sources cited accurately and completely?** Accurate citations are one indication that the original literature is being used and support the accuracy of the interpretation of the data. Incomplete or incorrectly cited references take away from the credibility and usefulness of the resource.

9. **Is the review well balanced and objective? Is there a conflict of interest (financial or otherwise) relative to the outcome of the safety evaluation?** Conflicts of interest should lead the user to be more skeptical in interpreting the review's assessment of safety as unbiased and appropriate. In considering the objectivity of a particular evaluation, the starting assumptions should be identified. For example, there is a difference between concluding that a substance can be consumed without safety concerns because the data reviewed included relevant safety information and it was determined to be of little concern, compared with concluding that a substance can be consumed without concern but not having any data that provided information related to safety. Guidelines for authors of scientific journals include the importance of disclosing financial relationships (Campbell, 2001), underscoring the importance of full disclosure relative to the information included in the review

10. **Do the authors have the depth and breadth of expertise necessary to assess the primary sources, weigh the data, and make conclusions as to the adequacy of the data for safety assessment?** Persons knowledgeable in safety assessment should be included in the evaluations. In addition, particular types of expertise may be needed depending on the safety issues being considered for the particular supplement.

11. **Was the authored information peer-reviewed by knowledgeable experts?** A good safety review will utilize the expertise of a variety of appropriate experts. Peer review is an essential component and, as such, the review should be critically reviewed by experts from a variety of disciplines. As the National Research Council (NRC, 1998) has stated, "External experts often can be more open, frank, and challenging to the status quo than internal reviewers, who may feel constrained by organizational concerns. Evaluation by external reviewers thus can enhance the credibility of the peer review process by avoiding both the reality and the appearance of conflict of interest."

12. **If appropriate, is variability of specific preparations addressed or acknowledged? Do reviewers address or acknowledge the limitations in**

extrapolating across different parts of a botanical (i.e., roots, stems, flowers, and leaves) in the safety assessment? A safety review should attempt to explain different dietary supplement ingredient preparations and how those different preparations might change the safety assessment. For some ingredients that are well characterized this is not an issue, but for many botanical ingredients it is important to understand the plant part used, as well as the effect of different methods of preparation that may concentrate active compounds or otherwise alter the activity of the ingredient.

13. Does the review focus on the safety of a particular standardized product? Frequently, reviews from another country describe the safety of standardized preparations of supplements available in that country; however, the relevance of such reviews to the safety of nonstandardized products consumed in the United States should be addressed for such reviews to be considered relevant to U.S. consumers. Reviews describing the safety of a standardized product are helpful in understanding some safety concerns inherent in the ingredient, but less relevant to safety concerns that vary with preparation. Similarly, good reviews will convey limitations inherent in extrapolating from studies suggesting safety of one standardized product to other products of the same ingredient. That is, they acknowledge that extrapolation to other products to mitigate safety concerns may be inappropriate.

14. Is the ingested amount (or range of ingested amounts) under consideration specified in the review? Does the review address the relevance of the amount used in the evaluated research studies and published data to the amount commonly ingested or recommended for ingestion? Given the basic tenet of toxicology, "the dose makes the poison," a good review of safety will describe the relevance of ingredient levels that produce safety concerns to the ingredient levels commonly consumed by or recommended to humans. (Many resources available to consumers specify recommendations for consumption, even if the labeling *per se* does not include recommended ingestion levels.)

15. Does the review consider the relevance of data that describes results of non-oral administration of the ingredient? While safety issues with oral consumption are obviously the most relevant, some safety issues that come to light with other routes of administration may also be relevant. The relevance of such issues should be considered on a case-by-case basis, but expressly disregarding any safety information derived from non-oral exposure is not appropriate for some dietary supplement ingredients, especially when sufficient, quality data about oral ingestion are lacking. A review that considers non-oral data in its evaluation will have more value to FDA than one that ignores this type of information regardless of relevance. In many of the resources described, it was not evident whether non-oral data were considered.

16. Does the review address the possible biological activity or mechanism of action of the ingredient and its implications for human safety? Knowledge of the mechanism of action may be useful in understanding the biological basis for possible harm.

17. Does the review address whether the ingredient might pose safety problems for specific groups within the general population? Does the review address specific concerns related to pregnant or lactating women, children, the aged, or those with specific diseases or other physiological conditions? A good review will address vulnerable populations and may be helpful in targeting safety concerns that may apply to a subpopulation, but that may not cause a significant safety concern for the general population (see Chapter 9).

18. Does the review address the potential for interaction with other supplements, drugs, foods, or other medical interventions? A useful review will address potential interactions (see Chapter 8) and explain whether possible interactions have actually been observed from human use, or if interactions described are predicted based on other types of information (e.g., *in vitro* assays, chemical structure). Inclusion of both demonstrated and theoretical interaction information is important to understanding the safety profile of an ingredient. If considering potential interactions is not within the authors' expertise or capabilities, then the review should acknowledge that the potential for interactions with other substances was not evaluated.

Strengths and Weaknesses of Available Dietary Supplement Resources

Table 2-1 provides an overview of many of the available resources that address dietary supplements and characterizes each based on the considerations listed in the previous section. The summaries following the table[1] provide a general description based on the general information reviewed. As is apparent from the table, the resources vary in their relevance to FDA's mission of identifying dietary supplements that would present risk of significant or unreasonable harm.

Of the resources that do sufficiently focus on safety, some are not ideally transparent or unbiased. Other resources fall short in other areas. Nevertheless, the different resources are valuable even when their conclusions are less relevant to FDA's task—they can serve as starting points of information about concerns and as sources of primary literature references.

In preparing Table 2-1, it was difficult to provide descriptions for some

[1]The descriptive summaries and Table 2-1 are largely based on information from the resource itself via websites or books, or descriptions written by others (Barrett, 1998); they are not based on verification of the statements included in those resources.

TABLE 2-1 Brief Characterization of 13 Secondary Resources and How They Meet the Described Considerations

	Resource	
Considerations	Agency for Healthcare Research and Quality (AHRQ) (AHRQ, 2000a, 2000b, 2002b, 2003a)	American Herbal Pharmacopoeia (AHP, 2002, 2004a, 2004b; Upton, 1997, 1999) (Reviewed St. Johns Wort and Valerian Root monographs)
Type of organization responsible for resource	U.S. government	Private, nonprofit organization
Substances reviewed	Many health care techniques, practices, and substances, including several dietary supplements	Botanicals commonly used in the United States; selections are based on recommendations of a prioritization committee or monograph sponsorship from interested organizations or companies
Product/endpoint	Meta-analysis published when completed	Summary monographs
Focus on safety/risk	Both efficacy and safety are considered	Identification, handling, standardization, and analytical methods are discussed; safety and efficacy information are considered
Reliance on primary data	Primary sources are cited, including foreign language sources	Primary and secondary sources are used, including foreign language articles
Use of nonhuman data	Only human data are considered in the examples reviewed	Human, animal, and *in vitro* information are used in efficacy assessment; however, from the examples reviewed, it is not clear the degree to which various types of information are generally used
Description of limitations	Limitations are described: a summary of challenges in conducting and interpreting the research is given, difficulties in obtaining and interpreting adverse events are explained	The material examined includes limitations as described by the authors of the primary sources

continued

TABLE 2-1 Continued

Description of literature search strategy	Well-defined search strategy, including databases and key words used	Strategy was not described in detail
Use of current literature	Examples reviewed were very current at time of publication, no explanation of updates	Monographs published periodically since 1997; older publications, as well as citations within 5 years of publication, were included
Starting assumptions/ appearance of impartiality		A lack of information appears to be interpreted as safety
Use of peer review	Peer reviewed	Outside peer reviewers are used
Focus on a particular standardized product and discussion of preparation impact on safety	Discusses different preparations and where effect of preparation on safety issues is unclear	Preparations are described, but impact of preparation on safety is not specifically described
Description of consumption levels considered	Ingested amount under consideration is described	Recommended levels are described; it is assumed that the safety conclusions are based on these levels
Consideration of data from non-oral routes of exposure	No mention is made of how non-oral data were handled; in the example reviewed, non-oral data were referred to in some sections, but it is not clear if these data are considered as possibly relevant for safety of oral consumption of the ingredient	Non-oral data are referred to in some sections, but it is not clear if these data are considered as possibly relevant for safety of oral consumption of the ingredient
Discussion of biological activity or possible mechanism of action	Addressed	Discussion is included, but implication for safety is not discussed
Discussion of specific groups within the general population, if appropriate	No recommendations for specific groups in the examples reviewed; for ephedra, the panel was asked to consider safety in children, adolescents, young athletes, and adults, but conclusions on safety are not specific for these groups	Precautions for pregnant and lactating women are given in the examples reviewed, but not for children or other groups

TABLE 2-1 Continued

Interaction with other interventions	Interaction with caffeine discussed extensively in the ephedra report; not discussed in other examples reviewed	Interactions discussed in the examples reviewed
Other comments and considerations for using this resource	AHRQ reviews are extensive reviews of health care practices Thorough resource for those supplements considered; less useful due to small number of supplements included to date: garlic, milk thistle, SAMe (S-adenosyl-L-methionine), and ephedra	Only 18 monographs are available to date; starting assumption appears to be one of safety, therefore a lack of information appears to be interpreted as safe This is a useful resource to understand use levels, stability, and analytical methods, but the literature search on safety information may not be sufficiently comprehensive for all ingredients considered

	Resource	
Considerations	American Herbal Products Association Botanical Safety Handbook (McGuffin et al., 1997)	Institute of Medicine (IOM) Dietary Reference Intakes—Tolerable Upper Intake Levels (ULs) (IOM, 1997, 1998a, 1998b, 2000, 2001, 2002, 2004)
Type of organization responsible for resource	Nonprofit trade association representing the herbal products industry	Prepared by expert panels assembled by the IOM of the National Academies (Nonprofit organization chartered to give advice to the government)
Substances reviewed	Botanicals sold in North America	Essential vitamins, minerals, and electrolytes, as well as macronutrients and water
Product/endpoint	Book; safety classifications of botanicals	Chapter sections; component of Dietary Reference Intakes publications
Focus on safety/risk	Safety is primary focus	Safety is primary focus; specifically, determining the level at which nutrient intake may cause adverse effects

continued

TABLE 2-1 Continued

Reliance on primary data	30 references are cited for over 500 botanicals; most are secondary sources of information	Primary sources are used, including foreign language articles
Use of nonhuman data	Cannot be determined due to limited use of primary data	Human data primarily, although animal data are used on occasion
Description of limitations	Limitations of primary data for specific ingredients are generally not described, authors classify some botanicals as "Insufficient Data for Classification"	Limitations regarding studies used and the review were well described
Description of literature search strategy	Not described	Not described
Use of current literature	Published in 1997; secondary sources cited are mostly late 1980s to early 1990s	The ULs have been published from 1997 to 2004 in groups of nutrients; at the time of their publication, the authors considered the most recent literature; when and if they will be updated has not been determined
Starting assumptions/ appearance of impartiality	Not possible to discern due to reliance on secondary sources	Caution regarding excess intakes is given when no UL is provided
Use of peer review	Reviewers are listed in text	External peer reviewers were used and are listed in the report
Focus on a particular standardized product and discussion of preparation impact on safety	Some different preparations, including different plant parts, are considered (e.g., cooked/ raw, stems/leaves)	Focuses on nutrients present in foods or as concentrates, some of which may be various structural forms; when UL relates to one or more specific forms, discussed in text which forms and why
Description of consumption levels considered	For some substances, a "common therapeutic dose" is included, so safety conclusions are assumed to be based on these ingestion levels; however, many substances lack	Detailed description included on amounts consumed; how the amount ingested will impact the safety is considered, as the purpose is to derive a UL

TABLE 2-1 Continued

	information on the common doses to which safety conclusions are relevant	
Consideration of data from non-oral routes of exposure	According to the text, "Information associated with other forms of administration were reviewed but was not considered as a sole basis for classification"	Only oral routes of administration were considered in safety evaluations; evidence of adverse effects related to other routes of exposure may be mentioned
Discussion of biological activity or possible mechanism of action	Not discussed	Biological activity and mechanisms for possible harms are discussed
Discussion of specific groups within the general population, if appropriate	Pregnant and lactating women, as well as children, are discussed; however, only 34 of 600 botanicals are classified as "not for use during lactation"	Age, gender, pregnancy, lactation, and sensitive subpopulations are discussed
Interaction with other interventions	Information on some ingredients includes comments about interactions, but a discussion of possible interactions is not included for each substance	Overall model for review includes section on interaction with other nutrients; some ULs are based on their known interaction with other nutrients (e.g., zinc)
Other comments and considerations for using this resource	Working assumption is that "safety concerns for herbal products need not be extrapolated from constituent profiles with any more alarm than is appropriate for foods" Botanicals are classified as: Class 1, which can be safely consumed when used appropriately; Class 2, for which certain restrictions apply; Class 3, for which significant data exist to recommend special labeling; and Class 4, for which there is insufficient data	Limited to nutrients Uses a risk-assessment methodology related to chronic intake; does not give guidance related to acute ingestion Useful for assessing safety of specific nutrient levels used as supplements Useful in examining specific subpopulations that may be sensitive or at risk

continued

TABLE 2-1 Continued

	Classification may be helpful for identifying some potential problems, but there is no class that is "Unsafe" Safety classifications need more justification; the fact that a botanical does not appear on one of the restricted use lists for particular conditions does not indicate that it is safe for the particular condition	

	Resource	
Considerations	Translation of the German Commission E (Blumenthal et al., 1998)	Expanded German Commission E (Blumenthal et al., 2000)
Type of organization responsible for resource	Commission E, which wrote the original monographs in German, is a German government organization; American Botanical Council (ABC), which translated the Commission E monographs for this resource, is a nonprofit member organization (including corporate members) that promotes herbal medicines	ABC expanded upon the original Commission E monographs in this text
Substances reviewed	380 medicinal plants and phytomedicines in the German marketplace	107 medicinal plants and phytomedicines common to the United States; largely derived from those in the German marketplace
Product/endpoint	Book of brief monographs	Book of monographs
Focus on safety/risk	Safety and efficacy are considered	Safety and efficacy are considered
Reliance on primary data	Some primary and many secondary sources were reported to be used, but the sources are not cited or available	Primary and secondary sources are cited in the text

TABLE 2-1 Continued

Use of nonhuman data	—*a*	Appeared to rely mostly on human data, although some animal data are mentioned
Description of limitations	—*a*	—*a*
Description of literature search strategy	General types of sources are described, but specifics of the search strategy are not	General types of sources are described but specifics of the search strategy are not
Use of current literature	Original Commission E monographs were completed in 1994; assessment of literature used is not possible because it is not cited	Includes references from the year 2000
Starting assumptions/ appearance of impartiality	Translation sponsored by ABC (including corporate members), but it is assumed to replicate the original Commission E findings	Sponsored by ABC (including corporate members)
Use of peer review	—*a*	Text indicates "streamlined peer review process" was employed, but also indicates additional information provided in the expanded text was not subject to the level of review conducted by Commission E
Focus on a particular standardized product and discussion of preparation impact on safety	Preparation impact on safety is not specifically discussed; safety conclusions are assumed to be based on standardizations described because conclusions were made for the German marketplace	Specific preparations were not addressed except for two botanicals (Echinacea and hawthorne), where confusion existed from Commission E; safety conclusions are based on products standardized for the German marketplace
Description of consumption levels considered	Recommendations for therapeutic doses are included, so it is assumed that these are the intake levels on which safety judgments are made	Recommendations for therapeutic doses as in the Commission E translation, so it is assumed that these are the intake levels on which safety judgments are made

continued

TABLE 2-1 Continued

Consideration of data from non-oral routes of exposure	No mention of how non-oral data were handled	No mention of how non-oral data were handled
Discussion of biological activity or possible mechanism of action	Not discussed in detail	Discussed somewhat
Discussion of specific groups within the general population addressed, if appropriate	Pregnancy and lactation are considered	Pregnancy and lactation are considered, as are contraindications, side effects, and interactions with other drugs
Interaction with other interventions	Discussed	Limited to drug interactions, but the statement "none known" is generally used
Other comments and considerations for using this resource	Medicinal plants only Safety is considered in light of potential benefit because this was part of a review of all medicines on the German market Categorized into three classes: Approved, Unapproved-negative (safety concerns outweighed benefit), and Unapproved-null (no risk, but also no substantiated efficacy) Lack of references and ability to distinguish reasons for Negative review in the text limit this resource's usefulness; it may be useful for understanding recommended doses, Table 13 may be useful for identifying botanicals of suspected risk (but inclusion of well-known spices in the table without indication of dose is not useful) Usefulness of conclusions depends on similarity of German products to products consumed in the United States	Updated review of selected German Commission E monographs Limited in terms of in-depth evaluation of safety, toxicology, adverse effects, or drug interactions The "quick look" cross-references included may be useful in establishing a list of supplements for which safety concerns may arise

TABLE 2-1 Continued

Considerations	Resource: European Scientific Cooperative on Phytotherapy (ESCOP) Monographs on the Medicinal Uses of Plant Drugs (ESCOP, 1996, 1997, 2001) (Reviewed St. John's Wort and Valerian Root)	Resource: Natural Medicines Comprehensive Database (NMCD) (NMCD, 2002) (Reviewed St. John's Wort and Valerian)
Type of organization responsible for resource	Coalition of international trade associations	Therapeutic Research Center, publisher of the *Pharmacist's Letter* and the *Prescriber's Letter*; a for-profit organization
Substances reviewed	Botanicals used within the European community	Botanicals, vitamins, minerals, amino acids, glandular products; over 1,000 entries
Product/endpoint	Groups of monographs (Fascicules)	Website and book
Focus on safety/risk	Includes safety data, but primarily designed for efficacy assessment by regulatory authorities	Safety and efficacy are considered; describes circumstances in which the supplement is Likely to be Safe, Possibly Safe, Possibly Unsafe, Likely to be Unsafe, Unsafe
Reliance on primary data	Primary sources are cited, including many foreign language sources	Primary and secondary sources are cited, including foreign language sources
Use of nonhuman data	Animal and *in vitro* experiments are used	Safety information is generally derived from human data
Description of limitations	—*a*	Limitations in interpreting human data are presented
Description of literature search strategy	Not described	Not described in database, but some aspects of strategy are described in description below, from personal communication
Use of current literature	Late 1990s literature cited	Very current; according to the publisher, individual supplements are updated about every 6 months; the book is updated annually
Starting assumptions/ appearance of impartiality	The stated purpose is to "advance the scientific status of phytomedicines";	

continued

TABLE 2-1 Continued

	ESCOP is an umbrella organization for phytotherapy trade associations, thus conflict of interest cannot be ruled out	
Use of peer review	Peer reviewed	Personal communication with NMCD indicated that peer review is conducted
Focus on a particular standardized product and discussion of preparation impact on safety	Appears to focus on a standardized product; one monograph compares the effects of the root preparation with the syrup on driving impairment	Generally does not focus on specific products or impact of preparation on safety
Description of consumption levels considered	The level at which adverse effects were reported is described	Doses used are described; impact of dose on safety is discussed
Consideration of data from non-oral routes of exposure	—[a]	Non-oral data are referred to in some sections, but it is not clear if these data were considered as possibly relevant for safety of oral consumption of the ingredient
Discussion of biological activity or possible mechanism of action	Addressed, but not necessarily with safety in mind	Discussed
Discussion of specific groups within the general population, if appropriate	Considers pregnancy and lactation	Pregnancy and lactation are always included in the safety assessment, children are sometimes included; secondary sources are largely used for this discussion
Interaction with other interventions	Sections for interactions are included, but both examples examined stated "none reported"	Describes information for other supplements, drugs, and foods, and other medical conditions; discusses side effects or contraindications observed in the literature, as well as those that might be theorized based on knowledge of the mechanism of action
Other comments and considerations for using this resource	Emphasis on European botanical products that may not resemble	Comprehensive in terms of the human clinical literature and the number

TABLE 2-1 Continued

	products sold in the United States Sponsorship by trade association organization Starting assumptions of safety; lack of information appears to be interpreted as safety Preclinical safety data section may be useful for individual botanicals	of supplements that are covered; describes a wide range of dietary supplements A useful cross-reference to brand names is included The continuum of safety classifications considered is helpful, as is the attention paid to formulation, plant part, and species

	Resource	
Considerations	Natural Standard (Natural Standard, 2003) (Reviewed Black Cohosh)	Physican's Desk Reference (PDR) for Herbal Medicines (Medical Economics, 1998, 2000)
Type of organization responsible for resource	For-profit, not supported by any interest group, professional organization, or pharmaceutical manufacturer	For-profit organization
Substances reviewed	Covers alternative therapies and complementary medicines, including nutrient and nonnutrient dietary supplements	Over 700 botanicals
Product/endpoint	Online monograph	Book of brief monographs
Focus on safety/risk	Safety and efficacy are considered	Both safety and efficacy are considered
Reliance on primary data	Mostly primary sources, some abstracts, including foreign language articles	Primary sources are cited, including foreign language sources
Use of nonhuman data	Mostly human data, some *in vitro* data and a limited number of animal studies are considered	Mostly human data; however, some animal and *in vitro* data are considered
Description of limitations	Limitations are described	Limitations are somewhat described
Description of literature search strategy	Described thoroughly	Search strategy is not described; many monographs appear to be based upon the Commission E translation

continued

TABLE 2-1 Continued

Use of current literature	Current literature, updated every 3–18 months	Mostly current, some historical information
Starting assumptions/ appearance of impartiality		Appears to give favorable consideration toward the approved German Commission E monographs (the basis for about half of the monographs) as "approved by the Commission E," without critical evaluation
Use of peer review	Introductory information describes an evidenced-based, consensus-based, peer review	No indication of peer review found
Focus on a particular standardized product and discussion of preparation impact on safety	Does not appear to focus on specific preparations	A number of different preparations are described, impact on safety is described for some; for monographs based on conclusions of Commission E, usefulness of conclusions depends on similarities of German products to products consumed in the United States
Description of consumption levels considered	A recommended use amount is described; it is assumed that safety conclusions are based on this amount	Recommended doses are described
Consideration of data from non-oral routes of exposure	No mention is made of how non-oral data were handled in the example reviewed	No mention is made of how non-oral data were handled
Discussion of biological activity or possible mechanism of action	Discussed	Addressed, but not necessarily with safety in mind
Discussion of specific groups within the general population, if appropriate	Pregnant and lactating women are addressed	Second edition has separate indexes for herbs not for use during pregnancy or lactation or for use only under supervision
Interaction with other interventions	Thorough section on interactions with conventional therapies, drugs, other herbs, and supplements	Interactions discussed and a Drug/Herb Interaction Guide is included

TABLE 2-1 Continued

Other comments and considerations for using this resource	Brief safety summary describes the situations in which the supplement would be considered Likely Safe, Possibly Safe, Possibly Unsafe, Likely Unsafe Comprehensive in terms of clinical literature and number of supplements considered Useful resource to gain understanding of historical uses	Useful cross-reference index of common and scientific names and glossary Inconsistent reference use Appears to be a summary of information and not a committee-authored or peer-reviewed activity Concerns about possible inaccuracies, such as example cited by Chambliss et al. (2002): PDR entry for English hawthorne monograph indicates Commission E approval, but Commission E approved only the leaf with the flower, not the berries, leaf, extracts, powders, etc., as suggested by the PDR

	Resource	
Considerations	PDR for Nutritional Supplements (Medical Economics, 2001)	American Pharmaceutical Association Practical Guide to Natural Medicines (Peirce, 1999)
Type of organization responsible for resource	For-profit organization	Nonprofit organization
Substances reviewed	Vitamins, minerals, amino acids, and other nonbotanical dietary supplements	Botanicals
Product/endpoint	Book	Book
Focus on safety/risk	Safety and efficacy are considered	Safety and efficacy are considered
Reliance on primary data	Many primary sources, some secondary, including foreign language articles	Mostly secondary sources
Use of nonhuman data	Some *in vitro* and animal data are used	Cannot be determined due to reliance on secondary data
Description of limitations	Limitations are generally not discussed	Describes insufficiencies in amount of available data, but discussion of primary data is limited

continued

TABLE 2-1 Continued

Description of literature search strategy	Search strategy not described	Description limited to indication that the "National Library of Medicine's biomedical literature, Medline, and NAPRALERT" were used
Use of current literature	Current for some supplements, less so for others	Some current sources, as well as secondary sources, are used
Starting assumptions/ appearance of impartiality		
Use of peer review	No indication of peer review found	Board of Reviewers listed
Focus on a particular standardized product and discussion of preparation impact on safety	Impact of preparation on safety is not particularly addressed; however, it is focused on nutrients preparations, which are often USP-standardized; for other natural products, does not focus on particular standardized products	Describes different forms available, but impact on safety is not specifically discussed; does not describe characteristics of the products to which comments about safety apply
Description of consumption levels considered	Usual ingested amounts and how substances are supplied is described; it is assumed that the safety conclusions are based on these ingested amounts	Usual ingested amounts are described; it is assumed that the safety conclusions are based on these ingested amounts
Consideration of data from non-oral routes of exposure	No mention is made of how non-oral data were handled	—[a]
Discussion of biological activity or possible mechanism of action	Discussed for substances for which the information was known	Discussed for most substances
Discussion of specific groups within the general population, if appropriate	Discussed	Pregnancy and lactation issues are discussed when considered relevant
Interaction with other interventions	Discussed, when available, for other supplements, drugs, and botanicals	Interactions are discussed in some places
Other comments and considerations for using this resource	Comprehensive in terms of the number and range of supplements described Limitations in the comprehensiveness of the literature	Book was developed largely for the consumer, limited citations Lack of comprehensive literature search limits usefulness

TABLE 2-1 Continued

	Table of side effects and interactions guide may be helpful Useful cross-references and indexes

Considerations	Resource World Health Organization (WHO) Monographs (WHO, 1999, 2001, 2003) (Reviewed Radix Valerianae, Radix Ginseng, Herba Echinaceae Purpureae)
Type of organization responsible for resource	International, nonprofit organization
Substances reviewed	Major medicinal plants; selection based on extent of use, worldwide importance, and availability of data
Product/endpoint	Book of summary monographs
Focus on safety/risk	Safety, efficacy, and quality control are considered
Reliance on primary data	Some primary and some secondary sources are cited, including foreign language articles
Use of nonhuman data	All types of data are considered
Description of limitations	Data limitations are described for efficacy, but not for safety
Description of literature search strategy	Describes sources of information searched and timeline of scientific literature search
Use of current literature	Several volumes have been published since 1999; additional safety concerns may arise well after the review was prepared, due to the length of time it takes to get agreement on a monograph and print it
Starting assumptions/ appearance of impartiality	
Use of peer review	Extensive peer review

continued

TABLE 2-1 Continued

Focus on a particular standardized product and discussion of preparation impact on safety	Defines the medicinal plant and describes compounds to standardize a product; adverse reaction description discusses preparation
Description of consumption levels considered	Dose is specified in relation to adverse effects; although one monograph only states that "large doses may...," many specify how much was associated with the adverse reaction
Consideration of data from non-oral routes of exposure	Non-oral data are referred to in some sections, but it is not clear if these data were considered as possibly relevant
Discussion of biological activity or possible mechanism of action	Discussed
Discussion of specific groups within the general population, if appropriate	Pregnancy, lactation, and children are considered
Interaction with other interventions	Interactions with drugs are mentioned, if known; many entries say "None reported"
Other comments and considerations for using this resource	The section on medicinal uses is divided into three parts: Uses Supported by Clinical Data; Uses Described in Traditional Medical Systems, and Uses Described in Folklore; thus, may be a good resource for historic information
	Some of the safety data references the German Commission E
	Useful in that the standardized product is carefully defined and adverse reactions are viewed in this context
	Additional safety concerns may arise well after the review was prepared, due to the length of time it takes to get agreement on a monograph and print it

[a] This question could not be answered due to limitations in the analysis or lack of description in the available material.

of the criteria because (1) information in the material reviewed was insufficient to determine the extent to which a criterion was generally met, and (2) available information was likely to vary from ingredient to ingredient or the available information required in-depth analysis beyond the scope of this report. For example, it is necessary to know what safety data are available and *should* have been considered to determine whether the authors or organizations paid appropriate attention to all the relevant information when providing a safety conclusion in the resource. Empty cells in the table should be considered limitations in this examination, not in the resource itself.

Several examples of questions that are difficult to answer warrant explanation. Question 4, for example, was not answered at all because conclusions about whether data were weighed appropriately require knowledge of what type of information is available on a particular ingredient and may vary significantly from ingredient to ingredient, especially in the resources that were comprised of monographs authored by different individuals. Of note, however, was the Agency for Healthcare Research and Quality (AHRQ) process, which described in detail how data were analyzed.

Table 2-1 answers Question 7 ("How current is the information?") by examining whether current literature was cited, but the importance of using current literature will depend on the ingredient being considered and whether there is new information that also should be considered. Question 8 regarding the use of accurate citations cannot be answered until one tries to locate the citations and determine whether they exist and, if so, whether they document the information attributed to them. Question 9, regarding balance and objectivity, was answered for some resources by considering whether there was a tendency toward assuming that an ingredient was safe unless information to the contrary was available. Clearly, there are other aspects of balance and objectivity that will become apparent as more information about a particular ingredient is known.

Question 10 was not answered because it was not possible to assess the backgrounds of those involved in the production of the resources or individual monographs within a resource. Information about advanced degrees was helpful, but usually did not indicate whether the individuals had the knowledge needed to conduct a safety evaluation or to evaluate the various types of concerns raised for an ingredient. It may be unrealistic to expect that individuals with in-depth knowledge and expertise in the safety of all dietary supplement ingredients, or even all botanicals, exist. While some experts in botanicals may be knowledgeable about historical and current use of botanicals, they may not know enough about the particular safety concerns raised by animal or *in vitro* studies to be considered an expert in this specific area.

For Question 11, the table indicates whether peer review was conducted; most resources indicated that they were. As with Question 10, however, it was not possible to determine if the peer reviewers had adequate expertise in the safety issues raised. It was also not possible to determine the degree to which reviewers' comments were considered.

Questions 12 and 13, regarding the impact of preparation and focus on particular products, were answered together. The answer varies in importance, depending on whether the preparation of the ingredient varies significantly.

Question 14 asks whether ingested amounts under consideration were specified in the review. As indicated in the table, the committee assumed that specified "recommended" or "typical" ingestion levels were the basis of safety comments, but for resources that made conclusions, it would be useful for the reviews to explicitly state the amounts to which the conclusions apply.

Resources Related to Dietary Supplement Safety

A number of resources are available that have potential use for aiding in the evaluation of the safety of dietary supplement ingredients. The description of the resources that follow are based on information available from the organizations responsible or in published descriptions of the resources. Thus, the descriptions have not been verified further, and their inclusion in this report does not constitute endorsement of the approaches used or the information provided. While readily available resources are included, there are other resources and thus this group should not be considered inclusive of all efforts to consider safety, efficacy, or quality of dietary supplements.

Agency for Healthcare Research and Quality

AHRQ of the U.S. Department of Health and Human Services is authorized to sponsor, conduct, and disseminate research to improve the quality and effectiveness of health care (AHRQ, 2001). Other federal agencies, private sector agencies, and Congress periodically ask AHRQ to review and evaluate the scientific information on specified topics; their reviews are then used as the basis for clinical guidelines, performance measures, and other quality improvement tools. AHRQ administers the Evidence-based Practice Centers (EPCs), which have produced evidence reports requested by other federal agencies on the effectiveness and safety of a limited number of dietary supplements. The San Antonio EPC at the University of Texas Health Sciences Center, working under contract to AHRQ, has completed reports on garlic and milk thistle at the request of the National Center for Complementary and Alternative Medicine (NCCAM) of the National Institutes of Health (NIH) (AHRQ, 2000a, 2000b). The Southern California EPC/RAND completed an evidence-based report on S-adenosyl-L-methionine (SAMe) in 2002 for NCCAM (AHRQ, 2002b), and an evidence-based report on ephedra, released in February 2003, for NIH's Office of Dietary Supplements and NCCAM (AHRQ, 2003a).

The EPC reports are based on a systematic analysis of the relevant scientific data (AHRQ, 2002c). The analyses are based on a weighting and ranking methodology and are dependent on judgments based on well-defined criteria. The reports are designed to differentiate the types and strength of evidence (AHRQ, 2002c). Due to the exhaustive nature of the reports, they are resource intensive.

The first step of an AHRQ review is to identify relevant citations following an exhaustive search of the literature in a variety of electronic databases. Additional citations are identified from bibliographies, manufacturers, and technical experts. Both English and non-English references are included in the search. In general, only published full articles are used, but additional unpublished information provided by authors of published studies may also be included (AHRQ, 2000a, 2000b).

Independent reviewers on the EPC staff read the titles and abstracts of all the identified citations and exclude those citations that do not meet defined selection criteria on types of participants, interventions, control groups, outcomes, and study designs. To assess adverse clinical events, all types of human studies are used (e.g., randomized controlled trials, prospective trials, and case-control and cohort studies). Data are abstracted from the literature and analyzed by independent reviewers with clinical and methodological expertise. The analysis includes an assessment of the internal validity and quality of the studies. The data analysis includes generation of evidence tables, graphical summaries, statistical tests, and meta-analyses. The results and conclusions of the analysis are summarized in an evidence report that contains conclusions on the current knowledge on the efficacy and adverse effects of the substance and provides recommendations for future research (AHRQ, 2000a, 2000b).

Nominations for clinical topics to be reviewed by an EPC are solicited through notices in the *Federal Register*. Topics must meet specific selection criteria including, "high incidence or prevalence in the general population and in special populations . . . ; significance for the needs of Medicare, Medicaid, and other federal health programs; high cost associated with a condition, procedure, treatment, or technology, whether due to the number of people needing care, high unit cost of care, or high indirect costs; controversy or uncertainty about the effectiveness or relative effectiveness of available clinical strategies or technologies and availability of scientific data to support the systematic review and analysis of the topic" (AHRQ, 2002a). Based on this process, the dietary supplements milk thistle, ephedra, garlic, and SAMe, in addition to over 80 other nondietary supplement topics, had been reviewed as of 2003 (AHRQ, 2003b).

American Herbal Pharmacopoeia

The American Herbal Pharmacopoeia (AHP), a nonprofit organization, develops monographs on the quality, effectiveness, and safety of botanical medicines commonly used in the United States. The monographs include information on traditional use and information from scientific sources (Barrett, 1998). They are designed to provide consumers, health professionals, and botanical manufacturers with the knowledge required for using and manufacturing botanical products safely and effectively, and to provide regulatory bodies and researchers with guidance for integrating botanical products into the health care system (AHP, 2004b).

Botanicals are selected for monograph development based on judgment about the extent of use, the unique value of the botanical, and sponsorship by other interested organizations or companies (AHP, 2004b). Selection of a botanical for monograph development can be made by three methods. The first method is through a prioritization committee consisting of professional herbalists, botanical industry representatives, and herbal educators, which produces a list of priority botanicals based on the extent of their use or their unique values. A second method is through monograph sponsorship. Because AHP seeks funding and technical support for development of monographs from interested organizations or companies, a sponsored botanical may be given higher priority than was assigned by the prioritization committee (AHP, 2004b). Third, AHP considers what other groups have done. If there is an existing monograph of a botanical on the prioritization list, AHP may use relevant sections of that monograph as a starting point for its own monograph development (AHP, 2004b).

The monographs include botanicals with origins in Ayurvedic, Chinese, and Western traditions and include information from both traditional and scientific sources (AHP, 2002; Barrett, 1998). AHP monographs are relatively detailed compared with monographs produced by other organizations. They are released individually as they are completed, and 18 have been released since 1997 (AHP, 2004a).

In preparing the monographs, literature searches are conducted in order to review all reported side effects, contraindications, and negative interactions of the botanical (AHP, 2004b). According to AHP, primary literature is preferred, but secondary literature, such as review articles, may be used if considered acceptable or necessary. The search is not limited to English-language references. According to AHP, a review of the toxicological literature is done to address the safety of the botanical and includes data on acute and chronic toxicity; use during pregnancy, lactation, and fetal development; use during operation of motor vehicles; mutagenicity; teratogenicity; and carcinogenicity.

Next, each section of the monograph is assigned to a writer with expertise in the topic of the section, and the writer is provided with the results of the literature search. Once the sections are drafted, the AHP editor and at least one other expert in the specific field review them. The sections are then incorporated into an initial monograph draft. This draft is then circulated to a peer-review committee of botanists, chemists, herbalists, pharmacists, pharmacologists, pharmacognosists, and physicians (AHP, 2004b). Reviewer comments are incorporated into the draft and the initial authors review and approve their sections. Before it is finalized for publication, the monograph is reviewed by an expert of either the botanical under review or the physiological system that the botanical affects (AHP, 2004b).

American Herbal Products Association

The American Herbal Products Association (AHPA) is a national trade association for the botanical products industry. In response to passage of the Dietary Supplement and Health Education Act (DSHEA), AHPA convened a special subcommittee of its standards committee to address the need for a comprehensive review of safety data for botanical ingredients sold in North America. The committee was made up of natural products scientists and practicing herbalists. According to AHPA, the goal of this committee was to critically evaluate safety and categorize botanicals based on safety. These evaluations are published as *The Botanical Safety Handbook* (McGuffin et al., 1997).

The committee reviewed over 500 botanicals that were available in the United States, identified primarily by reviewing *Herbs of Commerce*, another AHPA publication (Foster et al., 1992). After identifying which botanicals to include, AHPA reported that its committee reviewed the available scientific literature for data on human and animal toxicity, traditional use, regulatory status in numerous countries, and current usage of herbs in the United States, China, India, Europe, and Australia. The committee also relied on its own and others' expertise and clinical experience for the evaluations.

There was no formal weighting of the data used for the evaluations; however, there were some exclusionary criteria. The monographs did not include the following data, conditions, or related products: ". . . excessive consumption, safety or toxicity concerns based on isolated constituents, toxicity data based solely on intravenous or intraperitoneal administration, traditional Chinese and Ayurvedic contraindications, gastrointestinal disturbances, potential drug interactions, idiosyncratic reactions, allergic reactions, contact dermatitis, well-known toxic plants that are not found in products in trade, homeopathic herbal preparations, essential oils, herbal products to which chemically-defined active substances had been added, or environmental factors, additives or contaminants" (McGuffin et al., 1997).

The AHPA review committee followed guidance from the World Health Organization's (WHO) Programme on Traditional Medicines (WHO, 1991), which states that regulatory action is not necessary for traditionally used products that have not been shown to be harmful unless new evidence necessitates a risk–benefit assessment. According to AHPA, the safety classification was based on an assumption of rational, informed use of botanicals and the committee reported that it carefully considered the intended use of the substance within the historical context of that use (McGuffin et al., 1997). As listed in the exclusionary criteria above, the committee also reported that it did not extrapolate toxicity data of isolated constituents and did not use data from studies that had excessive or irresponsible consumption patterns (McGuffin et al., 1997).

Once the committee reviewed all available information, the botanicals were assigned to one of four safety classes. Class 1 substances are botanicals that the AHPA committee believes can be used safely when used appropriately. Class 2 substances are botanicals for which certain restrictions apply (see subclasses) unless otherwise directed by an expert qualified in the use of the substance. Class 2a substances are botanicals only to be used externally. Class 2b substances are botanicals not to be used during pregnancy. Class 2c substances are botanicals not to be used while lactating. Class 2d substances are botanicals for which other use restrictions have been specified in the monograph. Class 3 substances are botanicals for which significant data exist to recommend special labeling: "To be used only under the supervision of an expert qualified in the appropriate use of this substance." Finally, class 4 substances are botanicals for which the AHPA committee found insufficient data for classification (McGuffin et al., 1997).

Institute of Medicine

In 1997 the Food and Nutrition Board, IOM, National Academies, published its first report on Dietary Reference Intakes (DRIs) (IOM, 1997), a set of reference values that grew out of the periodic editions of the Recommended Dietary Allowances (RDAs) for nutrients over the previous 50 years. The RDAs and now the DRIs are to be used as reference values in food and nutrition policy and programs. Included in the DRI set of reference values is the category of Tolerable Upper Intake Levels (ULs), defined as the highest levels of nutrient intake likely to pose no risk of adverse health effects for almost all individuals in a specified life stage group. As intake increases above the UL, the potential risk of adverse effects may increase.

While not recommended intakes, the ULs are based on published data on adverse effects of consuming excess levels of nutrients, usually demonstrated in humans, on a chronic basis over time. Using a risk assessment methodology (IOM, 1998a), uncertainty factors are applied to develop the UL, and depend on the availability of a dataset with dose-response information. In some cases, ULs have not been set where information on chronic ingestion was not available. The reviews are under the direction of an oversight committee of experts, as well as a subcommittee of experts in toxicology and risk assessment. To date, all essential vitamins, minerals, trace elements, macronutrients, and electrolytes have been reviewed (IOM, 1997, 1998b, 2000, 2001, 2002, 2004).

Commission E[2]

In 1978 the Second Medicines Act in the Republic of Germany went into effect, requiring a scientific review of all medicines in the pharmaceutical market, including conventional drugs, medicinal plants, and phytomedicines. This resulted in the formation of a series of scientific commissions. Commission E was established by the German Minister of Health to review botanical drugs and preparations from medicinal plants. This 24-member committee was made up of physicians, pharmacists, nonmedical practitioners, pharmacologists, toxicologists, and biostatisticians (Blumenthal et al., 1998). According to a Commission E member consulted, at least 60 percent of the commission members had practical experience with phytomedicines (Personal communication, H. Schilcher, Commission E, March 19, 2002). The Commission completed its monograph work in 1994; however, it has met since 1994 to review drug registrations (Blumenthal, 1997; Blumenthal et al., 2000). The monographs produced by Commission E were compiled and published in English in 1998 by the American Botanical Council (Blumenthal et al., 1998). A subsequent publication by the American Botanical Council, *Herbal Medicine: Expanded Commission E Monographs*, was published in 2000 (Blumenthal et al., 2000).

The stated objective of Commission E was to ensure that approved botanicals were reasonably safe when used according to the product label instructions and to remove unapproved botanicals from the market even if they only posed minor safety risks (Blumenthal et al., 1998). Commission E

[2]Translation of the German Commission E (1998) is a translation of German documents and describes the process used by Commission E. In addition to input from a member of the Commission E, it serves as the basis for this summary.

reviewed 378 botanicals used in German folk medicine for both safety and effectiveness (Blumenthal, 1997; Personal communication, H. Schilcher, Commission E, March 19, 2002). It was the manufacturer's responsibility to provide proof of quality (Blumenthal et al., 1998). Safety and effectiveness were assessed using published scientific literature. Approximately 100 to 200 worldwide references were consulted for each botanical (Personal communication, H. Schilcher, Commission E, March 19, 2002).

The Commission considered data on traditional use, chemical composition, pharmacology, and toxicology and used data from clinical studies, *in vitro* and *in vivo* studies, field studies, epidemiological studies, case reports, and unpublished proprietary data submitted by manufacturers that included chemical, toxicological, pharmacological, and clinical testing data. The Commission also reviewed summaries produced by Kooperation Phytopharmaka (an umbrella organization of about 120 pharmaceutical manufacturers). According to Blumenthal, these summaries were based on literature reviews and clinical experience, but did not contain any recommendations about the product under review (Blumenthal et al., 1998).

According to the American Botanical Council's description, controlled clinical studies appear to have been considered the most useful type of data (Blumenthal et al., 1998). If no controlled studies were available, safety was evaluated based on other types of data, such as well-documented review articles, older clinical trials, and well-documented knowledge of traditional usage (Blumenthal et al., 1998). Commission E did not accept long-term therapeutic or traditional use as sufficient evidence of safety without additional data, and field and case studies were used only when they had been evaluated according to scientific standards (Blumenthal et al., 1998).

Once the Commission finished drafting a monograph for a botanical medicine, it was published and comments were solicited from scientists and other experts. The Commission then prepared a final draft of the monograph. The resulting monographs do not include references. Unpublished justifications with relevant references for the monographs are kept; however, these justifications cannot be accessed except in cases of legal disputes (Blumenthal et al., 1998).

Each substance was assigned one of three approval ratings: (1) positive (approved), (2) negative (unapproved), or (3) negative-null (unapproved). Potential therapeutic benefit was taken into account in the assignment of ratings. Positive (approved) substances were considered reasonably safe when used according to the dosage, contraindications, and other warnings specified in the monograph. If safety concerns outweighed the potential benefits of a substance, the monograph was assigned a negative (unapproved) rating. No dosage recommendations were provided for substances assigned a negative rating, and the intent of the Commission was the immediate withdrawal from the market of substances receiving a negative rating.

If no risk was found, but also no substantiation of efficacy, the substance was designated as negative-null (unapproved). If manufacturers could later document the efficacy of such substances, the products could be approved; however, no new monographs would be produced (Blumenthal et al., 1998).

Expanded German Commission E

The American Botanical Council, which published the English translation of the original monographs from the German Commission E, subsequently expanded upon the original monographs by adding references, some of which were published after the 1994 review by Commission E, for 107 medicinal plants and phytomedicines common to the United States.[3] This was published as the book *Herbal Medicine: Expanded Commission E Monographs* (Blumenthal et al., 2000)

European Scientific Cooperative on Phytotherapy

The European Scientific Cooperative on Phytotherapy (ESCOP) was created in 1989 to promote the scientific status of phytomedicines and the harmonization of their regulatory status in Europe (ESCOP, 1996). ESCOP is an umbrella organization of national trade associations for phytotherapy from countries both within and beyond the European Union. According to ESCOP (2001), monographs are produced by a scientific committee of ESCOP, which consists of a subgroup of delegates from participating member countries with expertise in medicine, phytotherapy, pharmacognosy, pharmacology, and regulatory affairs. The goal is to compile monographs that provide information on the therapeutic uses and safety of botanicals that are widely used in European medicine and pharmacy (Blumenthal, 1997; ESCOP, 2001). Information on quality is not included in these monographs (Blumenthal, 1997).

The ESCOP scientific committee, with assistance from others who do research on specific plants, drafts a monograph by evaluating information from the published scientific literature (ESCOP, 2001). Once a monograph is drafted, it is reviewed by an independent board of supervising editors that consists of academic experts in phytotherapy and medicinal plants. The monographs are then published in groups, as fascicules, each containing 10 monographs; 60 monographs have been published to date (ESCOP, 1996, 1997, 2001).

---

[3]In response to interest in references, the American Botanical Council developed the book. The editors of this book have included references for statements and expanded the original monographs.

Natural Medicines Comprehensive Database

The publisher of *Pharmacist's Letter* and *Prescriber's Letter* created the *Natural Medicines Comprehensive Database* (NMCD) which is available online and in print (NMCD, 2002). This database reviews many "natural medicines" on the market in North America, and it reviews safety and efficacy for a large number of dietary supplement ingredients. Its goal is to bring together the consensus of the available data on natural medicines so that practitioners do not need to search multiple sources to find scientifically reliable and clinically practical information on botanical medicines and supplements (NMCD, 2002). NMCD reports that it covers nearly every natural medicine on the market in North America. New product reviews are prioritized based on market saturation and requests by health professionals (Personal communication, P. Gregory, NMCD, February 21, 2002).

For each product that is reviewed, a research team of pharmacists, physicians, and pharmacologists begins the process with a literature search. Initially, when the database was first being developed, the research team consulted reference textbooks, such as the *Commission E Monographs*, the *Physicians' Desk Reference (PDR)*, and AHPA's *Botanical Safety Handbook*, for their evaluation of the literature. However, the research team soon turned to the primary literature using electronic databases (e.g., MEDLINE and TOXLINE) to find the pertinent literature (Personal communication, P. Gregory, NMCD, February 21, 2002).

For the most part, the research team limits their search to English-language references. However, non-English articles of special significance are also included. For the safety evaluation, the team relies mainly on human data; animal data are rarely used (Personal communication, P. Gregory, NMCD, February 21, 2002).

After completion of the literature review, the information is evaluated, a consensus on any relevant issues is reached by the research team, and then a single author drafts the review. The draft is sent out for review to two or three pharmacists and physicians who are not on the research team. After this review, the final draft is added to the database (Personal communication, P. Gregory, NMCD, February 21, 2002).

Each product is rated according to specific criteria as: likely safe, possibly safe, possibly unsafe, likely unsafe, or unsafe. Natural products that are rated likely safe are those for which there is general agreement among reliable references that the product is safe when used appropriately or those for which a governmental body has approved their use. A product is rated possibly safe if the reputable references suggest that the product might be safe when used appropriately or there are human studies that report no serious adverse effects. A rating of possibly unsafe requires that there are some data suggesting product use might be unsafe. Likely unsafe indicates agreement among reputable references that the product can be harmful or there are reliable reports of harm to product users. A rating of unsafe is based on finding general agreement among reliable references that the product should not be used, reliable reports of clinically significant harm to product users, or safety warnings for the product issued by a reliable agency. Special mention is made if use during pregnancy, lactation, or in children presents special concerns (NMCD, 2002).

Natural Standard

Natural Standard was founded as a multi-institution initiative in January 2000 by clinicians and researchers to provide evidence-based information about complementary and alternative therapies (Natural Standard, 2003). It considers itself an impartial service and is not supported by any interest group, professional organization, or pharmaceutical manufacturer. Paid subscriptions to its website, NaturalStandard.com, are the only visible means of support.

According to Natural Standard, for each therapy (dietary supplement or other), a research team gathers scientific data and expert opinions. To prepare each monograph, electronic searches are conducted in several databases, including AMED, CANCERLIT, CINAHL, CISCOM, the Cochrane Library, EMBASE, HerbMed, International Pharmaceutical Abstracts, MEDLINE, and NAPRALERT, without restrictions on language or quality of publications. Additionally, industry warnings are regularly monitored. When clinically relevant new data emerge, best efforts are made to immediately update the content. In addition, regular updates with renewed searches occur every 3 to 18 months; the exact interval varies by topic.

Rating scales based on the Jadad scoring technique are used to evaluate the quality of the evidence (Jadad et al., 1996). Grading scales "reflect the level of available scientific evidence in support of the efficacy of a given therapy for a specific indication" (Natural Standard, 2003). In addition, "Expert opinion and folkloric precedent are not included in this assessment, and are reflected in a separate section of each monograph" (Natural Standard, 2003). Evidence of harm is considered separately and the grading applies only to evidence of benefit. Monographs undergo blinded peer review prior to inclusion in the database. In cases of editorial disagreement, a three-member panel addresses conflicts and consults experts when needed (Natural Standard, 2003).

Physicians' Desk Reference for Herbal Medicines

In 1998 the PDR organization broadened its scope from producing a widely used collection of information on prescription drugs to also producing a collection of information on botanical medicines. This publication was the first edition of the *PDR for Herbal Medicines* (Medical Economics, 1998). A second edition of *PDR for Herbal Medicines* was published in 2000 that provides monographs for approximately 700 medicinal herbs (Medical Economics, 2000). The monographs contain information on efficacy, safety, potential interactions, precautions, adverse reactions, and dosage. For 300 of these monographs, the findings and assessments were taken from the German Commission E report. There are useful cross-referencing indices for information such as names, indications, side effects, and interactions. This collection of monographs does not appear to be the product of direct committee effort or to involve a peer review in a consistent manner given the variety of origins of information included.

Physicians' Desk Reference for Nutritional Supplements

The *PDR for Nutritional Supplements* contains over 200 monographs of nearly 1,000 nutritional products, including amino acids, fatty acids, metabolites and cofactors, nucleic acids, proteins, glycosupplements, phytosupplements, hormonal products, and probiotics (Medical Economics, 2001). Crude botanicals or herbal medicines are not included in the 2001 book. Each monograph contains trade names, description, actions and pharmacology, indications and usage, research summary contraindications, interactions, warning signs of overdose, dosage and administration, how supplied, and literature cited. Inaccuracies and typographical errors were noted in some of the references. Like the *PDR for Herbal Medicines*, there are useful cross-referencing indices. This publication appears to be a summary of information rather than a committee-authored or peer-reviewed activity.

The American Pharmaceutical Association's Practical Guide to Natural Medicines

The American Pharmaceutical Association (APhA) is a national professional society of pharmacists that is dedicated to helping pharmacists help consumers. The book, *Practical Guide to Natural Medicine,* was written for the consumer by a writer for APhA (Peirce, 1999). It is a compilation of information on many substances (mostly botanicals), but includes other substances, such as melatonin. For each substance, the monograph describes what it is, what it is used for, the forms available, and the dosage commonly reported. Sections include, "Will it work for you? What the studies say"; and "Will it harm you? What the studies say" (Peirce, 1999). Given its orientation to the lay reader, the evaluation of the literature does not appear to be as extensive or rigorous as some of the other resources.

General sources and text citations are listed at the end of each monograph. Also included is a list of the board of reviewers for the book.

World Health Organization[4]

WHO has begun to develop international specifications for the most widely used medicinal plants in an effort to fill the need for current, authoritative information on their safety and efficacy (WHO, 1999). WHO published the first volume of monographs on selected medicinal plants in 1999 (WHO, 1999); second and third volumes were published in 2000 and 2003. The medicinal plants and products in each volume were selected by a WHO advisory group based on the extent of each plant's use and importance throughout the world and on the sufficiency of the data available to evaluate safety and efficacy. The goal is to include information on safety, effectiveness, and quality control of botanical medicines. The monographs present descriptive information, purity tests, chemical constituents, medicinal uses, clinical studies, pharmacology, contraindications, warnings, precautions, adverse reactions, and posology[5] (WHO, 1999).

Each monograph published to date was drafted under the direction of a team of experts in botanical medicines and medicinal plants. Information for the monographs was collected from a review of the literature, bibliographies, review articles, pharmacopoeias from several countries, reference books, and the NAPRALERT database.[6] Once drafted, the monographs were reviewed by a number of additional basic scientists, physicians, pharmacologists, pharmacognosists, and toxicologists throughout the world with expertise in traditional medicine, drug regulation, drug evaluation, and pharmaceutical sciences. WHO convenes a Consultation on Selected Medicinal Plants that consists of 16 experts in medicinal plants and drug regulation to give final approval, modification, or rejection of the proposed monographs. WHO plans to periodically supplement and update the monographs as new data are made available (WHO, 1999).

---

[4]As a matter of disclosure, the author of the WHO specifications is committee member Norman Farnsworth.

[5]From the Greek, *posos* (how much), representing the science or doctrine of dosing.

[6]NAPRALERT, an acronym for Natural Products ALERT, is a relational database of world literature describing the ethnomedical or traditional uses, chemistry, and pharmacology of plant, microbial, and animal (primarily marine) extracts. In addition, it contains considerable data on the chemistry and pharmacology (including human studies) of secondary metabolites of known structure, derived from natural sources. NAPRALERT is available by subscription from the University of Illinois (Farnsworth, 2003).

U.S. Pharmacopeia-National Formulary[7]

The U.S. Pharmacopeia-National Formulary (USP-NF), a nongovernmental, nonprofit organization, develops and provides standards of identity, strength, quality, purity, packaging, and labeling of drugs sold in the United States in the form of standards monographs; these monographs do not consider the inherent safety of the substance. The USP-NF standards were recognized by Congress in the Federal Food, Drug, and Cosmetic Act of 1938 (21 U.S.C. § 321 et seq.) as the official compendium of the United States, making its established standards for drugs essentially similar to federal regulations (USP, 2002a, 2002b).

In its first publication in 1820, the USP contained monographs for hundreds of botanicals; however, most of them were removed by the end of the 1930s due to diminishing use in medical practice following the appearance of synthetic medicinal compounds in the U.S. marketplace (Barrett, 1998; Blumenthal, 1997). In 1990, in response to a USP Convention Resolution, the USP Committee of Revision, an independent body of elected scientific experts representing industry, academia, and government agencies, established public standards for vitamins, minerals, and their combination products. These standards monographs, along with general chapters that include manufacturing practices for nutritional supplements, were grouped together and published within a separate section of the USP called *Nutritional Supplements* (Roll, 2002).

In 1995, after passage of DSHEA, the USP Convention, in recognition of the resurgence in the use of botanicals by the American public, adopted a resolution that encouraged the USP Committee of Revision to establish public standards for botanical dietary supplements. In response to the Convention resolution, the USP Committee of Revision generated a list of approximately 20 widely used botanicals for public standards monographs. Criteria for identification of these botanicals included lack of safety risk,

[7]Distinct from its development of the USP-NF monographs, USP launched the Dietary Supplement Verification Program (DSVP) in November 2001. Manufacturers sponsor products that are tested and reviewed by USP. If the product meets the DSVP requirements, the product is granted a USP certification mark. This mark is intended to signify that the product (1) contains the ingredients stated on the label in the declared amount and strength, (2) meets stringent standards for product purity, (3) meets specified limits on known contaminants, and (4) has been manufactured under good manufacturing practices according to the USP-NF General Chapter on Manufacturing Practices for Nutritional Supplements and the FDA's Advance Notice of Proposed Rulemaking for Good Manufacturing Practices (Personal communication, S. Srinivasan, USP, February 14, 2002; USP, 2004). Importantly, the DSVP certification mark is not intended to imply safety or efficacy of dietary supplement ingredients. The USP-DSVP is not included in Table 2-1 due to the program's emphasis on quality and label verification, rather than inherent ingredient safety. Similar work of NSF International and other organizations is not described for the same reason.

extent of use by consumers, interest from regulatory agencies, positive assessment by recognized pharmacognosists, and the ability of the botanical to meet typical requirements for USP monographs. History of traditional use and pharmacological action were also considered. According to USP, standards monographs are not developed for botanicals that USP believes may be associated with a significant safety risk (Roll, 2002).

Once a botanical has been approved for inclusion in the USP or the NF,[8] analytical methods are requested from several manufacturers and reviewed by the USP Expert Committee relating to dietary supplements. Before official adoption into USP-NF, public comment on proposed standards is generated by publicizing them in *Pharmacopoeia Forum* (Personal communication, V.S. Srinivasan, USP, February 11, 2002).

An evaluation of USP or USP-NF was not included in Table 2-1 due to the emphasis on ingredient quality rather than safety.

CONSIDERATION OF FRAMEWORKS FOR EVALUATING THE SAFETY OF OTHER SUBSTANCES

In the previous section, resources that address the safety of dietary supplements were considered. There are also numerous frameworks in place that the FDA and other organizations have used to evaluate the safety of other substances to which humans may be exposed. Assessment of the scope, characteristics, and processes used in other frameworks can aid in the development of a workable framework for dietary supplement safety evaluation. Frameworks that FDA already has in place to evaluate food additives and pharmaceuticals were reviewed, as well as mechanisms for considering the safety of cosmetic ingredients and of flavors and extracts. The Environmental Protection Agency (EPA) has also developed a system for considering possible human and environmental impacts of toxic substances. Detailed summaries of the different frameworks, as described by the organizations, are included in Appendix A.

Role of Premarket Approval and Postmarket Surveillance

Consideration of frameworks used to evaluate the safety of other substances contributed to an understanding of different types of "frameworks." For most of the frameworks that were evaluated, the scientific principles

[8]Whether a substance's monograph is admitted into the USP or its companion guide, the NF, currently depends on its approval status, as determined by USP. If the substance has an FDA- or USP-approved use, then standards are developed for it and it is published in the USP; otherwise, the standards for the substance are published by USP in the NF.

associated with the framework operate in a context that utilizes some aspects of premarket approval or requirements for postmarket surveillance. DSHEA does not include provisions for either of these conditions in its regulation of dietary supplement ingredients, although it provides the agency with the requirement for conducting postmarket review of dietary supplement safety (see Chapter 1). Consequently, the existing frameworks reviewed could not simply be adapted to dietary supplement ingredients; this resulted in the need to define the use of the scientific principles in the context of postmarket review of safety.

The postmarket versus premarket difference is apparent from reviewing the FDA process for approval of a new food additive. The *Redbook*, periodically published by FDA (OFAS, 2001, 2003), outlines the types of testing expected in order to receive food additive approval, thus specifically defining the types of premarket testing that must be conducted. No such requirement exists for dietary supplement ingredients. Likewise, the generally recognized as safe (GRAS) notification procedure (see Table 1-1) identifies certain types of information that a manufacturer must present in order for a food ingredient to be considered GRAS. In this context it is clear that manufacturers are responsible for demonstrating the safety of an additive before it is allowed in the marketplace. In contrast, DSHEA places the burden of proof on FDA to provide evidence that a dietary supplement ingredient currently on the market is associated with significant or unreasonable risk.

In the EPA new chemicals program, the manufacturer submits a premanufacturing notification. Often little or no data are available on the new substance, so an expert team considers the chemical structure and substructure to look for health-based "structural alerts," based on safety concerns of analogous chemicals. If a chemical is categorized in one of the structural alert categories, it is treated as if it causes the health effects of concern unless demonstrated otherwise.

Such a structure-based approach was considered difficult to adapt to the dietary supplement system as a whole because many of the dietary supplements, such as botanicals, are complex mixtures of many substances that may or may not be known, and health concerns may be very dependent on the level ingested. Nonetheless, aspects of this approach remain in the principles regarding structural relatedness (see Chapter 6).

Conceptualization of a Framework

Review of other resources on dietary supplements and consideration of other frameworks assisted in the development of the framework described in the next chapter. A working concept/definition of a framework for safety evaluation of dietary supplement ingredients was developed, having two basic elements that must work together: (1) principles for how to assess risk in a scientifically valid way, using the types of data and information that are likely to be available to FDA, and (2) a process by which FDA gathers this information and increases its level of scrutiny to make decisions of whether significant risk exists, overturning the assumption of safety and determining if regulatory action is needed.

SUMMARY

In reviewing the methods used by other expert bodies to consider dietary supplements and in reviewing the discussions with the sponsor and other interested representatives, the following attributes of a framework to evaluate the safety of dietary supplements were identified:

- It must be workable and able to be integrated into the agency's program of work and resources available.
- It should provide guidance on organizing diverse information that is already available.
- It should provide for the scientifically valid categorization, based on priority, of the diverse substances classified as dietary supplements.
- It should establish a database for the collection of information regarding potential safety concerns that can be updated as new information becomes available.
- It should provide a method to integrate diverse information into a priority-setting scheme so that efforts and resources can be maximally directed toward those dietary supplement ingredients with the greatest safety concerns.
- It should provide a mechanism for public input.
- It should be consistent with the provisions of DSHEA.

Once the definition and key attributes of a safety framework were identified, a framework that focused on the safety of dietary supplements was developed. This approach is described in the following chapter, with the basis for the scientific principles incorporated into the framework discussed in detail in the succeeding chapters.

REFERENCES

AHP (American Herbal Pharmacopoeia). 2002. *Mission Statement: The American Herbal Pharmacopoeia*. Online. Available at http://www.herbal-ahp.org/mission.html. Accessed November 20, 2002.

AHP. 2004a. *Monographs: American Herbal Pharmacopoeia and Therapeutic Compendium: Standards of Analysis, Quality Control, and Therapeutics*. Online. Available at http://www.herbal-ahp.org/. Accessed February 12, 2004.

AHP. 2004b. *Monographs Defined. Developing Quality Control and Therapeutic Monographs: Monograph Prioritization, Development, Review, Finalization and the Value of Monographs to Health Professionals, Industry, and Consumers.* Online. Available at http://www.herbal-ahp.org/mgdefine.html. Accessed February 12, 2004.

AHRQ (Agency for Healthcare Research and Quality). 2000a. *Garlic: Effects on Cardiovascular Risks and Disease, Protective Effects against Cancer, and Clinical Adverse Effects. Evidence Report/Technology Assessment Number 20.* Available at http://www.ahrq.gov/clinic/tp/garlictp.htm. Accessed March 2, 2004.

AHRQ. 2000b. *Milk Thistle: Effects on Liver Disease and Cirrhosis and Clinical Adverse Effects. Evidence Report/Technology Assessment Number 21.* Available at http://www.ahrq.gov/clinic/tp/milkttp.htm. Accessed March 2, 2004.

AHRQ. 2001. *AHRQ Profile: Quality Research for Quality Health Care.* Available at http://www.ahrq.gov/about/profile.htm. Accessed February 16, 2004.

AHRQ. 2002a. Nominations of topics for evidence-based practice centers. *Fed Regis* 67:6933–6936.

AHRQ. 2002b. *S-Adenosyl-L-Methionine for Treatment of Depression, Osteoarthritis, and Liver Disease. Evidence Report/Technology Assessment Number 64.* Available at http://www.ahrq.gov/clinic/tp/sametp.htm. Accessed March 2, 2004.

AHRQ. 2002c. *System to Rate the Strength of Scientific Evidence. Evidence Report/Technology Assessment Number 47.* Available at http://www.ahrq.gov/clinic/tp/strengthtp.htm. Accessed March 2, 2004.

AHRQ. 2003a. *Ephedra and Ephedrine for Weight Loss and Athletic Performance. Clinical Efficacy and Side Effects. Evidence Report/Technology Assessment* No. 76. Available at http://www.ahrq.gov/clinic/tp/ephedtp.htm. Accessed March 2, 2004.

AHRQ. 2003b. *Evidence-Based Practice Centers.* Available at http://www.ahrq.gov/clinic/epc. Accessed February 16, 2004.

Barrett M. 1998. *Council for Responsible Nutrition Reference on Evaluating Botanicals.* Washington, DC: Council for Responsible Nutrition.

Blumenthal M. 1997. Herbal monographs. *HerbalGram* 40:30–38.

Blumenthal M, Busse WR, Goldberg A, Gruenwald J, Hall T, Riggins CW, Rister RS, eds. 1998. *The Complete German Commission E Monographs: Therapeutic Guide to Herbal Medicines.* Austin, TX: American Botanical Council.

Blumenthal M, Goldberg A, Brinckmann J, eds. 2000. *Herbal Medicine: Expanded Commission E Monographs.* Austin, TX: American Botanical Council.

Campbell P. 2001. Declaration of financial interests. *Nature* 412:751.

Chambliss WG, Hufford CD, Flagg ML, Glisson JK. 2002. Assessment of the quality of reference books on botanical dietary supplements. *J Am Pharm Assoc* 42:723–734.

Ernst E. 2000. *Herbal Medicine: A Concise Overview for Professionals.* Boston: Butterworth-Heinemann Medical.

ESCOP (European Scientific Cooperative on Phytotherapy). 1996. *Monographs on the Medicinal Uses of Plant Drugs. Fascicules 1–2.* Devon, UK: ESCOP.

ESCOP. 1997. *Monographs on the Medicinal Uses of Plant Drugs. Fascicules 3–5.* Devon, UK: ESCOP.

ESCOP. 2001. ESCOP *Publications. ESCOP Monographs and the ESCOP Scientific Committee.* Online. Available at http://www.escop.com/publications.htm. Accessed November 12, 2001.

Farnsworth NR. 2003. *NAPRALERT (Natural Products ALERT) Database.* Chicago: University of Chicago.

Foster S, Tyler VE. 1999. *Tyler's Honest Herbal. A Sensible Guide to the Use of Herbs and Related Remedies.* 4th ed. New York: Haworth Herbal Press.

Foster S, Moley T, Awang D. 1992. *Herbs of Commerce*. Austin, TX: American Herbal Products Association.

Grieve M. 1996. *A Modern Herbal: The Medicinal, Culinary, Cosmetic, and Economic Properties, Cultivation, and Folklore of Herbs, Grasses, Fungi, Shrubs, and Trees with all Their Modern Scientific Uses*. New York: Barnes and Noble.

IOM (Institute of Medicine). 1997. *Dietary Reference Intakes for Calcium, Phosphorus, Magnesium, Vitamin D, and Fluoride*. Washington, DC: National Academy Press.

IOM. 1998a. *Dietary Reference Intakes: A Risk Assessment Model for Establishing Upper Intake Levels for Nutrients*. Washington, DC: National Academy Press.

IOM. 1998b. *Dietary Reference Intakes for Thiamin, Riboflavin, Niacin, Vitamin B6, Folate, Vitamin B12, Pantothenic Acid, Biotin, and Choline*. Washington, DC: National Academy Press.

IOM. 2000. *Dietary Reference Intakes for Vitamin C, Vitamin E, Selenium, and Carotenoids*. Washington, DC: National Academy Press.

IOM. 2001. *Dietary Reference Intakes for Vitamin A, Vitamin K, Arsenic, Boron, Chromium, Copper, Iodine, Iron, Manganese, Molybdenum, Nickel, Silicon, Vanadium, and Zinc*. Washington, DC: National Academy Press.

IOM. 2002. *Dietary Reference Intakes for Energy, Carbohydrate, Fiber, Fat, Fatty Acids, Cholesterol, Protein, and Amino Acids*. Washington, DC: National Academy Press.

IOM. 2004. *Dietary Reference Intakes for Water, Potassium, Sodium, Chloride, and Sulfate*. Washington, DC: The National Academies Press.

Jadad AR, Moore RA, Carroll D, Jenkinson C, Reynolds DJ, Gavaghan DJ, McQuay HJ. 1996. Assessing the quality of reports of randomized clinical trials: Is blinding necessary? *Control Clin Trials* 17:1–12.

McGuffin M, Hobbs C, Upton R, Goldberg A. 1997. *American Herbal Product Association's Botanical Safety Handbook*. Boca Raton, FL: CRC Press.

Medical Economics. 1998. *PDR for Herbal Medicines. 1st Ed.* Montvale, NJ: Medical Economics.

Medical Economics. 2000. *PDR for Herbal Medicines. 2nd Ed.* Montvale, NJ: Medical Economics.

Medical Economics. 2001. *PDR for Nutritional Supplements. 1st Ed.* Montvale, NJ: Medical Economics.

Natural Standard. 2003. *About Natural Standard*. Online. Available at http://www.naturalstandard.com/. Accessed May 30, 2003.

NMCD (Natural Medicines Comprehensive Database). 2002. *About the Database*. Online. Available at http://www.naturaldatabase.com/aboutdb.asp. Accessed January 7, 2002.

NRC (National Research Council). 1998. *Peer Review in Environmental Technology Development Programs*. Washington, DC: National Academy Press.

OFAS (Office of Food Additive Safety). 2001. *Toxicological Principles for the Safety Assessment of Direct Food Additives and Color Additives Used in Food. Redbook II Draft.* Washington, DC: OFAS, Food and Drug Administration.

OFAS. 2003. *Redbook 2000. Toxicological Principles for the Safety of Food Ingredients.* Online. Center for Food Safety and Applied Nutrition, Food and Drug Administration. Available at http://www.cfsan.fda.gov/~redbook/red-toca.html. Accessed June 19, 2003.

Peirce A. 1999. *The American Pharmaceutical Association Practical Guide to Natural Medicines*. New York: William Morrow and Company.

Roll D. 2002. *Statement of Dr. David Roll, Director, Dietary Supplements, United States Pharmacopeia*. Presentation given at the Institute of Medicine Committee on the Framework for Evaluating the Safety of Dietary Supplements' Open Session on the Proposed Framework for Evaluating the Safety of Dietary Supplements, Washington, DC, September 26.

Upton R, ed. 1997. *American Herbal Pharmacopoeia and Therapeutic Compendium. St. John's Wort, Hypericum perforatum. Quality Control, Analytical and Therapeutic Monograph*. Santa Cruz, CA: AHP.

Upton R, ed. 1999. *American Herbal Pharmacopoeia and Therapeutic Compendium. Valerian Root, Valerian officinalis. Analytical, Quality Control, and Therapeutic Monograph*. Santa Cruz, CA: AHP.

USP. 2002a. *The United States Pharmacopeia. The National Formulary. USP 25-NF 20.* Rockville, MD: USP.

USP. 2002b. *USP Fact Sheet.* Online. Available at http://www.usp.org. Accessed June 18, 2002.

USP. 2004. *Overview: USP's Dietary Supplement Verification Program.* Online. Available at http://www.uspverified.org/pinfo/overview.html. Accessed March 10, 2004.

WHO (World Health Organization). 1991. *Report of the Consultation to Review the Draft Guidelines for the Assessment of Herbal Remedies. Munich, Germany, June 19–21, 1991*. Geneva: WHO.

WHO. 1999. *WHO Monographs on Selected Medicinal Plants. Vol. I.* Geneva: WHO.

WHO. 2001. *WHO Monographs of Selected Medicinal Plants. Vol. II.* Geneva: WHO.

WHO. 2003. *WHO Monographs of Selected Medicinal Plants. Vol. III.* Geneva: WHO.

3

The Framework

Under the provisions of the Dietary Supplement Health and Education Act (DSHEA), dietary supplements are to be considered as foods and assumed safe unless the Food and Drug Administration (FDA) has evidence that the supplement or one of its ingredients presents "a significant or unreasonable risk of illness or injury" when used as directed on the label or under normal conditions of use. Since the FDA is not authorized to require or impose premarket safety evaluations for dietary supplement ingredients marketed for use in the United States before October 15, 1994, FDA itself must monitor safety data and gather and assess existing information on safety to determine if a significant or unreasonable risk is present.

Thus the purpose of the Framework[1] described in this chapter is to provide a process for FDA to translate the results of their scientific review into a decision regarding regulatory action needed to protect the health of the public.

CONSIDERATIONS IN DESIGNING THE FRAMEWORK

The Framework consists of two components: (1) a process for prioritizing, evaluating, and describing available information to establish risk of

[1]A "framework" for safety evaluation of dietary supplement ingredients is characterized by the application of generally accepted scientific principles relating to adverse effects in order to make decisions of whether significant or unreasonable risk exists, thus overturning the *a priori* assumption of safety.

harm, and (2) a set of science-based principles that serve as guidelines for evaluating risk to human health.

For the Framework to be useful, FDA must have adequate resources for implementation. To be credible, it must be scientifically based and include guidelines for obtaining and integrating the totality of the information from many areas of science. The Framework should allow FDA to react to information, as well as to proactively gather information. It needs to be efficient and provide a system for updating information as new information becomes available. In providing a scientific infrastructure for the evaluation of the safety of dietary supplement ingredients, the framework must facilitate decision-making regarding a dietary supplement's potential to cause harm when uncertainty exists. Adequate staff with appropriate expertise must be available within FDA to administer the process and evaluate the information.

The Framework described here characterizes the nature of the scientific evidence that FDA is likely to encounter and describes a process for organizing this evidence to assess where a dietary supplement ingredient lies on a spectrum of concern[2] (see Figure 3-1). As the level of concern increases, so does the potential for a "significant or unreasonable risk," the standard warranting regulation under the Food, Drug, and Cosmetic Act (FDCA), as amended by DSHEA.

I. THE PROCESS

The process comprises three major components:

- Signal detection,
- Initial review of the signal, and
- Integrative evaluation.

Signal Detection

According to the DSHEA, it is assumed that dietary supplements are generally safe; given the large number of dietary supplement ingredients, it is unlikely that FDA will have the resources or the need to evaluate each ingredient uniformly to determine if it presents an unreasonable risk of illness or injury. Thus, at least initially, it is assumed that some "signal" will indicate that an ingredient's safety may need to be reviewed. When a signal is detected, it is up to FDA to decide the next step once the credibility of the

[2]The use of the term "concern" denotes a need for further investigation and inquiry by FDA based on a relative level of interest arising from initial information.

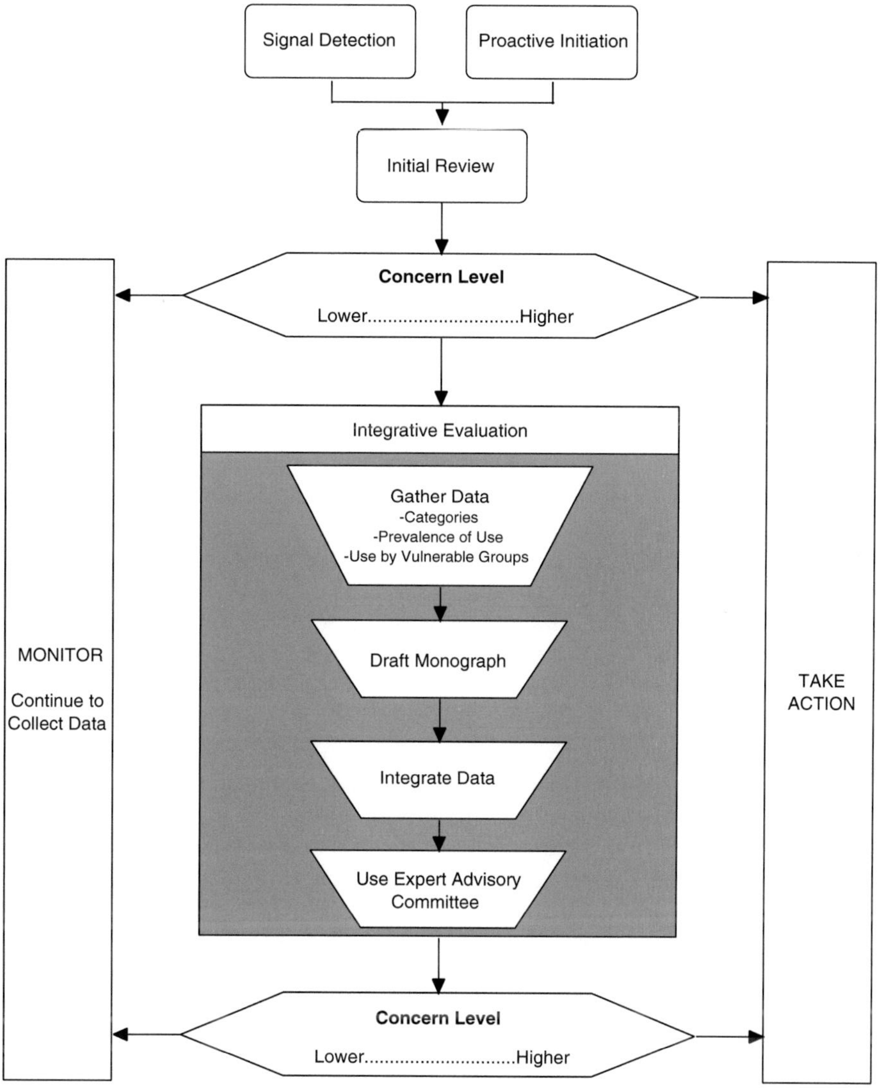

FIGURE 3-1 Diagram of the three components of the Safety Framework: signal detection, identification of level of concern in an initial review, and integrative evaluation, as well as how these components feed into FDA's decision to take action.

signal is evaluated and to determine the possibility that the ingredient caused the adverse effect noted (using the guiding principles outlined later in this chapter and discussed in detail in the chapters that follow).

What Constitutes a Signal?

FDA is likely to receive or become aware of a variety of signals suggesting potential risks to human health with the use of a dietary supplement ingredient. Signals may come to FDA's attention and thus be "detected" through notice of regulatory action taken by other countries regarding a specific dietary supplement, through routine monitoring of medical and scientific literature, directly through it's own Special Nutrition/Adverse Event Monitoring System, or through consultation with experts. FDA may also become aware of signals indirectly through reports in the media, through new data from animal experiments suggesting a specific risk, or through information provided by consumer protection advocacy groups. Signals can thus come from many sources and originate from many different types of scientific data. Given the significant number of dietary supplement ingredients, **FDA's attention should focus on signals that indicate a serious[3] health problem may result from ingestion of a dietary supplement ingredient.**

Quality of the Signal

In this first component little is done to evaluate the quality of the data because the focus is simply on signal detection. While some signals may result from concerns expressed by other expert bodies, such as those described in Chapter 2, or by case reports of adverse effects, the quality of the signal is not reviewed until the second component of the process (initial review of available information). The quality of the information behind the signals detected will be highly variable and in some cases may provide only weak evidence or be of little use or credence. Nonetheless, detecting these signals requires the attention of qualified professional staff at FDA and will result in a reaction by FDA (even if the reaction is only to consider the signal of little importance, as described in the next component).

[3]"Serious" is defined as any experience resulting in any of the following outcomes: death, a life-threatening adverse experience, inpatient hospitalization or prolongation of existing hospitalization, a persistent or significant disability/incapacity, or a congenital anomaly/birth defect. Important medical events that may not result in death, be life-threatening, or require hospitalization may be considered serious when, based upon appropriate medical judgment, they may jeopardize the individual and may require medical or surgical intervention to prevent one of the outcomes previously listed (in accordance with 21 C.F.R. § 600.80 [2002] and 21 C.F.R. § 314.80 [2002]).

Proactive Initiation of Review

In contrast to reaction based on detecting a signal, FDA may decide to proactively initiate a review of a dietary supplement ingredient due to high prevalence of use in the general population, high prevalence of use by a particularly vulnerable population, or other factors. More than likely, however, a signal indicating possible concerns will be the instigating factor in further review of a substance.

Prioritization for Review

One of the requirements of the study was to develop a framework that would include criteria for how the review of safety of dietary supplements and ingredients should be prioritized. It was suggested that a scheme to initially identify dietary supplement ingredients considered of higher priority for subsequent review based on only one criterion, such as end-organ toxicity in animal studies or the structure of one or more known compounds present in the ingredient be devised and applied to all dietary supplement ingredients. However, given the wide variety of dietary supplement ingredients available, the multiple forms of a specific ingredient that are sold, the voluntary and thus varying nature of the data available on an ingredient, and the wide variety of adverse effects that are possible for dietary supplements and the dependence of such effects on exposure levels, such a scheme is not feasible nor scientifically defensible.

This is not to say that the availability of data from only one category is not enough to determine a higher level of concern. As emphasized in the following chapters on the various types of data, any one category of information can raise concern to a level that requires action by FDA. A hierarchy of adverse effects that warrant greater concern than others based on collective judgment is provided in Chapters 4 through 7; however, a formulaic or algorithmic approach that considers all the important variables—such as the dose at which such effects may occur, the relevance of the information, the information available suggesting the ingredient may be safe—is not useful given the multidimensional matrix that would be needed.

The signal detection step, followed by an initial review of the information, should serve to identify those dietary supplement ingredients that are in need of further review and evaluation via an integrated evaluation.

Initial Review of Available Information

The second component of the Framework is to conduct an initial review of available information. First, the nature of the information generating the signal is examined to determine the appropriate level of concern regarding a risk to human health. This component is not envisioned as a detailed analysis of data, but rather as an assessment of the concern level warranted by the nature of the evidence (e.g., quality of the report, applicability to humans, route of exposure) and whether the information raises questions that require further examination.

Second, some effort can be made to gather easily available data to place the detected signal in context; such additional information may come from many sources, including other categories of data. Thus this initial review of the signal information need not be limited to reviewing only the information associated with the signal. For example, if the signal is a case report suggesting a possible problem in an elderly woman and clinical trials of the ingredient exist, these should be considered during the initial review.

Level of Concern

The outcome of the initial review is a determination of the initial overall level of concern to decide if an integrative evaluation is needed. Higher concerns warrant an integrative evaluation; lower concerns do not.[4] A decision about an ingredient with a moderate concern level should be made after a review of other information to see if other signals are apparent; for example, if the initial signal is animal data that warrant moderate concern, a cursory literature search on the substance or a review of FDA's adverse event monitoring system could be conducted to determine if other data about the ingredient raise concerns as well, leading to the need for further evaluation.

Assuming that sufficient evidence may not be available from just one type or category of data to cause a higher level of concern, it is important for FDA to consider data from other categories to determine if a higher level of concern may exist.

Decisions Possible Based on Initial Review

When the initial review of the nature of the evidence available indicates a higher level of concern, FDA would then initiate an integrative evaluation process or possibly decide to take immediate action, if the concern is serious enough and the data are strong. If the level of concern is categorized as relatively low, FDA would continue to monitor signals and incorporate the

[4]"Higher" level of concern is relative to the level of concern warranted by other evidence. The terms "higher" and "lower" are used to indicate that the level of concern is relative, rather than categorical.

information obtained into a monitoring database for future use if new data regarding the ingredient become available.

Maintaining a database of specific issues to monitor would allow FDA staff familiar with the criteria outlined in Chapters 4 through 8 to systematically look for information that may address the data gaps. Similarly, data collected should be saved in case a decision is made to move to an integrative evaluation. If a decision is made to conduct an integrative evaluation, but a monograph is not subsequently prepared, then information and a summary of the thought processes involved in the integrative evaluation should be noted and filed for future consideration. Making data gaps and unanswered questions available to other interested parties such as the National Toxicology Program of the National Institute of Environmental Health Sciences (NIEHS) or the Office of Dietary Supplements, both part of the National Institutes of Health (NIH), Department of Health and Human Services, would allow them to incorporate these data needs on specific dietary supplement ingredients into their programs of work.

In summary, once the initial level of concern based on the initial review of the signal is determined, FDA might decide that continued routine monitoring is needed, or it could decide to proceed with an integrative evaluation. This depends on the level of concern raised by the signal: ingredients provoking higher concern should proceed to the integrative evaluation; ingredients resulting in lower levels of concern would generally not proceed; and ingredients with moderate concerns might proceed after considering additional information not necessarily related to the initial signal, such as prevalence of use or concern related to a specific vulnerable population group. Since it is assumed by the DSHEA that dietary supplements are safe, there should be relatively few dietary supplement ingredients that will be categorized as of higher concern after the initial review and thus warrant further examination. This allows FDA to focus its efforts on dietary supplement ingredients that are strong candidates for regulation.

Integrative Evaluation

The third component of the Framework is to conduct an integrative evaluation for those dietary supplement ingredients that are deemed to warrant further investigation, based on the preliminary data reviewed in the second component and the resulting relative placement on the spectra of concern continuums. There are four aspects to the Integrative Evaluation component (see Figure 3-1): in-depth literature search and review, drafting a safety monograph based on this information, integrating the available data into an analysis to complete the monograph, and possibly referring the draft monograph and accompanying information to an expert committee for additional input prior to determining whether to take regulatory action.

Reviewing the Literature

A critical review of the literature is a three-part process. First, multiple databases are searched for information on the dietary supplement ingredient and other substances with similar taxonomical, structural, or functional properties. Such searches are broad-based, and include information on safety and biological activity of the ingredients, including human data, animal data, and *in vitro* data.

Second, each primary research paper is reviewed for internal consistency; for example, are proper methodologies used? Do data fit the conclusions? Are the associations real? Is appropriate information included? Are there chance, bias, confounding variables, a lack of coherence, or other significant internal issues or limitations that should be taken into account?

Third, the external consistency of the research papers must be judged as a group. Are the studies coherent as a whole? Is there strength in the associations, general agreement, etc.? Studies can then be sorted into those that suggest that there is little risk of illness or injury when consuming the supplement ingredient, those that indicate a relevant concern for risk of illness or injury, and those that have equivocal results. Each should then be examined for flaws and strengths in accordance with the principles and concepts discussed in the subsequent chapters on each general category of data (Chapters 4 through 7).

Focused Versus Broad-Based Evaluation. An integrative evaluation might be reactive to the signal and focused in nature, in that it is conducted to examine a specific moderate- or high-level concern about an ingredient, or it might be more proactive and broad-based, in that it is looking for any risk associated with use of the dietary supplement ingredient. As described above in the description of the signal detection component, a proactive integrative evaluation might be initiated simply because a large percentage of the population is using the ingredient, rather than as a reaction to a particular safety concern.

The amount of information gathered depends on the nature of the harmful effect that is the focus of concern. If a focused evaluation is conducted, it is assumed that less information will be reviewed. However, the relative importance of an individual study is established in conjunction with an evaluation of other relevant literature. Clearly, data or information outside the primary safety concern may include information that has a direct bearing on the overall evaluation of the safety concern identified in the signal component. Thus a comprehensive review can provide information that may raise concerns in other areas not relevant to the focus, but which should not be ignored in a safety monograph.

Relevancy of Data. Gathering data and reviewing it for relevance provides the scientific base upon which FDA can substantiate its conclusions. Data that are not relevant to safety or to the concern in a focused integrated evaluation need not be incorporated into the report; however, acknowledging that it was considered and deemed irrelevant will be helpful if the information has been characterized by others as substantiating safety.

Drafting a Safety Monograph

In most cases, the integrative evaluation will be documented in a monograph[5] that summarizes the categories of data available and their use in drawing conclusions about the potential risk associated with use of the ingredient. Evidence obtained either from only one category of data or from integrating all the categories that results in an increased level of concern should result in a higher priority for development of a safety monograph.

A monograph need not be developed for every dietary supplement ingredient, as it is assumed that only those ingredients with moderate or higher concern levels following the initial review will be subject to an integrative evaluation (essential nutrients represent a special case; see Annex 3-1). The monograph may not need to cover every concern, in which case a focused integrative evaluation and resulting monograph would be completed. In a few cases, where available information obtained in the initial review results in a highly significant level of concern, it may be necessary to undertake regulatory action prior to or without developing a monograph. The development of a monograph may be resource and time intensive, especially when initiated proactively and thus with a much broader focus.

However, the development of a monograph provides a method to document in a systematic format the evidence on which FDA can base a regulatory decision. The science-based guiding principles described in the following sections of this chapter, and explained in detail in the following chapters, should be used to reach a decision regarding whether there is an unreasonable risk of illness or injury.

The general types of information to be collected and used in the integrative evaluation and thus collated in a monograph are listed in Box 3-1 and include a description of the ingredient (e.g., constituents, different types of preparations, typical intake amount and duration, historical use) and available information about toxicities and safety (human data, animal data, data describing risks associated with related substances, and *in vitro* data). In most cases, this information will be gathered from the medical and

---

[5]A monograph is defined as a "learned treatise on a small area of knowledge" (Merriam-Webster, 2001).

BOX 3-1
Safety Monograph

I. Description of the Ingredient

- Constituents as appropriate: chemical classification and structure; for a botanical ingredient, genus, species, part of plant; for an animal ingredient, genus, species, part of body
- Description of individual components, alternative forms or secondary constituents
- Descriptions of different dietary supplement preparations, how they may differ in constituents, and amounts ingested in ordinary use

II. Safety Information (in narrative form, referencing data tables)

- Human safety data (serious and nonserious adverse effects): historical use, if applicable; adverse effects from clinical trials, clinical case reports, and adverse event reports; interactions (i.e., drug interactions); consequences of unusually large intake and/or chronic cumulative use
- Animal studies
- *In vitro* studies
- Biological activity of related substances (structurally, taxonomically, and functionally related)

III. Other Relevant Information (if known and applicable)

- Sources of ingredient
- Conditions of use suggested or recommended in labeling or other marketing material
- Cautions about use from historical use, labeling, or other marketing material
- Usage patterns (prevalence of use in the general population, use by vulnerable groups)
- Information on regulatory actions, including those of regulatory agencies in other countries
- Available information on physiological and biochemical aspects (bioavailability, distribution, metabolism)

IV. Summary and Conclusions

- Summary
- Conclusions about the safety of the ingredient, based on the strength of the scientific evidence
- Unresolved issues and uncertainties in the available data
- Data gaps and future research recommended

V. Literature Search Strategy

VI. Literature Cited

VII. Tables of Key Data Evaluated

scientific literature. However, additional information may be obtained by requesting information from clinical investigators who have published reports about the particular ingredient, as well as by requesting information from industry (e.g., distributors and manufacturers) and other stakeholders. The collected information should be collated into a draft safety monograph. The monograph should be prepared using a standard format to summarize all the data collected on the ingredient (see Annex 3-2 to this chapter for a more detailed discussion of monograph preparation).

Integrating the Data to Determine Risk

The data evaluation component of the integrative evaluation should be conducted on the initial assumption that consumption of the supplement should not present an unreasonable risk of illness or injury, as is assumed in DSHEA. To overturn this assumption, the end result of the review should demonstrate that there is an unreasonable risk of illness or injury to the consumer.

When evidence on a dietary supplement ingredient presents a moderate or higher level of concern relative to this risk, data from other categories should be considered to evaluate biological plausibility and consistency. Integration within and across the other categories of data will help determine if an unreasonable risk exists by looking at the overall picture. Such an analysis can be represented by creating a causal model diagram—a tool to organize the data to visualize how the different types of available data link together to establish risk (described in Chapter 10). For example, in reviewing the potential for concern in the use of saw palmetto for the prototype monograph described in this report, data from all categories were integrated to make a conclusion about risk (see Chapter 11 and Appendix H).

The principles described for considering the various types of data and modifying factors (Chapters 4 through 9), as well as the principles described for how to integrate among and within categories of data (Chapter 10), are applied in the integrative evaluation. They should be followed in assessing and weighing the different types of evidence that enter into the decision. They are summarized in the conclusions in the safety monograph. The conclusions should describe:

- The relevance of the evidence;
- How the dose, manner of use, and product affect conclusions about risk;
- The seriousness of the potential harm suggested by the evidence; and
- The quality and strength of the evidence.

Review of the information does not need to prove toxicity, only that there is an unreasonable risk of its occurrence (see Box 3-2). Such an analysis is captured in the monograph. The evaluation of the totality of the scientific evidence is thus summarized in conclusions about risk based on the high level of concern resulting from the in-depth review and analysis of the available information.

To guide those making conclusions about risk as a result of the integrative evaluation component, it might be possible to develop a taxonomy of levels of risk—such as "no basis for concern," "some grounds for further monitoring," "some basis for concern about risk," or "presents a risk that warrants regulation under the FDCA as amended by DSHEA." This was not done in this report because the definitions might become too prescriptive given the variety of information and types of dietary supplement ingre-

BOX 3-2
Safety in the Context of Dietary Supplements

It has been said that the ". . . dose differentiates a poison from a remedy." Even essential substances for humans, such as oxygen and water, can be toxic in high concentration or if imbibed in large amounts. Thus no substance is completely "safe." Safety is a qualitative term that is applied to a variety of situations or environmental factors and is related to the context in which it is evaluated. What is safe in one situation (e.g., driving 50 mph) might be considered unsafe in another. In relation to ingested substances, in some cases it is possible that concerns related to adverse effects resulting from consumption may be mitigated by benefits derived from the substance when ingested.

For drugs and medical devices, safety is evaluated as a measure of potential harm relative to benefit (see Chapter 1). For food additives, safety is defined as the reasonable certainty of no harm, without consideration of benefit beyond that of improving the functional characteristics of the resulting food product, such as retarding microbial growth or maintaining texture. The DSHEA classifies dietary supplements similarly to food, and therefore supplements are considered, like conventional foods, to be reasonably safe.

While dietary supplements are biologically active substances that may have desirable health benefits, they may also cause adverse health outcomes. DSHEA requires that the FDA determine that a dietary supplement ingredient is unsafe (i.e., consumption results in unreasonable risk of illness or injury at recommended intake levels) rather than requiring that a manufacturer provide data supporting its safety, as it does for food additives, drugs, and medical devices.

Since FDA's authority is limited to evaluating a dietary supplement ingredient for potential to cause illness or injury, but it cannot take into account possible beneficial effects on health, any safety framework for a dietary supplement ingredient must depend on (1) the accumulation of evidence indicating potential for harm and (2) the determination of when this accumulated evidence raises concern to a point that a significant or unreasonable risk exists.

dients. Thus this Framework, while qualitatively providing descriptions of points on a continuum of relative concern about risk derived for the various types of data, does not include a metric for categorization of risk.

Referring Review to an External Advisory Committee

After considering the conclusions about risk in the draft monograph, FDA should make a decision to (1) take regulatory action, (2) not take regulatory action and continue to monitor for new data regarding safety, or (3) refer the dietary supplement ingredient to an advisory committee of multidisciplinary experts for a safety review.

It is expected that FDA may want further input from an advisory committee on many of the dietary supplement ingredients undergoing an integrative evaluation because only ingredients with significant potential for concern are likely to reach this stage, and outside evaluation may be critical to ensure that all relevant information was reviewed. Also, in cases where FDA does not have internal scientists with the appropriate expertise, it may be cost-effective to create an external advisory committee to provide further input on the safety of the dietary supplement ingredient. This could be an activity under the existing Food Advisory Committee of the Center for Food Safety and Applied Nutrition of FDA, or it could be an additional committee, either standing or *ad hoc*, depending on the ingredients to be reviewed. See Annex 3-2 for additional discussion of the composition of an advisory committee.

Where the data and thus conclusions are not clear-cut, an external advisory committee would thus be constituted for the following reasons:

- While there may be credible evidence that the ingredient may cause harm, further review may be needed by consultants with specific knowledge about the ingredient, as well as by consultants with specific knowledge about the safety issues raised, to interpret the totality of the data and derive conclusions and recommendations.
- The available evidence may be of questionable scientific basis or it may be difficult to interpret.
- Insufficient data may be available to allow the rationale for the decision to be clearly established.
- It provides a mechanism for public input.

These reasons are only examples, as many other circumstances may trigger the need for external advisory committee review (See Annex 3-3 for committee composition).

After reviewing the information collected in the draft monograph and in the public information sessions envisioned as part of their deliberations, the external advisory committee should provide input to FDA regarding revisions in the draft monograph, as needed, to create as complete a picture of the available scientific information on safety as possible, within the resources made available to FDA. The advisory committee should evaluate the ingredient based on the weight of the scientific evidence as described in the previous section.

The advisory committee's report should include comments about the risks and hazards that may be associated with use by the general population, as well as risks that may be particular to subgroups of the population. As much as possible, the advisory committee should describe how its review of the safety depends on how the ingredient is used—the dose, manner, and form.

The advisory committee may conclude that there is inadequate evidence within the available information to suspect a hazard to the public when the ingredient is used at the levels recommended on the label or at levels that might reasonably be expected. If current use does not demonstrate a hazard, the advisory committee may decide to comment on whether it is possible to foresee that a significant increase in consumption would constitute a hazard. If there is not enough information available to conduct a scientific evaluation of the safety of the dietary supplement, the advisory committee should indicate this.

In cases where the data are insufficient to determine whether a hazard exists, conclusions should also be accompanied by a brief description of additional research that would be most useful in forming science based decisions.

Decision to Take Action

After the advisory committee's review is shared with FDA, the completed monograph and the advisory committee's comments should be posted on FDA's website. One of the important components of DSHEA was that the public should be educated about dietary supplements. FDA thus has a responsibility to educate consumers about the safety of supplement ingredients, and the public availability of the completed monographs can be an important aspect of the educational process. The monographs can provide the public with a reputable summary of the available information and scientific uncertainties about the inherent safety of the supplement ingredient whose safety has been questioned.[6] Importantly, public access to infor-

---

[6]Monographs made available to the public should make clear the type of monograph—focused or broad-based—and the fact that monographs are developed for those dietary supplement ingredients where serious concerns have been evaluated, unlike other available monographs, where "safety" may be presumed if a monograph is published.

mation from an advisory committee will add to the quality and strength of the available scientific literature.

The decision to refer a dietary supplement ingredient to an external advisory committee rests with FDA. As with other federal advisory committees, while the external advisory committee opinions or conclusions should be based on the information and data presented, the decision on whether to follow the determinations of the external advisory committee rests with FDA, as it alone possesses regulatory authority in these matters. If FDA decided to take an action, it would initiate a judicial enforcement proceeding, such as a seizure, suit for injunction, or prosecution, designed to elicit a court ruling that the supplement was unsafe. In order to justify the use of FDA's resources to the extent envisioned by the Framework, the results of the integrative evaluation should play a pivotal role in establishing that a supplement ingredient is unsafe.

As a result of the integrative evaluation, it is quite possible that FDA will decide to take action, declaring that a dietary supplement ingredient presents a significant or unreasonable risk of illness or injury. It is also possible that, more selectively, concerns related to the use of a supplement by a vulnerable group within the population may be highlighted, so that specific action related to the use by specific groups is possible where warranted, even though the general population may not be at the same level of risk.

An added benefit of making monographs easily available to the public is that industry and publicly funded scientists may choose to conduct studies that address the concerns raised, thereby increasing the knowledge base regarding the safety of dietary supplements. The general public, as well as industry, pharmacists, health care providers, and distributors, will benefit from the publicly available information and individually can decide whether to use, sell, or recommend the dietary supplement ingredient in question, regardless of whether FDA decides to take action or not.

Decision to Continue to Monitor

When the review of information, either at the initial review step or as a result of an integrative evaluation, indicates a lower level of concern, FDA should continue to monitor information it receives relative to the dietary supplement ingredient. Monitoring consists of either passively watching for new signals of other concerns about the ingredient or developing search strategies to routinely search the scientific literature for new data to address specific concerns. (See Chapter 12 for how monitoring might be approached for some of the dietary supplement ingredients reviewed in the prototypes.) Monitoring might also include working with the National Toxicology Program at NIEHS or the Office of Dietary Supplements at the NIH to initiate research addressing unanswered questions relative to some of the signals detected.

II. APPLYING SCIENCE-BASED PRINCIPLES TO ESTABLISH RISK

In outlining the task, FDA requested that the Framework include a method based on safety concerns to categorize and prioritize dietary supplement ingredients sold in the United States. Given the variety of types of information that are likely to be available, the Framework classifies scientific information into four broad categories for use in determining the potential for serious harm for a specific dietary supplement ingredient. These categories of data include:

- Human data,
- Animal studies,
- *In vitro* experiments, and
- Information on related substances.

Subsequent chapters describe the types of information that may be available in each category of data and the strengths and weaknesses of these different data sources in evaluating the potential of a dietary supplement ingredient to cause harm (Chapters 4 through 7). Also described are how to consider the potential for dietary supplement interactions with drugs and other xenobiotics[7] (Chapter 8), important considerations that should be factored into evaluations when vulnerable populations consume dietary supplements or when supplements are widely consumed (Chapter 9), and considerations for integrating the available data from various sources to determine an overall level of concern (Chapter 10) using a causal model diagram. The level of concern appropriate for a specific piece of information within a particular data category (i.e., human, animal, *in vitro*, or related substances information) is summarized in diagrams that relate the available evidence to show the level of concern when consuming a dietary supplement ingredient.

Evidence that results in a higher level of concern indicates a more immediate priority for further investigation to determine if an unreasonable risk to public health exists. In contrast, a single piece of information resulting in a lower level of concern may suggest that continued routine monitoring for new evidence is warranted—evidence that might elevate the level of concern and thus its priority for increased scrutiny.

---

[7]A chemical substance or compound that is foreign to the human body or to other living organisms.

Although each chapter strives to describe all types of information that may be available, it is important to recognize that for most dietary supplement ingredients, it will be difficult, if not impossible, to find useful information from all data categories. The following section provides an overview of the types of information that may be encountered and summarizes general scientific guidelines for assessing the relevance and quality of the available information from each data category (Box 3-3). More specific information and details are provided in Chapters 4 through 9.

Spectra of Concern

As briefly outlined in the process description earlier in this chapter, included in the Framework is a qualitative method to evaluate the nature of the evidence for a specific piece of information within a particular data category (i.e., human, animal, *in vitro*, or information about related substances). Distinguishing characteristics of evidence determine where a piece of information falls on the continuum of lower to higher level of concern. This is summarized in diagrams referred to as *spectra of concern*. Evidence that results in a higher level of concern indicates a more immediate priority for investigating further whether an unreasonable risk to public health exists, because a higher level of concern suggests a potential risk to public health. In contrast, a single piece of information resulting in a lower level of concern may suggest continued routine monitoring for new evidence that might elevate the level of concern and thus initiate increased scrutiny.

Human Data

Information about human use of dietary supplement ingredients may be in the form of formal studies, such as clinical studies or trials and epidemiological studies; in the form of spontaneously reported adverse event reports or literature case reports; or in the form of information about historical use of the ingredient. Because there is no requirement that dietary supplement ingredients undergo formal studies prior to marketing, formal study data on a dietary supplement ingredient will be less commonly available than spontaneous adverse event reports and information about historical use. The lack of such data, however, does not diminish their importance.

Data about human intake can be useful either as indicators of possible risk or, conversely, as mitigators of concerns raised by other categories of data. Within each type of human data, questions can be asked about the nature and quality of the scientific information to determine whether the information raises the level of concern regarding the probability to cause harm. While discussed in detail in Chapter 4, the general spectra of concern

BOX 3-3
Guiding Principles for Evaluating Data to Determine Unreasonable Risk

- General principles

— Absence of evidence of risk does not indicate that there is no risk.

— Proof of causality or proof of harm is not necessary to determine unreasonable or significant risk.

— Integration of data across different categories of information and types of study design can enhance biological plausibility and identify consistencies, leading to conclusions regarding levels of concern for an adverse event that may be associated with use of a dietary supplement.

- Human data

— A credible report or study finding of a serious adverse event in humans raises concern about the ingredient's safety and requires further information gathering and evaluation; final judgment, however, will require consideration of the totality of the evidence.

— Historical use should not be used as *prima facie* evidence that the ingredient does not cause harm.

— Considerable weight can be given to a lack of adverse events in large, high-quality, randomized clinical trials or epidemiological studies that are adequately powered and designed to detect adverse effects.

- Animal data

— Even in the absence of information on adverse events in humans, evidence of harm from animal studies is often indicative of potential harm to humans.

- Related substances

— Scientific evidence for risk can be obtained by considering if the plant constituents are compounds with established toxicity, are closely related in structure to compounds with established toxicity, or the plant source of the botanical dietary supplement itself is a toxic plant or is taxonomically related to a known toxic plant.

— Supplement ingredients that are endogenous substances or that may be related to endogenous substances should be evaluated to determine if their activities are likely to lead to serious effects. Considerations should include the substance's ability to raise the steady-state concentration of biologically active metabolites in tissues and whether the effect of such increases would be linked to a serious health effect.

- *In vitro* data

— Validated[a] *in vitro* studies can stand alone as independent indicators of risk to human health if a comparable exposure is attained in humans and the *in vitro* effects correlate with a specific adverse health effect in humans or animals.

---

[a]In this report, *in vitro* assays are considered validated when their results have been proven to predict a specific effect in animals and/or humans with reasonable certainty (not necessarily universally accepted or without detractors).

related to human data are identified in Tables 3-1 through 3-5. An important concept in Chapter 4 that is not captured in the spectra of concern tables is that historical use information becomes less relevant as difference from traditional use increases. Changes in historical versus modern use may arise from new methods of preparation (e.g., plant part used or extraction process) or new patterns of use (e.g., higher intake level, route of administration, duration and frequency of consumption, indication for use).

Animal Data

Information about animal exposure to dietary supplement ingredients may be in the form of formal studies, such as traditional toxicity studies, safety pharmacology data, or observations from clinical veterinary medicine. Because dietary supplement ingredients are not required to undergo formal animal toxicity testing before marketing, extensive toxicity studies are uncommon, but limited amounts of animal data for a number of dietary supplement ingredients are available in the scientific literature. Despite the challenges of dealing with incomplete data, available animal data warrant attention when assessing risk of dietary supplement ingredients.

Animal studies are powerful because controlled studies can be conducted to predict effects that might not be detected from customary use by humans until they result in overt harmful effects. Animal studies are especially useful in detecting effects of chronic exposures and effects on reproductive and developmental processes because epidemiological methods of studying humans are especially problematic in these areas. The ability to administer agents to animals during their entire lifespan enables scientists to ascertain the potential toxic effects that may arise for long-term (chronic) exposure. Animal studies thus serve as important hypothesis generators and may be sufficient to indicate potentially unreasonable risk to human health, which justifies their use in evaluating the risks of dietary supplement ingredients to humans.

In general, adverse effects observed in well-designed and conducted animal studies should be treated as if they occur in at least some members of the human population, assuming humans receive a sufficiently high dose. With some notable and important exceptions, the biological factors affecting the capacity of chemical substances to cause toxicity are broadly similar across mammalian species. While discussed in detail in Chapter 5, the general spectrum of concern related to animal data is described in Table 3-6, based on the relative seriousness of adverse effects seen in animal studies (Box 3-4).

TABLE 3-1 Relative Spectrum of Concern for Individual Spontaneous Adverse Event Reports

Increasing Concern →		
Describes a serious adverse event with less information than would justify moderate or strong concern, and/or with prominent confounding factors (e.g., multiple concomitant substances and/or conditions)	Describes a serious adverse event with some, but not all, characteristics associated with strong concern	Describes a well-documented serious adverse event with plasma levels (if available) at a relevant range and demonstrates dechallenge and rechallenge (if possible), temporality, and strong attribution

TABLE 3-2 Relative Spectrum of Concern for Case Series of Spontaneous Adverse Event Reports

Increasing Concern →		
Describes a series of serious adverse events, with less information than would justify moderate or strong concern, and/or prominent confounding factors (e.g., multiple concomitant substances and/or conditions)	Describes a series of serious adverse events, with some, but not all, characteristics associated with strong concern	Describes a series of well-documented cases demonstrating consistent serious adverse events and clinical findings, and dechallenge (if possible), temporality, and strong attribution

TABLE 3-3 Relative Spectrum of Concern Raised by Historical Evidence of Toxicity

Increasing Concern →		
Traditional cautions (contraindications) exist regarding use in certain populations or circumstances	Traditional cautions (contraindications) exist regarding use in certain populations or circumstances that, if ignored, might be associated with a serious adverse effect (e.g., do not use during pregnancy)	There is clear evidence that traditional use causes conditions considered to be serious adverse events (e.g., hallucination, lethal poisoning)

TABLE 3-4 Spectrum of Relative Concerns with Clinical Studies Data

Increasing Concern →		
Describes a serious adverse event, but with less information than would justify moderate or strong concern, and/or the interpretation of the clinical study is hampered by the presence of prominent confounding factors (e.g., multiple concomitant substances and/or conditions) that could not be controlled by balancing AND/OR Prominent methodological concerns (e.g., unexplained high level of dropouts, lack of control groups)	Nonsignificant, but clinically important, trend of a higher rate of a serious adverse event OR Abnormalities in clinical laboratory values OR Other abnormalities, such as electrocardiographic findings in the dietary supplement ingredient group	A significantly higher incidence of a serious adverse event OR Other potentially dangerous abnormalities, such as in clinical laboratory values that are associated with risk of serious adverse events OR Other abnormalities, such as electrocardiographic findings in the dietary supplement ingredient group

TABLE 3-5 Spectrum of Relative Concerns with Epidemiological Data

Increasing Concern →		
Case-control or cohort study (including registries), with small,[a] but statistically significant, relative risk or odds ratio of a serious adverse event OR Large relative risk or odds ratio of a serious adverse event that is not statistically significant OR Poorly conducted studies with large or significant effects	Case-control or cohort study (including registries), with moderate, statistically significant relative risk or odds ratio of a serious adverse event OR Moderate relative risk or odds ratio of a serious adverse event that is not statistically significant but that implies a trend	Well-conducted case-control or cohort study (including registries), with large, statistically significant relative risk or odds ratio of a serious adverse event

[a] In short, 2 or less is generally considered weak association, and 3 or more is considered strong, but this is only a very general "rule of thumb" guidance, which is somewhat debatable.

TABLE 3-6 Relative Spectrum of Concern: Guidelines for Types of Evidence from Animal Studies[a]

Increasing Concern →		
At least one acceptable, quality study showing effects of Category A at Dose > 1,000× Human Intake OR At least one acceptable, quality study showing effects of Category B at Dose > 100× Human Intake OR At least one acceptable, quality study showing effects of Category C at Dose > 10× Human Intake OR Studies showing adverse effects, but which cannot be interpreted because of deficiencies in design, conduct, or reporting OR Acceptable, quality non-oral studies indicating adverse effect from Category A, B, or C	At least one acceptable, quality study showing effects of Category A at Dose > 100 to < 1,000× Human Intake OR At least one acceptable, quality study showing effects of Category B at Dose > 10 to < 100× Human Intake OR At least one acceptable, quality study showing effects of Category C at Dose > 1 to < 10× Human Intake	At least one acceptable, quality study showing effects of Category A at Dose < 100× Human Intake OR At least one acceptable, quality study showing effects of Category B at Dose < 10× Human Intake OR At least one acceptable, quality study showing effects of Category C at Dose ≤ 1× Human Intake

[a] Categories A, B, and C refer to relative seriousness of a variety of adverse effects identified in animal studies, ranging from reproductive failure (A) to reduced food consumption (C). See Box 3-4 for further examples.

Information About Related Substances

Information about substances related to the dietary supplement ingredient of interest may be useful when predicting risk to human health. Such substances may be related to dietary supplement ingredients in one of several ways, such as:

- Chemical relatedness—the ingredient or constituent of an ingredient is similar to known toxic chemicals, or is known to contain chemicals similar in structure to known toxicophores;[8]

[8]Chemical structures associated with potential adverse effects.

BOX 3-4
Guidelines for Relative Seriousness for Selected Examples of Adverse Effects Obtained from Animal Studies

Category A (most serious)

- Neoplasia (including genotoxic and nongenotoxic carcinogens), teratogenesis, mortality
- Severe target organ toxicity
  - — Necrosis, dysplasia
  - — Reproductive failure, fetotoxicity, severe developmental effects
  - — Severe neurobehavioral changes

Category B (moderately serious)

- Moderate target organ toxicity
  - — Atrophy, hyperplasia
  - — Reduced reproductive capacity, moderate developmental effects
  - — Moderate Neurobehavioral Changes
  - — Clinical chemistry changes associated with histological lesions outside reference value ranges

Category C (less serious)

- Reduced body-weight gain
- Body weight/organ weight ratios
- Reduced food consumption
- Enzyme changes, other biochemical and toxicity biomarker alterations accompanied by histological changes
- Reversible degenerative changes

- Taxonomic relatedness—the ingredient is from the same classification as a known toxic plant species, genera, or family;
- Functional relatedness—the ingredient or chemical constituent shares a common biological target or mechanism of action that is clearly tied to a toxic effect demonstrated with another substance. This includes endogenous substances and mimetics of endogenous substances, when the effect of increasing the amount of an endogenous substance is linked to an adverse health effect.

Taken together, the value and utility of this information to predict risk depends on the type of dietary supplement ingredient that is being considered. A concern may be raised about a botanical dietary supplement based on information about risk associated with known chemical constituents, as well as information about risk associated with related toxic plants. Similarly, pure single chemical compounds may be of concern based on comparison to known risk-associated chemical compounds and chemical moieties (toxicophores) that raise concern of safety. Substances that are normally present in the human body (endogenous substances) may be of concern based on knowledge of what the substances do in the body at normal concentrations, and an understanding of what might occur if the normal concentrations are exceeded. For dietary supplements for which the chemical composition is undefined,[9] but for which information about biological activity is available, it may be helpful and it is appropriate to consider whether the exhibited biological activity is the basis for safety concerns of other substances that are considered potentially harmful. While discussed in detail in Chapter 6, the general spectrum of concern regarding related substances is described in Table 3-7, based on knowledge of the relative seriousness of adverse effects seen with ingestion of related substances.

In Vitro Studies

A range of *in vitro* experimental systems are used to gain insight into the risk of adverse effects of compounds. These systems include isolated organs, isolated cells, microorganisms, subcellular organelles, and molecular entities such as enzymes, receptors, transport proteins, isolated membranes, and genes or gene fragments. A primary advantage of conducting *in vitro* studies is that their reductionist (non-whole-organism) approach allows insight into a compound's mechanisms of action that might be more difficult to obtain in a whole-animal study. The control possible with *in vitro* experiments enables examination of the effect on the target process or structure in isolation from confounding factors. For example, control over the concentration of the chemical of interest or of one or more of its metabolites enables the interactions among chemicals or metabolites to be studied. *In vitro* experiments are also generally more rapid and less expensive to conduct than *in vivo* studies; thus, *in vitro* studies are more likely than *in vivo* studies to be available for assessment of dietary supplement safety.

Some experiments are specifically designed to examine safety endpoints while the information provided by other experiments is less specific about an ingredient's biological activity. Because no battery of tests is required on dietary supplement ingredients, results from safety tests common to other chemicals are not widely available. When they are available, these "validated" *in vitro* assays—assays that are accepted for use in predicting effects on whole organisms—can be of significant use. In such studies, the serious-

[9]An example of a nonbotanical dietary supplement with undefined chemical composition might be a preparation from a living organism or otherwise complex substance; shark cartilage is an example.

ness of harm can be predicted by a given assay. While discussed in detail in Chapter 7, the general spectrum of concern regarding *in vitro* data is described in Table 3-8 and is based on the predictability that adverse effects may occur in vivo.

Interactions

One of the major concerns about the safety of dietary supplement ingredients is that interactions between a supplement and other ingested substances (drugs, other dietary supplement ingredients, conventional foods) will result in adverse clinical outcomes due to an increase or decrease in the level of the dietary supplement in the organism, an increase or decrease in the level of other xenobiotics, or combined toxicities.

Interactions can be detected with human, animal, or *in vitro* studies or predicted on the basis of how related substances behave. There are numerous mechanisms for interactions among xenobiotics, but most can be categorized as direct chemical-chemical, pharmacodynamic, or pharmacokinetic interactions. In direct chemical-chemical interactions, the action of one or both chemicals is modified by taking them within a relatively short time of each other. With pharmacodynamic interactions, there is a change in response to either the dietary supplement ingredient or the xenobiotic, but with no change in plasma concentration in either. Pharmacokinetic interactions, which occur when one substance affects the absorption, distribution, metabolism, or excretion of the other, result in altered levels of one of the substances or its metabolites. *In vitro* and *in vivo* experimental methods for identifying ingredients that may cause such interactions are available. While discussed in detail in Chapter 8, the general spectrum of concern regarding interactions among dietary supplement ingredients and other dietary supplements, foods, or drugs is described in Table 3-9, based on prediction of serious adverse events. It should be noted that the potential seriousness of these interactions varies.

Prevalence of Use and Vulnerable Groups in the Population

The scientific bases for evaluating the safety of dietary supplement ingredients described in this section are critical in determining which dietary supplement ingredient warrants the most immediate attention (i.e., in setting priorities). However, it is also appropriate to take other information into consideration when setting priorities. That is, given *similar* degrees of concern about risk, attention from FDA is more appropriately directed towards a supplement that is being used by a greater portion of the population. It is also important to consider the safety of the most sensitive groups. These two factors are discussed in detail in Chapter 9.

TABLE 3-7 Relative Spectrum of Concern for Relatedness Information

Type of Information	Increasing Concern →		
Botanical chemical constituents of concern	Plant contains constituents that are known to be toxic to humans, but the constituents are commonly consumed in similar amounts in conventional food products	Plant contains constituents that are known to be toxic to humans at low concentrations, but the concentration of these substances in the plant part used for the supplement is *not* characterized OR Plant *part* used for the supplement contains constituents that are toxic to humans, but there is credible reason to believe that the constituent may not cause serious adverse effects at the amount typically ingested	Plant contains constituents that are known to be toxic to humans at low concentrations and the concentration of substances found in the plant *part* used for formulating the supplement has been characterized
Taxonomic relationship to other botanicals of concern	In a plant family that contains known toxic genera, but the supplement is not in a genus known to be toxic AND	Same genus known to be toxic to humans or animals OR In a plant family that is known to contain toxic plants but	Same species as a known toxic plant that is not ingested as a food

	It has a history of use as a food in a preparation and method similar to its current use	not in a genus known as a food plant OR In a plant family that is known to contain toxic plants, and in a genus that may have a history of food use, but supplement is either a concentrated extract or from a different plant part than is ingested as a food	
Chemical structure	Structurally similar to, or likely contains, a chemical compound known to be toxic to humans or animals when ingested in high doses	Supplement contains chemical constituent known to be toxic to humans or animals	Supplement contains chemical constituent known to be toxic at very low doses to humans
Endogenous substances or mimetics of endogenous substances	*May result* in tissue concentrations that would be expected to cause biological effects (either because homeostasis is disrupted or because the substance has potent biological activities), but the seriousness of the biological effect is not definite	Results seen in tissue concentrations that would be expected to cause biological effects (either because homeostasis is disrupted or because the substance has potent biological activities), but the seriousness of the biological effect is not definite	Results seen in tissue concentrations that would be expected to cause biological effects (either because homeostasis is disrupted or because the substance has potent biological activities) that are considered serious

TABLE 3-8 Relative Spectrum of Concern for *In Vitro* Data

Increasing Concern →		
Standardized[a] subcellular and cellular assays validated for the purpose of establishing *in vivo* toxic effect AND Multiple different assays suggesting the same pathological condition or endpoint AND Poor consistency/ reproducibility in response AND No knowledge about concentration of toxicant in blood or tissue	Standardized subcellular and cellular assays validated for the purpose of establishing *in vivo* toxic effect AND Multiple different assays suggesting the same pathological condition or endpoint AND Consistency in response AND No knowledge about concentration of toxicant in blood or tissue	Standardized subcellular and cellular assays validated for the purpose of establishing *in vivo* toxic effect AND Multiple different assays suggesting the same pathological condition or endpoint AND Knowledge of presence of toxicant in blood or tissue enhanced by knowledge of concentrations comparable with those causing toxicity *in vitro*
OR	OR	OR
Standardized assays validated for the purpose of establishing organ toxicity AND Multiple different assays suggesting the same pathological condition or endpoint	Standardized assays validated for the purpose of establishing organ toxicity AND Multiple different assays suggesting the same pathological condition or endpoint	Standardized assays validated for the purpose of establishing organ toxicity AND Multiple different assays suggesting the same pathological condition or endpoint

Vulnerable subpopulations can be defined as groups of individuals who are more likely to experience an adverse event related to the use of a particular dietary supplement ingredient or individuals in whom the specific adverse effects identified are more likely to be *serious* in comparison with the general population. Characteristics that contribute to such vulnerability may be physiological (including genetic predisposition) and include age, developmental stage (e.g., pregnancy or fetal period), presence of other diseases, or concurrent use of medications or other therapeutic practices.

When evaluating risk and reviewing data, it is important to ask if ingredients are more likely to cause harmful effects to particular subgroups of the population, especially if those subgroups are known to consume the particular ingredient of concern. Vulnerability of a population subgroup is

TABLE 3-8 Continued

Increasing Concern →		
AND Poor consistency/reproducibility in response AND No knowledge about concentration of toxicant in blood or tissue OR Results obtained with nonstandardized, nonvalidated assays OR Results from microarray experiments show a gene expression pattern predictive of dangerous compounds[b]	AND Consistency in response AND No knowledge about concentration of toxicant in blood or tissue	AND Knowledge of presence of toxicant in blood or tissue at concentrations comparable with those causing toxicity *in vitro*

[a] Standardized in this context means that the assay is performed consistently across laboratories and often is officially promulgated by a standardization body, such as AOAC International (formerly the Association of Official Analytical Chemists), or the protocol is specified by a regulatory agency.

[b] Toxicogenomics is a relatively new field, the impact of which is not possible to predict at this point. However, these types of data may become more important as the field progresses. If the value of genomics, proteomics, and other new technologies in identifying dangerous compounds is demonstrated in the future, then such results may warrant more concern than is indicated in this figure.

TABLE 3-9 Spectrum of Concern for Interactions

Increasing Concern →		
Pharmacokinetic and/or pharmacodynamic data suggesting a supplement-drug/food/other dietary supplement interaction that might lead to a serious adverse event and/or identifying a population at risk for a serious adverse event	Pharmacokinetic and/or pharmacodynamic data documenting a supplement-drug/food/other dietary supplement interaction that might lead to a serious adverse event and/or identifying a population at risk for a serious adverse event	Pharmacokinetic and/or pharmacodynamic data documenting a supplement-drug/food/other dietary supplement interaction that leads to a serious adverse event

described as a modifying factor, in that whether identifiable subpopulations are particularly susceptible to harm should always be taken into consideration when setting priorities for review.

GENERAL PRINCIPLES AND CONCEPTS WHEN CONSIDERING DATA

The principles for evaluating specific types of information are described above, but some concepts are more global in nature, because they are applicable to all types of data or because they are principles for integrating different types of data that may or may not be consistent.

Concentration of Substances at the Site of Action

A critical factor in determining toxicity of a compound in a dietary supplement is not necessarily the ingested amount, but rather the unbound (free) concentration of an active ingredient at its receptor site. Once absorbed, distribution of the ingredient is via the systemic circulation to its receptor site.

Bioavailability (i.e., the rate and extent, or fraction, of delivery of a compound to the systemic circulation) has a significant effect on the concentration achieved. Bioavailability is greatly affected by the composition of the dosage form, first pass metabolism in the intestines and liver, and physiological factors, such as the rate of gastric emptying. Bioavailability and the rates of metabolism and excretion are the major determinants of serum concentration of a given dose of product.

Knowing the concentration of the unbound fraction of a compound in plasma will assist in assessing the relevance of *in vitro* data. Also, the plasma concentration can assist in comparing data across animal species (note that the concentration of the parent compound and/or any active metabolite is frequently used when the unbound fraction is unknown). Knowing the concentration of the unbound compound in plasma may be used as a surrogate marker for toxicity potential if a relationship has been established between the concentration and toxicity. For example, studies evaluating barbiturate sleep time illustrate a similar effect for a given plasma concentration across animal species; barbiturate sleep times may vary among species, but each species appears to awaken at approximately the same barbiturate plasma concentration (Gillette, 1976).

When judging whether the concentration will reach levels of concern in humans in the absence of information relating dose to systemic concentration, conservative assumptions should be used. In the absence of specific data about an ingredient in humans, one should assume rapid absorption and 100 percent bioavailability and divide the dose administered by the plasma volume[10] to estimate the maximum achievable concentration from a single dose. These assumptions may not be accurate, but they do provide a reasonable basis for making decisions.

Bioavailability is further discussed in Chapter 5 as it relates to route of exposure when considering exposure of animals through non-oral routes. It is also discussed in Chapter 6, when looking at concentrations of substances that are similar to endogenous substances. In Chapter 10, the concept is discussed in terms of integrating data that may appear inconsistent.

Proof of Harm

To evaluate the safety of dietary supplements, it is necessary to determine if an unreasonable or significant risk exists—not to have complete evidence that a dietary supplement ingredient causes a serious adverse event—which is a lower standard than conclusive proof. The difference between proof of harm and risk of harm should be considered when judgment rather than strict interpretation of facts needs to be made.

Absence of Evidence

Absence of evidence of risk does not indicate that there is no risk. In some cases, some data will indicate a risk, while other data will not suggest the risk exists, producing what could be interpreted as an inconsistency. Even if a study showing lack of adverse effects is reported, if the study is not adequately designed to identify risk (e.g., not sufficiently powered, incompletely reported, does not include positive controls, or otherwise has inadequate mechanisms for detecting adverse events), it is not scientifically valid to use such information to mitigate suggested risk from other sources. This concept is discussed in Chapter 4, as it relates to comparing different types of human data. It is also discussed in Chapter 10, as it relates to comparing human and animal data.

Considering Consistency and Biological Plausibility

In many circumstances, data will need to be collated within the same category or across several categories to determine the appropriate overall level of concern. In integrating observations across categories of data, *consistency* and evidence of biological *plausibility* should raise the level of

---

[10]Plasma volume is used when actual volume of distribution is unknown. If the substance is known to distribute across the cell membrane or into a different distribution space, division by body water volume or other volume would be appropriate.

concern. This weaving together of available information can be facilitated, and conceptually illustrated, by the use of causal evidence models. A causal evidence model (see Figure 3-2) provides a structure to help interpret available data from a number of sources in order to address a specific safety question, and is explained in detail in Chapter 10. The model describes the relationship among a dietary supplement ingredient, potential adverse health effects, and biological effects by depicting the relationship as linkages illustrated with arrows. The type of arrow illustrates the type of evidence: convincing data are depicted by solid arrows, and weak or less conclusive data are depicted by dashed arrows. The path between a dietary supplement ingredient and an adverse health effect illustrates the strength of their potential relationship. When the available information is integrated, multiple links between the dietary supplement ingredient and a given health outcome are illustrated by multiple arrows. Evidence from all types of study designs may form linkages to aid in determining the extent of association between dietary supplement exposure and adverse health effects or outcomes. Causal models are useful when a single type of evidence is weak or does not illustrate a relationship, but other related information is available, as may often be the case with dietary supplement ingredients.

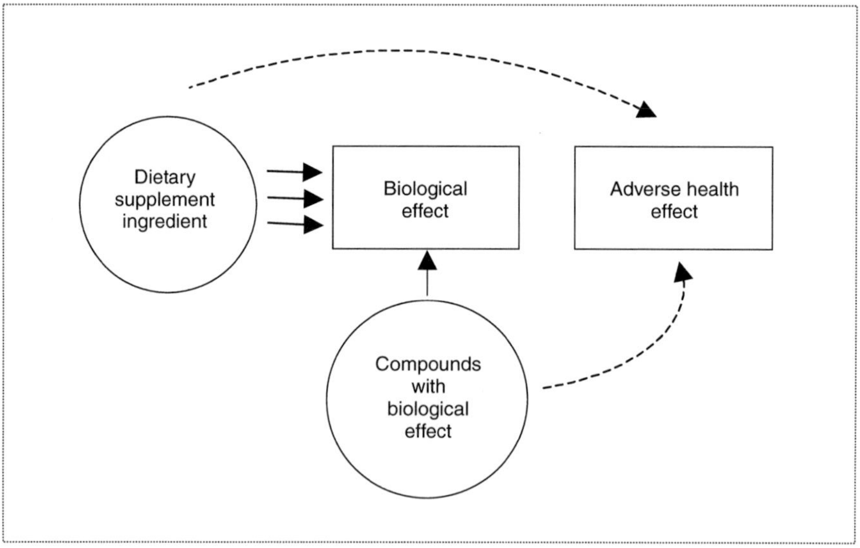

FIGURE 3-2 Diagram of causal model relating information to an adverse health effect.

UTILIZING THE FRAMEWORK

The request from FDA to develop a framework for evaluating the safety of dietary supplement ingredients also included a request that prototype monographs for six dietary supplement ingredients be developed as examples of how the Framework should be applied. Chapter 11 provides case studies of how the available evidence for six dietary supplement ingredients could be evaluated using the spectra of concern discussed in this chapter and described in detail in the following chapters.

Given the fact that these are prototype monographs, they should not be considered as representing findings related to these six dietary supplement ingredients. Rather, they are examples of how to approach reviewing and evaluating the various types of available information on dietary ingredients. Appendixes D through I contain summaries of the six prototype monographs. (The full prototype monographs are available on the web, at www.iom.edu/fnb.) Appendixes J and K contains examples of two focused prototype monographs to show how FDA could focus on determining a level of concern related to one specific adverse effect or outcome when identified. Conducting a broad-based comprehensive assessment would typically identify all data about the dietary supplement ingredient and would lead to a description and evaluation of other adverse effects—which would be a resource-intensive process.

SUMMARY

This chapter outlines a system for conducting a review of the safety of dietary supplement ingredients. Conducting the safety evaluation consists of three components: signal detection, an initial review of the available information, and, when needed, an integrative evaluation. Based on detection of a signal or a proactively initiated review of a dietary supplement ingredient, FDA evaluates the detected signal by conducting a brief initial review of readily available information to determine whether there is a need for a comprehensive review, termed an integrative evaluation. When an integrative evaluation is undertaken, FDA, or a contractor of FDA, prepares the initial draft monograph that is a collection and review of available safety information. In some cases, the integrative evaluation process, during which a draft monograph is developed, may provide sufficient evidence for FDA to decide on a course of action without use of an external advisory committee or public input. However, it is expected that when the data are not sufficiently definitive for FDA to make a decision about whether to take action, it will request the assistance of an advisory committee to review the information.

The external advisory committee, if constituted, reviews the draft monograph, determines if additional information should be collected, and holds sessions for input from the public. It then recommends modifications to the draft monograph as appropriate and summarizes concerns based on the evidence. The completed monograph, with input from the external advisory committee, is then made public in an easily accessible format.

In any scientific evaluation, at least four categories of information can be considered informative for evaluating the risk of ingesting chemicals, including dietary supplements: human data, animal data, *in vitro* data, and information about related substances. Evidence in any one of these four major categories can provide considerable guidance regarding the ingredient's safety. The chapters that follow provide detailed information on the use of this information, and how to integrate the available data to determine the extent to which an unreasonable risk of illness or injury from ingestion of a dietary supplement exists.

ANNEX 3-1
APPLYING THE SAFETY FRAMEWORK TO REQUIRED NUTRIENTS

Essential nutrients (i.e., vitamins and mineral elements) are unique compared to many other categories of dietary supplements in that much more data regarding adverse effects of overconsumption in humans are available. Structures of the vitamins have been elucidated, relative activity of closely related compounds determined, and, at least at physiologic doses, biological activities for these compounds are reasonably well characterized. Most have been characterized in terms of potency in standards such as those produced by the U.S. Pharmacopoeia, as is required by law when monograph standards are available for them. Several nutrients are regulated as generally recognized as safe substances, approved food additives, and as over-the-counter and prescription drugs. **It is for this reason that the essential nutrients are considered differently within the Framework than other types of dietary supplement ingredients.**

As summarized in Chapter 2, a system for reviewing data about the safety of vitamins and essential elements already exists. Since 1940, the Food and Nutrition Board of the National Academies has been commissioned by federal agencies to set Recommended Dietary Allowances (RDAs) for nutrients; more recently this was expanded to include other reference intake levels for nutrients, now collectively termed Dietary Reference Intakes (DRIs) (IOM, 1994, 1997). With the exception of only a few nutrients, scientific data on all vitamins and mineral elements, and some other nutrients, have been reviewed recently through the DRI process (IOM, 1997, 1998b, 2000, 2001, 2002, 2004).

While the RDAs are designed to be recommendations for intake to ensure that the needs of almost all apparently healthy individuals in a population group (such as women over 70 years of age or adolescent boys) are met in order to avoid nutrient deficiencies and to decrease risk of chronic disease, other reference values included as part of the new DRIs provide upper levels of intake for vitamins and mineral elements that, if consumed below the specified level on a continuing basis, should not cause specific identified adverse effects of overconsumption (IOM, 1998a). These upper levels of intake are called "tolerable upper intake levels," or ULs.

For the vitamins and the mineral elements that have been established as required by humans, a considerable amount of primary data relating to animal or experimental studies, human studies, and *in vitro* studies are available, and these data have been reviewed as part of the DRI consideration of the UL. The DRI review can thus provide substantial data and background information for an FDA evaluation; the process for incorporating this information is provided in the following sections.

Signal Detection for Nutrients

When nutrients present in dietary supplements are suggested for use at levels greater than established ULs, it is appropriate to be concerned, and thus this is an initial "signal" analogous to that described for other dietary supplement ingredients. However, the initial review in response to the signal should be focused on the DRI review of the serious adverse effects that were identified as potentially occurring at high intake levels, recognizing that there has been an uncertainty factor applied to ensure that few, if any, individuals will be adversely affected at the UL level. New information (post-DRI review) on adverse effects of consuming a nutrient also serves as an initial signal. In summary, it is appropriate to *a priori* consider any marketing of nutrients as dietary supplements above the UL to be potentially of some risk, but whether the risk is unreasonable will depend on the data available. Nonetheless, vitamins and mineral elements are not innocuous substances. Consumption at high levels of some nutrients is associated with illnesses and death as documented in the DRI reports (IOM, 1997, 1998b, 2000, 2001, 2002, 2004).

Initial Review for a Nutrient

Whenever the safety of a vitamin or mineral is considered, the first step should be to consult the results of the DRI UL process. It is possible that a UL was not established for a nutrient when the data were reviewed, but the review process and the data considered are included in the specific DRI report and serve as a credible, nonbiased review of the scientific data available at the time of review. If a UL was established for the vitamin or mineral under question, it is important to consider the following:

- Was the information suggesting concern available before the publication of the most recent DRI review, and were these data considered in the evaluation of ULs?

One limitation is that the reviews are conducted at specified intervals, so it is possible that safety issues relating to dietary supplements that are essential nutrients might be newly identified within the time period after the last DRI review and prior to an upcoming updated review.

- Is the ingredient in use the same formulation or is the dosage outside the ranges previously reviewed, and thus beyond the coverage of the most recent DRI review?
- Was the intake level under question addressed in the DRI report? There is increasing use of very high doses of nutrients in dietary supplements, so various biological activities, toxicities, and adverse effects may have been incompletely addressed (or not verified) in the most recent DRI review. These reviews necessarily must cover issues related to intakes over a wide range, looking for the lowest intake level at which adverse effects are noted, so that the issues at the highest levels of intake are not the sole (or primary) focus of the reviews.
- What was the critical endpoint or adverse effect used to set the UL? Was it a benign reversible adverse event or a serious and irreversible condition?
- Is concern about consumption above the UL directed primarily at specific populations, or does it apply widely? If a higher level of concern is directed primarily at specific populations, it may be appropriate for the integrative evaluation to focus on that concern as it relates to that population group.

It is necessary to consider the basis for the UL, with less concern being warranted for non-life-threatening or self-limiting effects, as well as the recommended dose of the supplement to determine the level of concern. The conclusions of the DRI review should be given much greater weight than other data available at the time of the review but not considered in it. This allows an immediate determination of the level of concern and thus a fairly rapid determination of the need to go forward with an integrated evaluation, following similar procedures to that of other dietary supplement ingredients (as described in earlier sections of this chapter).

Integrative Evaluation for a Nutrient

It is quite possible that situations will arise where, due to information which becomes available after the DRI review on the severity of the adverse effect, or the vulnerability of a population at risk, there will be a higher level of concern and thus a need to go further than the DRI review to determine if a significant or unreasonable risk of illness or injury exists when consuming a nutrient as a dietary supplement at its suggested level of intake. This is the integrative evaluation component.

An integrative evaluation should use as its basis the DRI review and analysis, recognizing that for some nutrients (i.e., vitamin K, β-carotene, arsenic, chromium, silicon, thiamin, riboflavin, vitamin B_{12}, pantothenic acid, biotin, potassium, and sulfate) the available data, while reviewed in the DRI series, were deemed insufficient to develop a UL based on requirements of the model of risk assessment used. This does not indicate that high intakes pose no risk of adverse effects (IOM, 1998a, 2000, 2001, 2004), but that a thorough review by an expert group could not identify dose- response evidence from chronic intakes that would provide a basis for establishing the level at which adverse effects might occur.

If a UL was not established for the vitamin or mineral element under question, it is important to consider the following:

- Was the substance reviewed by the DRI process, even if a UL was not established?
- Is there new evidence suggesting risk that was not available at the time of the DRI review?
- Was significant concern about serious harm expressed in the DRI review, even if a DRI could not be established because of limits in the data or acuteness of the adverse effect (e.g., arsenic)?

It is assumed that the integrative evaluation for a nutrient would contain the same general components as for other dietary supplement ingredients, with the exception that significant information is already captured by virtue of the DRI process and its reports. In situations where new data or information indicate that higher concern is warranted, the nutrient would enter the evaluation in the same manner as other supplement ingredients. Nutrients are usually well-characterized chemically and thus there is less concern about active ingredient identification and function.

ANNEX 3-2
MONOGRAPH PREPARATION AND PUBLIC ACCESS

Preparation of Draft Monographs

In evaluating evidence indicating that an ingredient may present an unreasonable risk to human health, a comprehensive examination of the literature is required, recognizing that not all studies are relevant to ascertaining the safety of a dietary supplement ingredient. The initial step in preparing a monograph is to gather as much information as possible from the published literature and other sources regarding the potential hazards of consuming the supplement. Multiple comprehensive databases, such as MEDLINE (NLM, 2003a), TOXLINE (NLM, 2003b), and EMBASE should be searched (Elsevier, 2003). In addition, NAPRALERT (Farnsworth, 2003) can be searched if the supplement is a natural product or botanical. To search for potential ingredient-drug or ingredient-ingredient interactions, the Metabolism and Transport Drug Interaction Database (UW, 2003) is a useful tool.

Abstracts and titles should be reviewed for relevance to the adverse event or harmful effect of concern. Although review articles may be useful for the purpose of providing literature references and an overview of the data, review of the original articles from the peer-reviewed literature is essential to obviate any bias or unsubstantiated opinion of the authors of the review. Information in other non-peer-reviewed literature that raises concerns about adverse effects should not be ignored. In order to get as much information as possible, FDA should request the voluntary submission of safety data information from industry and other stakeholders. This request may be made through notice in the *Federal Register* and through the FDA website. FDA should also request information directly from manufacturers and distributors of the ingredient under consideration, if they are known.

Collecting descriptive and safety information and organizing and summarizing the information into a draft safety monograph will require significant expertise and resources. Time and other resources required for completion of the draft monographs are likely to vary, depending on the amount and complexity of safety-related information available for the ingredient under consideration, as well as the focus of the monograph. FDA may choose to prepare monographs internally, or it may choose to contract the work out to organizations, individuals, or both.

The extent of time and effort devoted to preparation of monographs on dietary supplement ingredients will depend on FDA's prioritization of need. FDA could set priorities and develop a complete list of substances warranting monographs first. Alternatively, it could retain one or more individuals or groups to develop monographs and determine the need for individual monographs on an ongoing basis as priority setting proceeds or as new needs emerge. The former approach may be more cost effective to implement, given that the latter approach might not provide continuity in workload. However, preparing monographs for substances considered of high priority will require more resources up front if given to contractors and will be dependent on information available at the time high-priority substances are identified.

As discussed previously, monographs, whether prepared internally or by a contract organization, should be evaluated to determine if the conclusions could be improved by input from additional expert judgment. The decision to undertake a monograph internally or by contract to an outside group will depend on FDA's resources and internal expertise.

The monographs developed should not be considered static documents. New information should be added as it becomes available, and an organized process for adding information should be developed. The process should also include periodic reviews of monographs to determine if additional external reviews are appropriate.

Public Access to the Monograph

After the advisory committee's summary is shared with FDA, the revised monograph and the advisory committee's summary should be posted on FDA's website. One of the important components of DSHEA is that the public should be educated about dietary supplements. FDA thus has a responsibility to educate consumers about the safety of dietary supplement ingredients, and the public availability of the final monographs can be an important aspect of the educational process. The monographs can provide the public with a reputable summary of the available information and scientific uncertainties about the inherent safety of the supplement ingredient. Importantly, public access to information from an advisory committee will add to the quality and strength of the available scientific literature.

ANNEX 3-3
THE USE OF AN EXTERNAL ADVISORY COMMITTEE

The decision to refer a dietary supplement ingredient to an external advisory committee rests with FDA, which has the authority to refer to such a committee for any reason deemed necessary, as discussed in the text.

The external advisory committee needs to include experts in critical key disciplines. FDA has significant experience in establishing advisory committees and already has rules regarding membership (e.g., conflict of interest) in place. Possible approaches that FDA may wish to consider include:

- A standing committee of about seven persons, with the option to add one or two scientists with special expertise, as needed, for the review of individual substances.
- A standing committee of five scientists representing core disciplines, and the addition of three or four special experts depending on the nature of the ingredient, the data to be evaluated, and whether a focused or broad-based evaluation was required. The presence of individuals with expertise in either the ingredient under review or the purported adverse effect of the

ingredient is critical to providing a well-documented review of the literature where the data are equivocal.

To ensure that the critical evaluation of the information contained in the monograph and related information is as free of conflict of interest and as objective as possible, the external advisory committee should be composed of expert scientists who have appropriate training, education, and experience. Whether as a result of the appointment of a committee by FDA or by contract with a scientifically based, nonprofit organization, examples of expertise to be included are toxicology, preferably with expertise in safety evaluation; pharmacognosy; clinical pharmacology; nutritional science; epidemiology; biostatistics; clinical trials; medicinal chemistry and structure–activity relationships; pharmacokinetics; consumer behavior related to dietary supplement use; and public health, as well as *ad hoc* consultants with expertise in specific fields on an as-needed basis (e.g., specialists needed to evaluate particular ingredients, such as experts on oriental medicine, herbalists, veterinary toxicologists, or clinicians with relevant experience). Advisory committee members should be selected based on their disciplinary expertise rather than as representatives of stakeholder viewpoints, and they should not have a financial stake in the outcome of the process or otherwise have a real or perceived conflict of interest.

After the external advisory committee is assembled, a draft monograph should be released, and the public should be provided with an opportunity to comment on the completeness of the data included, as well as on the strength and relevance to humans of the different types of evidence. Industry and other stakeholders should be given time during meetings of the external advisory committee to provide input into the process. The external advisory committee should provide advice on the further refinement of the draft monograph as it reviews all the data and summarizes its conclusions.

REFERENCES

Elsevier. 2003. *EMBASE (Excerpta Medica Database)*. Online. Available at http://www.elsevier.nl/homepage/sah/spd/site/locate_embase.html. Accessed March 13, 2004.

Farnsworth NR. 2003. *NAPRALERT (Natural Products ALERT) Database*. Chicago: University of Illinois at Chicago.

Gillette JR. 1976. Application of pharmacokinetic principles in the extrapolation of animal data to humans. *Clin Toxicol* 9:709–722.

IOM (Institute of Medicine). 1994. *How Should the Recommended Dietary Allowances be Revised?* Washington, DC: National Academy Press.

IOM. 1997. *Dietary Reference Intakes for Calcium, Phosphorus, Magnesium, Vitamin D, and Fluoride*. Washington, DC: National Academy Press.

IOM. 1998a. *Dietary Reference Intakes: A Risk Assessment Model for Establishing Upper Intake Levels for Nutrients*. Washington, DC: National Academy Press.

IOM. 1998b. *Dietary Reference Intakes for Thiamin, Riboflavin, Niacin, Vitamin B6, Folate, Vitamin B12, Pantothenic Acid, Biotin, and Choline*. Washington, DC: National Academy Press.

IOM. 2000. *Dietary Reference Intakes for Vitamin C, Vitamin E, Selenium, and Carotenoids*. Washington, DC: National Academy Press.

IOM. 2001. *Dietary Reference Intakes for Vitamin A, Vitamin K, Arsenic, Boron, Chromium, Copper, Iodine, Iron, Manganese, Molybdenum, Nickel, Silicon, Vanadium, and Zinc*. Washington, DC: National Academy Press.

IOM. 2002. *Dietary Reference Intakes for Energy, Carbohydrate, Fiber, Fat, Fatty Acids, Cholesterol, Protein, and Amino Acids*. Washington, DC: National Academy Press.

IOM. 2004. *Dietary Reference Intakes for Water, Sodium, Potassium, Chloride, and Sulfate*. Washington, DC: The National Academies Press.

Merriam-Webster. 2001. *Merriam-Webster's Collegiate Dictionary*. 10th ed. Springfield, MA: Merriam-Webster.

NLM (National Library of Medicine). 2003a. *PubMed*. Online. Available at http://www.ncbi.nlm.nih.gov/entrez/query.fcgi. Accessed March 13, 2004.

NLM 2003b. *Toxline*. Online. Available at http://toxnet.nlm.nih.gov/cgi-bin/sis/htmlgen?TOXLINE. Accessed March 13, 2004.

UW (University of Washington). 2003. *Metabolism and Transport Drug Interaction Database*. Online. Available at http://depts.washington.edu/didbase. Accessed September 24, 2004.

4

Categories of Scientific Evidence—Human Information and Data

GUIDING PRINCIPLES: *A credible report or study finding of a serious adverse event (or experience)*[1] *in humans that is associated with use of a dietary supplement ingredient raises concern about the ingredient's safety and requires further information gathering and evaluation. A final judgment, however, will require consideration of the totality of the evidence. In considering the evidence, historical use should not be used as* prima facie *evidence that the ingredient does not cause harm. It may be appropriate, however, to give considerable weight to a lack of adverse events in large, high-quality, randomized clinical trials or epidemiological studies that are adequately powered and designed to detect adverse effects, including those adverse effects with established serious risks for human morbidity or mortality and that are known to rarely occur* de novo *in the population.*

[1]"Serious Adverse Experience. Any adverse experience occurring at any dose that results in any of the following outcomes: Death, a life-threatening adverse experience, inpatient hospitalization or prolongation of existing hospitalization, a persistent or significant disability/incapacity, or a congenital anomaly/birth defect. Important medical events that may not result in death, be life-threatening, or require hospitalization may be considered a serious adverse experience when, based upon appropriate medical judgment, they may jeopardize the patient or subject and may require medical or surgical intervention to prevent one of the outcomes listed in this definition. Examples of such medical events include allergic broncho-

Information about human use of dietary supplement ingredients may be in the form of formal studies, such as clinical studies or trials and epidemiological studies; in the form of spontaneously reported adverse event reports and literature case reports; or in the form of information about historical use of the ingredient. Because dietary supplements are not required to undergo formal studies before marketing, formal study data available on dietary supplements are less commonly available than adverse event reports or information about historical use.

The different types of data about human use can be useful either as (1) an indicator of possible risk or (2) a mitigator of concerns raised by other data. For example, spontaneous reports are generally used to detect concerns, and historical use information is often presented as a mitigator of concern. Formal studies are less likely to be available, but if they are, they can be the source of information about adverse events in individuals, or they can be used to demonstrate an overall increase in risk of a particular adverse event associated with ingestion of an ingredient. Formal studies can also be used as mitigators of concern if they are adequately designed and powered to detect adverse events.

Within each type of human data, questions can be asked about the nature and quality of the scientific information to determine whether the information raises the level of concern regarding the probability to cause harm. In the sections that follow, the nature of evidence that increases concern is described and illustrated in a spectrum of concern figure. Information that independently raises a higher level of concern requires immediate attention to evaluate the potential of the ingredient to cause harm. For observations categorized as lower to moderate concern based on their placement on the spectrum, it is important to consider whether other types of human, animal, *in vitro*, or related data, as well as information about potential interactions (see Chapter 8), add to the level of concern. For many dietary supplement ingredients, human data regarding their safety or risk will not be available. A lack of data should not be interpreted as an absence of risk. Other types of data must be examined and weighed appropriately to understand the risk.

SPONTANEOUSLY REPORTED ADVERSE EVENTS

Adverse events associated with product use—whether reported directly to the Food and Drug Administration (FDA), manufacturers, distributors,

---

spasm requiring intensive treatment in an emergency room or at home, blood dyscrasias or convulsions that do not result in inpatient hospitalization, or the development of drug dependency or drug abuse" (21 C.F.R. § 600.80 [2002] and 21 C.F.R. § 314.80 [2002]).

or poison control centers—constitute important sources of safety information, along with published case reports and case series about adverse events. All unsolicited reports from health professionals or consumers received by FDA via either the voluntary or mandatory route are called spontaneous reports, so classified because they are clinical observations that originate outside of a formal study (Faich, 1986). The large-scale regulatory agency safety databases are composed of adverse event information generated by reporting from all sources, including scientific literature case reports and case series; each type of product (e.g., drug, biologic, device, and dietary supplement) is represented.

While different products have aspects unique to their specific type, the principles of postmarketing safety monitoring apply to all; thus, what has been, and what will be, learned from one product realm is generally globally applicable. Dietary supplements, many of which contain biologically active ingredients, are no exception; that the guiding scientific principles for postmarketing safety surveillance have predominantly resulted from experience with pharmaceuticals (drugs and biologics) in no way invalidates their applicability to other substances, such as dietary supplement ingredients.

However, while the underlying principles for safety monitoring are globally valid, the regulatory situation of dietary supplements impacts the use of their associated adverse event reports in several ways. Unlike drugs, biologics, and medical devices, dietary supplements do not undergo premarketing evaluation for safety and efficacy by FDA, and a formal benefit/risk assessment is not performed as part of an approval process. There is no evaluation of product quality (including purity, content uniformity, and stability) prior to marketing, and there is no requirement for manufacturers to collect or report adverse events to FDA. Yet, at the same time, the threshold for concern or action for a dietary supplement is lower than for regulated medical products, as under the applicable law they are considered to be similar to foods.

In this section, the strengths and limitations of using adverse event reports for medical products in general are described, as well as how significant differences in laws and regulations impact the evaluation of adverse event reports associated with dietary supplement use.

Strengths and Limitations

The limitations of spontaneous adverse event reporting systems are well recognized, and include subjectivity and imprecision of adverse event recognition (Karch et al., 1976; Koch-Weser et al., 1977), underreporting (Chen et al., 1994; Chyka and McCommon, 2000; Rawlins, 1995), reporting biases (Sachs and Bortnichak, 1986), lack of precise exposure data (Begaud et al., 1994), and variability in report quality (Goldman, 1998). In particular, the lack of precise numerator (number of cases) and denominator (number of patients exposed) data render the computation of incidence rates from spontaneous reports problematic (Begaud et al., 1994), if not totally unfeasible. In addition, as spontaneous reports originate under conditions of everyday use rather than under study conditions, there are possible confounding factors to be considered when evaluating reports, such as multiple concomitant medications (prescribed or over-the-counter [OTC]), multiple concomitant dietary supplements, concomitant medical devices, underlying disease states, or alcohol use.

At the same time, these systems entail considerable concomitant strengths. Large-scale and relatively inexpensive (Fletcher, 1991), spontaneous adverse event reporting systems serve as the basis for safety-related hypothesis generation (Strom and Tugwell, 1990) and foster suspicions (Finney, 1971) that generate signals of potential problems warranting further study, while enabling individuals (health professionals and consumers alike) to contribute to public health (Goldman, 1998). This sentinel signaling function is critical, and the appropriateness of using a spontaneous reporting system in this regard is well documented and scientifically accepted (Blum et al., 1994; Goldman, 1996; Rossi and Knapp, 1984).

The cases spontaneously reported to any surveillance program will generally represent only a small percentage of the number that have actually occurred.[2] However, **if the submitted reports are of high quality, irrespective of number, the effect of underreporting can be somewhat mitigated** (Goldman, 1998). In the particular case of dietary supplements, a recent FDA-commissioned study estimated that FDA receives reports on less than 1 percent of all adverse events associated with their use (Walker, 2000). (With the majority of dietary supplement adverse event reporting to FDA done by consumers rather than by health professionals, it is possible that consumers might be less likely to associate dietary supplements with untoward effects, as opposed to making such attribution with a drug product, either prescribed or OTC). In addition, it has been found that consumers often do not inform their physicians about their use of dietary supplements (Eisenberg et al., 1998). Hence, reporting by physicians and other health professionals of adverse events on these products may well be minimal.

[2]Concerning the extent of underreporting of drug-associated adverse events, a study performed in the United States before establishment of the FDA MedWatch adverse event reporting program (Kessler, 1993) estimated that the FDA received by direct report less than 1 percent of suspected serious adverse drug reactions (Scott et al., 1987), while rarely more than 10 percent of serious adverse drug reactions were estimated to be reported to the British spontaneous reporting program (Rawlins, 1995). This latter figure of 10 percent is consistent with other studies (Skjeldestad et al., 2000). It is not clear that these relative percentages hold for every serious adverse event and associated drug.

Challenges Particular to Dietary Supplements

Scientifically, the use of adverse event reports to assess the safety of dietary supplements should be very similar to how the safety of drug and other medical products are assessed, but the unique regulatory situation of dietary supplements provides some additional challenges. Beyond the limitations inherent in postmarketing surveillance systems, this unique regulatory environment renders the assessment of dietary supplement adverse event reports of greater complexity versus that performed on reports regarding drugs, biologics, or medical devices.

Because premarketing safety studies are not required for dietary supplements, standard drug premarketing data, such as clinical pharmacology studies, are not likely to be available. As a result, significant clinical information such as how the product is absorbed, metabolized, and excreted is generally not available, nor is the product evaluated for possible interactions with foods, drugs, biologics, or devices. The lack of such clinical information generally does not allow specific populations at possible increased risk for adverse effects (such as children, the elderly, or those with renal and/or hepatic dysfunction) to be identified in a systematic manner.

In further important distinction from medical products, there are no current FDA regulations establishing a baseline mandatory standard for dietary supplement manufacturing (CFSAN, 2001). As a result, the situation of multiple manufacturers of a specific dietary supplement can result in significant variation from product to product. An illustrative example is a study of the St. John's wort products available in Germany, which detailed wide differences among the content of hypericin and hyperforin products, and notable interbatch variability in some of the products (Wurglics et al., 2001). Thus, unlike the situation with prescription drugs, in which there is standardized quality control of the innovator product and generic versions in manufacturing, adverse event reports on a particular dietary supplement may entail several different products that can vary significantly in dietary ingredient concentration, both among and within individual products.

FDA's proposed rule to establish current good manufacturing practices for manufacturers, with respect to both the production and labeling of dietary supplements (FDA, 2003a), addresses some manufacturing issues, but not all aspects of product-to-product variability. According to FDA, this proposed rule "would, for the first time, establish standards to ensure that dietary supplements and dietary ingredients are not adulterated with contaminants or impurities, and are labeled to accurately to reflect the active ingredients and other ingredients in the product" (FDA, 2003b).

The challenge of underreporting adverse events was described above as a general challenge in using spontaneous adverse event reports. A factor particular to dietary supplements, however, is that, unlike drugs, biologics, and medical devices, dietary supplement manufacturers and distributors are not required to disclose to FDA the adverse event reports that they receive (CFSAN, 2001; OIG, 2001). As a result, an important established source of reports for medical products is not duplicated for dietary supplements, and the evolution of a concomitant culture of adverse event reporting among manufacturers and distributors is not encouraged.

The lack of manufacturer disclosure requirements is especially important given that consumers may be less likely to report adverse reactions to practitioners, a usual source of adverse event reports. A study sought to determine whether botanical remedy users would report adverse reactions to such products differently from similar adverse reactions experienced with the use of OTC medications (Barnes et al., 1998). While approximately 30 percent would consult their general practitioner irrespective of which type of ingested product was being used, and another 43 percent would not consult in either case, 26 percent would consult their general practitioner for a serious OTC-associated adverse reaction, but not for a similar adverse reaction associated with use of an herbal remedy.[3]

In summary, adverse event report assessment of dietary supplement ingredients is of heightened complexity and ambiguity compared with that of medical products.

Using Spontaneous Reports

Assessing the Strength of Association Between Event and Product

Spontaneous reports entail an assumed association between the denoted adverse event and product in question, but careful evaluation of accumulated cases is needed to assess the actual strength of the association. Achieving certain proof of causality is not necessary to determine that an unreasonable or significant risk exists, especially if other types of data support the same conclusion.

Regarding numbers of cases needed for such assessment, **when the medical product-adverse event relationship is stronger and the incidence of the adverse event occurring *de novo*/naturalistically is lower (i.e., the event**

[3]Of further significance is the international variation with respect to consumer reporting. The European Union regulatory agencies do not routinely accept drug adverse event reports from consumers that are not confirmed by a health professional, while few countries (the United States and Canada being notable exceptions) require pharmaceutical companies to submit consumer reports that they receive (CIOMS, 2001). In addition, while U.S. consumers are encouraged to report adverse events directly to FDA (FDA, 2003c), it is conceivable that the lack of encouragement for consumer reporting in other countries might negatively affect accumulation of dietary supplement-associated adverse event data on a global basis.

is rarer), fewer case reports are needed to perceive causality (Auriche and Loupi, 1993). For rare[4] serious adverse events, such as toxic epidermal necrolysis, coincidental medical product-event associations have been found to be so unlikely that they merit little concern in spontaneous reporting, with more than three reports seen to represent a signal necessitating further study (Begaud et al., 1994). Further, it has been suggested that the combination of a temporal relationship between medical product and adverse event, positive dechallenge, and rechallenge can make individual reports conclusive as to product-event association (Temple et al., 1979).

Notwithstanding, there is no definitive number of cases for generating a signal of safety concern. It is dependent on the characteristics of the individual adverse event itself, including such factors as clinical manifestations and severity, potential for significant morbidity (reversible and irreversible) or mortality, potential populations at risk, and the overall risk to public health.

In judging any association to be causal, biological plausibility and reasonable strength of association are useful (Rawlins, 1995). However, given the outlined limitations of spontaneous reports, achieving certain proof of causality through postmarketing surveillance is unusual (Auriche and Loupi, 1993). Attaining a prominent degree of suspicion is much more likely, and, given that it may be deemed an ample basis for regulatory decisions on drugs (Auriche and Loupi, 1993), it is an ample basis for regulatory decisions on dietary supplement ingredients.

Regarding factors that can be useful in assessing the strength of association between any medical product and a reported adverse event, international consensus produced the following list (CIOMS, 1990):

- The chronology of administration of agent, including beginning and ending of treatment and adverse event onset,
- The course of the adverse event when the suspected agent stopped (dechallenge) or continued,
- The etiologic roles of agents and diseases in regard to an adverse event,
- Response to readministration (rechallenge) of the agent, and
- Laboratory test results.

[4]The United States has no regulatory definition that explicitly delineates events as common, infrequent, or rare based on their frequency of occurrence; the Council of International Organizations of Medical Sciences (CIOMS) III/V working groups have recommended the following standard categories of frequency: common (frequent): > 1/100 and < 1/10 (> 1 and < 10 percent); uncommon (infrequent): > 1/1,000 and < 1/100 (> 0.1 percent and < 1 percent); rare: > 1/10,000 and < 1/,1000 (> 0.01 and < 0.1 percent) (CIOMS, 1999).

Considering the Nature of the Adverse Event

Beyond the factors listed above, the nature of the adverse event itself is an important consideration in assessing spontaneous reports. The nature of the adverse event encompasses knowledge about its naturalistic frequency of occurrence and its potential for significant morbidity or mortality.

As previously discussed, premarket clinical trials in humans have inherent limitations that significantly affect their ability to detect adverse events (Goldman et al., 1995); to have a 95 percent chance of detecting an adverse event that occurs in 1 in 1,000 people, 3,000 people must be exposed (Lewis, 1981). For adverse events that occur *de novo* even more rarely, such as 1 in 100,000, 300,000 people must be exposed for there to be a good chance of detection. Many of the most serious adverse events occur relatively infrequently; that is why spontaneous report systems, which are designed to cover entire populations, are able to detect rare, serious events not discovered during premarket testing.

This important outcome of spontaneous report systems for dietary supplement ingredients is the same as for other products. There are serious adverse events that by their very nature necessitate increased attention and scrutiny due to their potential for significant morbidity and/or mortality. FDA, in its recently published *Proposed Rule for Safety Reporting Requirements for Human Drug and Biological Products*, specifically addressed this issue by proposing a new designation, "Always Expedited Reports" for specific suspected adverse drug reactions (SADRs) of medical significance (FDA, 2003c). The following SADRs,[5] regardless of expectedness, would be subject to expedited reporting due to their very nature: "congenital anomalies, acute respiratory failure, ventricular fibrillation, torsades de pointe, malignant hypertension, seizure, agranulocytosis, aplastic anemia, toxic epidermal necrolysis, liver necrosis, acute liver failure, anaphylaxis, acute renal failure, sclerosing syndromes, pulmonary hypertension, pulmonary fibrosis, confirmed or suspected transmission of an infectious agent by a marketed drug or biological product, confirmed or suspected endotoxin shock" (FDA, 2003c). **Reporting of any of these adverse events in association with dietary supplement use should trigger the same degree of concern as for any other product, and the same heightened need for a timely assessment.**

[5]Also subjected to expedited reporting within this new designation are any other medically significant suspected adverse drug reactions that FDA determines to be the subject of an always expedited report (i.e., may jeopardize the patient and/or require medical or surgical intervention to treat the patient).

Considering the Amount Ingested

Some reports of adverse events are based on intakes that exceed the amount specified on the particular dietary supplement label for "intended use." A number of factors make it difficult, if not impossible, to determine the contribution of dose to the effects reported. The lack of adequate premarketing data to establish the validity of labeled dosing for many dietary supplements is coupled with significant variability in the amount of the particular dietary supplement constituents in different preparations. Known pharmacokinetic variability among individuals also makes it difficult, if not impossible, to determine the contribution of dose to the effects reported. However, in conclusion, if an adverse event report provides credible evidence that a serious adverse event is associated with a dietary supplement ingredient (see criteria in the earlier section), its utility in establishing a level of concern should not be discounted simply because the intake (resulting in adverse events) exceeds that specified in current dietary supplement labeling.

Summary of Spontaneous Report Use

In summary, **higher concern is warranted in situations where one or more well-documented serious adverse events manifests positive temporality, and other factors (e.g., positive dechallenge, biological plausibility, or laboratory results) combine to strengthen the perceived association between the dietary supplement ingested and the adverse event in question.** Given the inherent limitations of spontaneous reports (including report quality) in general, and those concerning dietary supplement ingredients in particular, not all of this information will be available in many cases.

Tables 4-1 and 4-2 illustrate the relative spectra of concern. The columns on the right describe situations that warrant higher concern because the greatest risk to public health exists, while situations described on the left are of lower concern. The level of concern increases in proportion to the completeness of information provided and the likelihood of confounding decreasing. However, with serious, unexpected adverse events, possible confounding in the associated reports should not automatically lessen the level of concern, but rather heighten the attempt to obtain more reports of the highest possible quality to maximize the signaling function of spontaneous report systems. In addition, the nature of the serious adverse event itself and its potential for significant harm should stimulate appropriate heightened concern.

The great utility of spontaneous reports lies in the generation of hypotheses about relationships between supplement ingredients and untoward effects, thus highlighting potential problems and signals that the agency may want to explore in greater depth. Evaluation of signals from

TABLE 4-1 Relative Spectrum of Concern for Individual Spontaneous Adverse Event Reports

Increasing Concern →		
Describes a serious adverse event with less information than would justify moderate or strong concern, and/or with prominent confounding factors (e.g., multiple concomitant substances and/or conditions)	Describes a serious adverse event with some, but not all, characteristics associated with strong concern	Describes a well-documented serious adverse event with plasma levels (if available) at a relevant range and demonstrates dechallenge and rechallenge (if possible), temporality, and strong attribution

TABLE 4-2 Relative Spectrum of Concern for Case Series of Spontaneous Adverse Event Reports

Increasing Concern →		
Describes a series of serious adverse events, with less information than would justify moderate or strong concern, and/or prominent confounding factors (e.g., multiple concomitant substances and/or conditions)	Describes a series of serious adverse events, with some, but not all, characteristics associated with strong concern	Describes a series of well-documented cases demonstrating consistent serious adverse events and clinical findings, and dechallenge (if possible), temporality, and strong attribution

spontaneous reports should entail use of supplementary information available about the substance, such as animal data, *in vitro* data, epidemiological studies, or clinical trials in which formal hypothesis testing can occur. Such studies can be used to further evaluate the strength of the association between the adverse event and dietary supplement in question because, as described in the previous paragraphs, establishing a definitive causal relationship solely through use of spontaneous reports is rarely possible. However, as noted, regulatory decisions that directly involve the safety of the public's health do not necessitate definitive proof.

In the specific case of dietary supplements, the threshold for action is clearly stated in the Dietary Supplement and Health Education Act: demonstration of a "significant or unreasonable risk of illness or injury." **Given the state of the art in adverse event report evaluation, pharmaco-**

vigilance, and risk management, and given the potential risk to the public entailed by serious adverse events, regulatory action can be justified on the basis of adverse event report analysis alone or as the predominant source of information. There is ample precedent for this approach from the realms of regulated medical products, such as drugs, biologics, and medical devices. Dietary supplements, as agents with biological activity, should be no exception.

HISTORICAL USE

Experience from generations of use by humans is often referred to as evidence of safety for modern dietary supplements that bear resemblance to substances used historically. Some botanicals, for example, have a long history of medicinal use in many cultures. It may be useful to consider that there is both ancient (thousands of years) and recent history (perhaps the last 100 years). Ancient history may include traditional Chinese, Ayurvedic, and Native American medicines. Information about the preparation and use of ancient remedies is more difficult to locate and verify.

Information about historical use is of less importance when relevant clinical, epidemiological, or animal toxicity data exist because if these types of data document harm, then this outweighs historical use that may show no harm. However, for many dietary supplement ingredients, the amount of scientific and experimental data are insufficient for a critical analysis of safety. **Recognizing that a full range of data are unlikely to be available for many dietary supplement ingredients, historical use may be taken into account as a surrogate measure for safety in the absence of relevant scientific and experimental data. In doing so, it is important to consider the relevance of the traditional use to the current use and, as such, FDA must have information regarding both the traditional use and the current use to determine if the traditional use sheds any light on the potential risk associated with current use.**

Identifying Historical Uses of a Related Substance

A starting place for obtaining information regarding traditional use of dietary supplement ingredients is secondary references. If secondary references suggest that the traditional use is similar to the current use and that the historical use has been without observed complications, then it is important to verify this information with primary sources before relying on it as even a weak surrogate indicator of safety. The quality of the original source of information should be considered before placing much value in secondary sources, as questionable information appears to be cited repeatedly, with problems in obtaining original information.

If the supplement ingredient is a botanical or medicinal plant, it may be of value to understand the medical system of use from which the information is derived. This information is found in a number of books and symposium reports (e.g., Bannerman et al., 1983; Chadwick and Marsh 1990; Dobelis, 1997; Griggs, 1997; Prance et al., 1994). Traditional or folkloric uses are extensively described for more than 15,000 species of flowering plants in NAPRALERT, as are *in vitro* data, *in vivo* data, and reports of human use of extracts of flowering plants (Farnsworth, 2003). Information regarding current conditions of use, such as duration and amount ingested, can be obtained from third-party literature, labeling, marketing data, and survey data.

Considering the Relevance of Historical Use

The discussion in this section focuses on questions to consider when assessing whether the information about traditional use is relevant to current use conditions. These questions are listed in Box 4-1 and are explained in more detail in the following paragraphs.

BOX 4-1
Questions to Be Answered When Considering Relevance of Information About Historical Use

- Is the supplement ingredient one that was commonly used within the context of a traditional medical system? Moreover, if there are traditional cautions in the use of the supplement ingredient, are these cautions typically heeded?
- How "safe" is the historical use? Were the adverse events in question capable of being detected by the practitioners and, if observed, would they have been recorded?
- Was the substance traditionally ingested?
- If the supplement ingredient is a botanical, is the part of the plant marketed the same as the part that was traditionally used?
- Are current intake levels or recommended intake levels clearly different from traditional use?
- How similar is the current preparation to that used traditionally? Is the preparation a crude preparation, extract, or concentrate; a selected fraction; an isolated compound; or a mixture of these? Is the substance currently formulated in a method that will allow greater consumption?
- Is the modern duration of use consistent with historical indications?
- Is the modern reason for using the substance consistent with historical indication for its use?
- Is the target population similar to that which used the substance historically? Is the current user population similar to that which used the substance historically?

• *Is the supplement ingredient one that was commonly used within the context of a traditional medical system? Moreover, if there are traditional cautions in the use of the supplement ingredient, are these cautions typically heeded?* Some dietary supplement ingredients, including some botanicals, were traditionally prescribed by practitioners knowledgeable about contraindications to their use. **It is scientifically appropriate to take contraindications in traditional use into account when considering the safety of the ingredient.** If, for example, an ingredient traditionally contraindicated for pregnant women is currently being marketed to pregnant women or is frequently consumed by pregnant women due to its expected effects, then FDA should be more concerned about the safety of this ingredient.

• *How "safe" is the historical use? Were the adverse events in question capable of being detected by the practitioners and, if observed, would they have been recorded?* **The fact that a substance was consumed over a number of years does not indicate that it was consumed without adverse effects.** This is especially true for effects that are not acutely apparent, but even acute adverse effects may have been tolerated with the medicinal use because better treatments options did not exist. In understanding the relevance of historical use to safe current use, it is thus helpful to have information documenting safe historical use.

• *Was the substance traditionally ingested?* **Safe administration by non-oral routes of administration should not be taken as an indication of safety via oral administration.**

• *If the supplement ingredient is a botanical, is the part of the plant marketed the same as the plant part that was traditionally used?* **Historical information is only useful if the product in question is not so far removed from the original substance as to constitute a distinct entity.** For example, a whole root extract that was traditionally used for three days to treat a cold is not comparable with a fraction of a leaf extract promoted for long-term use to treat cancer. Safety comparisons for botanicals can only be made when the same plant part used in traditional preparations is used in the modern preparation because seeds, roots, leaves, and other parts may have distinct safety profiles due to difference in composition, as is evidenced by the differential distribution of toxins in some uneaten parts of common food plants. In summary, indication of safe use of one plant part does not indicate that other plant parts might also be used safely.

• *Are current intake levels or recommended intake levels clearly different from traditional use?* A frequently quoted axiom of toxicology from Paracelsus is that "only the dose makes the poison." Unfortunately, differences in traditional and modern formulations render dose comparisons between traditional and modern formations difficult or even impossible. It is a rare case when the levels of potentially dangerous bioactive compounds in traditionally used formulations have been quantified and can be compared with modern formulations. In most cases, however, dosing comparisons are so imprecise that they should probably only be attempted when the modern formulation clearly provides doses that may be orders of magnitude higher than traditional doses. For example, consumption of a culinary botanical in small amounts is very different, and thus may have different effects, than consumption of large amounts of the same encapsulated botanical, rendering a safety extrapolation from culinary to supplemental use inappropriate. **In summary, if the current level of intake is significantly above what has been traditionally recommended, then the level of concern should be increased.**

- *How similar is the current preparation to that used traditionally? Is the preparation a crude preparation, extract, or concentrate; a selected fraction; an isolated compound; or a mixture of these?* As discussed above, the toxicity of a substance depends on the amount ingested. The method of preparation will impact the amount and types of chemical compounds ingested, thus potentially impacting an ingredient's safety. The different methods of preparation are most clearly illustrated with botanicals. Traditionally, many orally ingested medicinal botanicals were administered as crude aqueous extractions of plant parts that were soaked, steeped, or boiled in water. Today's supplement ingredients are often sold in a different form—as encapsulated dried botanicals, fluid extracts, solid extracts (e.g., capsules or tablets), or foodstuffs containing botanical extracts. The same plant can be used as an extract prepared from dried plant materials (an infusion) or as lyophilized plant made from whole fresh materials.

Whether a botanical with a history of benign use in infusions (teas) manifests new toxic effects when concentrated, lyophilized, or encapsulated will depend on where any toxic components are localized in the plant, their water solubility, their potency, and the likelihood that a person could consume enough of the active ingredients to cause an ill effect. Differences in safety profiles could also be expected for alcoholic versus aqueous extracts of plants with known toxic components. Alcohol and water extract different compounds, so alcohol extracts may contain a higher concentration of toxic compounds than aqueous extracts. Wormwood (*Artemisia absinthium*), for example, in an aqueous extract contains little thujone (a neurotoxin) (Tegtmeier and Harnischfeger, 1994), but may contain substantial amounts of thujone in alcohol extracts. In summary, **if the method of preparation concentrates the bioactive compounds to a degree not known to be consistent with safe historical use, the level of concern should be raised.**

In addition to preparations that might result in increased concentration of bioactives in the products ingested, it is also important to note that **modern formulations may simply make the same substances more likely to be ingested in excessive amounts, which should raise concern.** If a substance is compacted in a capsule where taste and sheer volume of the material does not limit consumption, then there is a greater likelihood of an adverse reaction compared with the same botanical that was traditionally ingested in smaller amounts.

- *Is the modern duration of use consistent with historical use patterns?* **The duration of use needs to be considered because acute, short-term, and long-term intakes all have different safety implications. A lack of adverse events reported for a botanical traditionally used only for a few days has little or no relevance to safety of the same botanical when it is chronically ingested.** When considering how the current duration of use compares with traditional duration of use, it may be helpful to also consider whether the modern day indication is consistent with traditional indications. The modern uses of some botanicals, especially for nonmedical indications such as memory enhancement and ergogenics, may lead consumers to chronically use dietary supplements that were never used chronically in traditional medicine. In summary, concern is increased if the substance is now used for longer duration than it was traditionally.
- *Is the modern reason for using the substance consistent with historical indication for its use?* The reason for using the substance does not in itself provide information about its safety as a dietary supplement, but comparing the modern and traditional indications may provide clues for comparing historical and modern use. For example, some indications are more consistent with external use versus ingestion. Similarly, some indications are more consistent with long-term use (e.g., to lose weight) compared with short-term use (e.g., to treat an asthma attack).
- *Is the target population similar to that which used the substance historically? Is the current user population similar to that which used the substance historically?* People vary in their response to bioactive compounds. Due to physiological condition or other reasons, particular subpopulations may be more likely to suffer a serious adverse reaction than other groups. Thus, **the modern use of a dietary supplement ingredient by populations that have not traditionally consumed the ingredients reduces the relevance of safe historical use information. A change in usage does not necessarily in and of itself raise the level of concern; however, if the supplement ingredient is now used by a subpopulation that may be more susceptible to adverse effects, concern may be warranted.**

Summary of Historical Data Use

The fact that a botanical or other dietary supplement ingredient has been used for centuries is not *prima facie* evidence that it is safe. If the current preparation concentrates constituents, if the current use is more frequent or of longer duration, if the substance was not historically in-

TABLE 4-3 Relative Spectrum of Concern Raised by Historical Evidence of Toxicity

Increasing Concern →		
Traditional cautions (contraindications) exist regarding use in certain populations or circumstances	Traditional cautions (contraindications) exist regarding use in certain populations or circumstances that, if ignored, might be associated with a serious adverse effect (e.g., do not use during pregnancy)	There is clear evidence that traditional use causes conditions considered to be serious adverse events (e.g., hallucination, lethal poisoning)

gested, if a different plant part is now used, if the ingredient is formulated or processed differently, or if a different population is using the substance, then the level of concern should be raised. It is clear from these questions that historical use of a substance, even widespread historical use without documented ill effects, is no guarantor of long-term safety.

Historical use information is very useful when it describes a relationship between untoward effects and an ingested substance, as illustrated in Table 4-3. It is less useful in predicting safe use, especially if there are other reasons to be concerned about the possibility of effects that do not occur immediately following exposure. However, in the absence of other data that raise concerns about the safety of the substance, information about safe historical use may provide indirect evidence for lack of serious acute harmful effects if its relevance to current use conditions is carefully considered.

Information about the historical use of an ingredient may be most useful if it suggests potential adverse effects that could be anticipated. It is also helpful to compare relevant historical use information with other types of information that suggest possible harm (e.g., *in vitro* data, animal data, other human data, or data about related substances). While the historical use information should not be considered as more important than the scientific evidence, it may be appropriate to take information about the history of use into account if years of previous use would be expected to uncover the adverse effect under consideration. In such cases, historical use information may mitigate concerns to some degree.

CLINICAL STUDIES

Clinical studies evaluate the efficacy and/or safety of health care interventions in humans. There are several types of clinical studies, which differ as to whether the study includes a control group, the methods used to assemble the comparison groups, the extent of blinding (if any) of investigators and subjects, and other measures taken to minimize biases.

Although the double-blinded, randomized controlled trial (RCT) is often considered the "gold standard" for evaluating *efficacy* of many health care interventions, such studies have a much smaller role regarding *safety* concerns because they are not ordinarily primarily designed for that purpose. While adverse events are required to be monitored, collected, and evaluated during the course of an RCT, their known limitations (i.e., relatively small sample size, relatively short duration, narrowness of population studied, and narrowness of indication studied) (Goldman et al., 1995) make it almost impossible for a serious adverse effect that occurs relatively infrequently to be detected during the course of such a study. There is no scientific reason to think that efficacy studies of dietary supplements would be any exception. Given their limitations and the highly controlled settings in which most randomized trials are conducted, they are inadequate to fully assess the potential for harm of an intervention when it is routinely used in the target population. It is impossible to study all interactions of an intervention with combinations of comorbidities and concurrent medications or dietary supplements that may be present in the real world using a limited number of randomized trials. In addition, because dietary supplements are considered similarly to food, even if randomized controlled trials were performed to assess their benefits, there may be fewer perceived concerns for their safety and therefore a reporting bias on the part of the subjects and/or the investigators.

If it existed, an RCT designed to evaluate safety of a dietary supplement would include a sufficiently large number of diverse subjects who were systematically monitored for a sufficient amount of time to detect a wide array of adverse effects or physiological changes that might warrant concern. The physiological parameters focused upon in monitoring human subjects would be determined, in part, by effects found in preclinical (animal) studies. Extensive preclinical studies, however, are not often completed for dietary supplements.

It is the usual practice in an RCT to query subjects for possible adverse events at defined intervals and to record and evaluate these events as "definitely," "probably," "possibly," or "not" related to the ingested substance (ICH, 1995). Randomization and use of control groups enable investigators to determine the likelihood that adverse effects are actually due to the substance rather than to confounding factors. However, as previously noted, many RCTs available for dietary supplements are designed to assess beneficial effects and thus would not be expected to provide complete information relative to the safety of the dietary supplement under evaluation. In health care intervention studies, perhaps due to the greater tendency for authors to report positive findings and perhaps due to limited amount of space in journal articles, efficacy results are more consistently reported and are reported in greater detail than safety data (Ioannidis and Lau, 2001). Although investigators conducting efficacy trials are expected to observe and report adverse reactions, the extent and detail of this reporting is highly variable (Ioannidis and Lau, 2001). In some cases, however, investigators may be able to supply unpublished data useful in the safety evaluation, as the published results may not contain all the available information about adverse events (Ioannidis et al., 2002).

While investigators may be able to provide additional unpublished data, characteristics of the study design itself may limit usefulness in predicting safety because even large studies may lack sufficient statistical power to detect adverse events of low incidence. Clinical trials generally are designed to detect one primary endpoint; thus secondary events, such as adverse effects, will frequently be inadequately reported (Ioannidis and Lau, 2001). A major cause of an inadequate safety evaluation is that an unexpected adverse event may not be noticed by the subject or detected by the investigator. For these reasons, a study to test the effects of a dietary supplement ingredient on mood, for example, may not detect potentially dangerous cardiovascular effects of the supplement if heart function is not monitored.

These known limitations of RCTs regarding safety limit their sensitivity to be able to detect adverse events that occur infrequently, only after extended exposure, or predominantly in subpopulations (Goldman et al., 1995). For example, events that occur at the rate of 1 in 1,000 would require a study with at least 3,000 subjects at risk to have a 95 percent chance of being detected (Lewis, 1981). Differences between the study and the target population and administration of the substance during the RCT compared with its actual use by the general population, coupled with the inability to exhaustively evaluate for all possible interactions with drugs and other dietary supplements in RCTs, limits the generalizability of results from these types of studies.

However, **while clinical trials can be limited in their sensitivity, they do provide valuable information when adverse events are detected.** Utility of information from clinical studies is strengthened by providing the following (Counsell, 1997; ICH, 1995; Moher et al., 2001):

- Demographic information on the study population,
- Inclusion and exclusion criteria to determine whether the results are generalizable,
- A description of the condition or disease and comorbidities of the study population,

- A description of the intervention (supplement ingredient [composition], dose, and duration of exposure),
- A list of prior and concomitant ingested substances, including dietary supplements and drugs, and
- A description of the adverse event, including temporal relationship to ingestion of supplement ingredient (i.e., response to dechallenge and rechallenge, where appropriate).

Clearly, RCTs cannot be relied upon as the sole source of information to assess the safety of a dietary supplement. Because there are no regulatory requirements to demonstrate the efficacy of dietary supplements and because studies are lengthy and expensive, it is unlikely that many well-conducted RCTs for dietary supplements will be available. Even if they do exist, the limitations discussed earlier in this section make RCTs inappropriate for detecting rare adverse events. Epidemiological studies and spontaneously reported adverse events are better suited in general to provide this important information, as are other types of nonhuman data, as described in the next chapter.

While RCTs may not reveal the entire range of possible adverse events and the occurrence of adverse events may not be adequately reported, on occurrence adverse events are reported in this type of study. Although uncommon, some RCTs have been specifically designed to assess adverse events as the primary outcome. Because an RCT uses a randomized comparison group to minimize confounders and biases in the assessment of outcomes, statistical differences in adverse events in the treatment group warrant a good deal of attention.

A statistically significant increased rate in adverse events indicates that a sufficiently large number of events have occurred to allow one to conclude that the observation is unlikely due to chance alone. The relative concern appropriate for the different types of information typical of a clinical study is described in Table 4-4. In general, the highest concern (the right column) is raised when there is a statistically significant higher rate of a serious adverse event or serious abnormalities in clinical laboratory or other diagnostic test values in the dietary supplement group when compared with the control population. Examples of serious abnormalities in clinical laboratory or other diagnostic test values might include, for example, aberrant electrocardiography findings or electrolyte changes that indicate a very high risk of serious cardiovascular or neurological consequences.

Even if an adverse event is truly associated with the use of a dietary supplement ingredient, sometimes only a nonstatistically significant trend toward increased serious adverse events is observed in RCTs. This situation

TABLE 4-4 Spectrum of Relative Concerns with Clinical Studies Data

Increasing Concern →

Describes a serious adverse event, but with less information than would justify moderate or strong concern, and/or the interpretation of the clinical study is hampered by the presence of prominent confounding factors (e.g., multiple concomitant substances and/or conditions) that could not be controlled by balancing AND/OR Prominent methodological concerns (e.g., unexplained high level of dropouts, lack of control groups)	Nonsignificant, but clinically important, trend of a higher rate of a serious adverse event OR Abnormalities in clinical laboratory values OR Other abnormalities, such as electrocardiographic findings in the dietary supplement ingredient group	A significantly higher incidence of a serious adverse event OR Other potentially dangerous abnormalities, such as in clinical laboratory values that are associated with risk of serious adverse events OR Other abnormalities, such as electrocardiographic findings in the dietary supplement ingredient group

may occur if the study is small, too few adverse events were observed, or the study is otherwise underpowered. For example, the appearance of liver enzyme abnormalities in two or three subjects taking a dietary supplement may not produce a statistically significant difference compared with the control group. Therefore, it cannot be concluded with confidence that the liver abnormality is due to the dietary supplement, but the information can be used to augment other data related to safety of the dietary supplement ingredient. However, **in populations and settings where no adverse event is expected, a nonsignificant trend also warrants attention.**

Finally, **a concern still exists even if there is not a trend that would justify a moderate or statistically significant concern.** This often occurs when a firm conclusion cannot be reached due to confounding factors. A frequent confounding factor with dietary supplements, for example, is the concomitant consumption of other xenobiotics. Single cases of serious adverse events, such as death or liver failure in the dietary supplement group, also warrant special attention.

EPIDEMIOLOGICAL STUDIES[6]

Value of Epidemiological Studies

Epidemiological studies that contain information on the use of dietary supplements, when available, are valuable sources of information for evaluating their safety. Data from these studies complement information from RCTs and adverse events reports. This type of data is rare; however, this is likely to change as additional research is conducted on dietary supplement use, efficacy, and safety. The considerations described below will be helpful in considering epidemiological studies to assess unreasonable or significant risk.

As discussed above, among the limitations inherent to many RCTs is that relatively small size and short duration limit sensitivity to detect adverse events (Goldman et al., 1995). Latent or delayed effects that occur long after exposure may not be detected. Information about these latent and infrequent effects often comes from epidemiological studies that retrospectively or prospectively examine the effects of ingested substances on large populations. Another benefit of epidemiological studies is that the number of individuals exposed to supplements is expanded to the general population. Data from these studies usually contain a large number of individuals compared with the number exposed in clinical trials.

Like RCTs, the value of epidemiological studies also depends on the endpoints examined. For example, if a study evaluates the incidence of cancer, death, or liver damage but does not evaluate anemia, the study is unlikely to detect interference with iron absorption.

The assessment of the level of concern regarding the safety of a dietary supplement ingredient is dependent on the quality of the study and analyses, the estimated risk or odds ratio, the clinical significance of the risk, and the statistical significance of the estimate. Situations in the right column of Table 4-5 indicate higher levels of concern.

---

[6] "Observational" and "epidemiological" studies are referred to here as "epidemiological studies." Thus the term here includes (1) investigations in which the researcher has little or no control over events, and the relationships between risk factors and outcome measures are studied without the intervention of the investigator (e.g., surveys), and (2) the study of the distribution and size of disease problems in human populations, in particular to identify etiological factors in the pathogenesis of disease and to provide the data essential for the management, evaluation, and planning of services for the prevention, control, and treatment of disease.

TABLE 4-5 Spectrum of Relative Concerns with Epidemiological Data

Increasing Concern →

Case-control or cohort study (including registries), with small,[a] but statistically significant, relative risk or odds ratio of a serious adverse event OR Large relative risk or odds ratio of a serious adverse event that is not statistically significant OR Poorly conducted studies with large or significant effects	Case-control or cohort study (including registries), with moderate, statistically significant relative risk or odds ratio of a serious adverse event OR Moderate relative risk or odds ratio of a serious adverse event that is not statistically significant but that implies a trend	Well-conducted case-control or cohort study (including registries), with large, statistically significant relative risk or odds ratio of a serious adverse event

[a] Two or less is generally considered a weak association, and 3 or more is considered strong, but this is only a very general "rule of thumb" guidance and somewhat debatable.

Using Epidemiological Data on Dietary Supplements

Assessing causality from epidemiological data requires the specific study designs that are described here, for example, case-control and cohort studies. However, other types of epidemiological studies often have been used in combination with other study designs (e.g., RCTs, case reports) to draw or strengthen conclusions (GAO, 1992).

For any type of epidemiological study, the quality of the study and the analyses depends on the quality of the data. Missing data or, in the case of surveys, poor participation may cause biased results. Quality also may be affected by a conflict of interest by an author or study sponsor. Safeguards should be in place to prevent biased reporting of study results or where a conflict of interest is present. Errors in design, data collection, and analyses can also lead to poor-quality studies. Possible flaws of epidemiological studies have been well described in the medical and health care literature (Altman, 1998; Gardner et al., 1986).

Cohort Studies

Cohort studies generally evaluate a group of individuals (either prospectively or retrospectively) and estimate incidence rates of an event in exposed and unexposed individuals. From this information, the risk of the event occurring in the exposed group relative to the risk for the unexposed group (the relative risk) can be estimated. Unlike well-conducted RCTs, results from cohort studies can be influenced by selection bias and confounding—if they exist. Selection bias occurs when there are unmeasured factors that are related to the outcome of safety and also affect selection for use or non-use of a supplement. Confounding can occur when use of a dietary supplement is strongly correlated to other characteristics of individuals that also affect the safety outcome. These two potential study design problems should be considered when adjusting the level of concern warranted by cohort studies.

Primarily due to their relative expense, greater need for dedicated personnel, and inability to detect rare, serious adverse events, cohort studies are likely to be used less frequently than case-control studies in a postmarketing environment. Expense of cohort studies decreases when computerized medical records can be used, and thus as more records include information about intake of dietary supplement ingredients, the availability of cohort studies for dietary supplements is likely to increase. Nonetheless, for identified rare, serious adverse events, case-control studies may be more common.

Case-Control Epidemiological Studies

Case-control epidemiological studies are uniquely useful at estimating the likelihood that an ingested substance causes an adverse event when the occurrence of the event is rare or occurs following a long latency period. In a case-control study, cases (persons with the event of interest) and controls (persons who do not have the event of interest) are identified. The exposure rates among cases and among controls are then estimated.[7] Using the estimated exposure (dose is rarely known) in the controls and in the cases, the odds of the event in the exposed group relative to that in the unexposed group (the odds ratio) is estimated. (The odds of an event are equal to the probability of the event divided by one minus this probability).

Case-control studies require information on fewer individuals than cohort studies (see next section). However, in case-control studies there is the potential for bias caused by inappropriate selection of the control group or

---

[7]When used in epidemiology, the word "exposure" often has a different meaning than in the field of toxicology. It is unusual for an epidemiological study to state exposure in the quantitative terms of dose. Rather, there may be some evidence, direct or indirect, that exposure to an agent of concern occurred without regard to consideration of the actual ingested dose. In toxicology studies, dosages are explicitly stated.

inaccurate assignment of exposure status. Most textbooks on epidemiology cover this topic in detail (e.g., Rothman and Greenland, 1998).

If exposure to a dietary supplement is widespread, case-control studies could be useful for assessing the association of the supplement with an adverse event—even if the adverse event is rare. However, a case-control study also will be useful when assessing risk from a dietary supplement even when use is not widespread if the adverse event rate among users is high. Both situations—wide exposure and a rare outcome and limited exposure with a common outcome—make case-control studies a useful tool for assessing safety of dietary supplements.

Clinical Significance of Estimated Relative Risk or Odds Ratios from Cohort and Case-Control Studies: Using the Statistics Values

Relative risk is a measure of the association between the exposure to some factor (in this case, a dietary supplement ingredient) and the risk of some outcome (e.g., a serious adverse event). It is calculated as the incidence rate of a serious adverse event among persons taking the dietary supplement ingredient divided by the incidence rate of the serious adverse event among persons not taking the ingredient. An incidence rate is the ratio of the number of events (e.g., of a serious adverse event) over a period of time and the number in the population being studied during the time period. For example, relative risk of 2.5 means that the group exposed to the ingredient is 2.5 times (or 150 percent) more likely to have a particular serious adverse event than those not exposed to the ingredient. A relative risk of 1.0 shows no additional risk in the exposed group while a relative risk < 1.0 indicates less risk in the exposed group. For example, a relative risk of 0.67 means the exposed group has 0.67 times the risk (two-thirds the risk or 33 percent less risk) of the event than does the unexposed group.

An odds ratio is approximately equal to the relative risk when the probability of the adverse event is small in both the exposed and unexposed groups. Therefore, odds ratios often are described and interpreted as if they were relative risk values.

If case-control or cohort studies on a dietary supplement ingredient have been completed, the reviewer should consider the magnitude of the odds ratio or relative risk values, p values, or confidence intervals (see below), *and* the seriousness and severity of the adverse event in question when determining the relative concern about the safety of a dietary supplement ingredient. In general, the reviewer should be alert to relative risks or odds ratios of greater than 2, as described in Table 4-5. That said, a numerical cutoff is not appropriate and greater sensitivity to low values may be appropriate as the seriousness of the adverse event and the number of individuals exposed increases. As a "rule of thumb," a relative risk or odds ratio of 3 or more generally represents a strong association, although choice of this cut-point is debatable (Stolley, 1990; Temple, 1999). Similarly, as a rule of thumb, a relative risk or odds ratio of 2 or less generally represents a weak association (Temple, 1999).

In addition to the relative risk or odds ratio values, a measurement of uncertainty (e.g., standard error) is needed to properly assess the level of concern that should be attached to a finding. Confidence intervals and *p* values use both the estimated relative risk or odds ratio and the standard error of these estimates in their calculations. In most medical, biological, and health services literature, a *p* value (the probability of the observed data if the null hypothesis is true) of 0.05 or less is considered statistically significant. This cut-point translates into incorrectly rejecting the null hypothesis 1 time or fewer out of 20, on average. Although a *p* value of ≤ 0.05 is commonly used to determine when a result warrants attention, in interpreting studies regarding safety, a cutoff point of $p < 0.05$ is often not appropriate because of its implications. Dietary supplements are regulated similarly to foods and are presumed to be safe (the null hypothesis). A *p* value under this null hypothesis reflects the probability of the observed data when assuming that the dietary supplement is safe. A *p* value of 0.05 means that on average, one would incorrectly reject the assumption that a supplement is safe 1 time out of 20. For serious adverse events, when there is a high prevalence of use or when the supplement is used in special populations, a *p* value greater that 0.05 might raise the level of concern substantially. A *p* value of 0.10 would mean that the probability of the observed number of adverse events is 0.10 if one assumes that the supplement is safe (i.e., on average one expects to see this number of adverse events 1 time out of 10 if the supplement is safe). This type of finding could be enough to raise the concern level. Knowledge that at this level one incorrectly rejects the hypothesis of safety 1 out of 10 times on average should enable this information to be appropriately integrated with other types of information (e.g., animal data).

Finally, confidence intervals of relative risks or odds ratios may be more useful than *p* values in interpreting results. A 95 percent confidence interval typically is used and means that 95 percent of the calculated confidence intervals are expected to contain the true relative risk if the estimation were repeated a large number of times in similar study settings. However, as with *p* values, the choice of the value 95 percent should be used with full understanding of its consequences and meaning. Studies where a 95 percent confidence interval for a relative risk or an odds ratio covers 1 (thus indicating lower significance statistically) may still offer important information about safety. A recent example where it was decided that there existed a high safety concern even without having statistical significance is the hormone replacement therapy randomized control trial designed to look at benefits of the therapy over time (Rossouw et al., 2002).

Assessing the Strength of Association with Epidemiological Studies

Epidemiologists tend to agree on characteristics of epidemiological studies that suggest an increasingly strong association between an adverse effect and an ingested substance, describing this in terms of establishing "causality" between a substance and an effect (Hennekens et al., 1987; Hill, 1971; Rothman and Greenland, 1998; Sackett et al., 1991). While these characteristics can certainly be used to demonstrate whether the threshold of causality has been met, meeting such a threshold is less important for dietary supplements for which it is only necessary to determine whether an unreasonable or significant risk exists.

For a dietary supplement ingredient studied in epidemiological studies, concern increases as more of the following criteria are met: large relative risk; consistency of findings in different studies or in different populations; association that "makes sense" because other plausible causes are ruled out and results are consistent with current knowledge of cause and effect in humans, animals, and cells *in vitro*; association that is limited to a single potential cause and a single type of adverse event;[8] a dose-response relationship[9] and temporality (i.e., the adverse event occurs after a dietary supplement is ingested). In the evaluation of safety of dietary supplements, one high-quality epidemiological study alone can cause a high level of concern, as shown on the right side of Table 4-5. Epidemiological studies that do not meet these criteria may be used to form hypotheses about safety or to strengthen or generalize the results from RCTs or other data.

SUMMARY

As described in the guiding principles, a credible report or study finding of a serious adverse event in humans that is associated with use of a dietary supplement ingredient raises concern about the ingredient's safety. While historical use should not be used as *prima facie* evidence that the ingredient does not cause harm, it may be appropriate to give considerable weight to a lack of adverse events in large, high-quality, randomized clinical trials or

---

[8]One example of this is thalidomide—no other drugs were associated with the particular birth defects and the type of birth defect was unique.

[9]For example, people who smoke more cigarettes per day have a greater likelihood of disease.

epidemiological studies that are adequately powered and designed to detect adverse effects.

The basis for this guiding principle is described in the sections of this chapter, as are the following important corollaries and specific guidance:

- There are significant limitations in using clinical efficacy trials to predict that an adverse event *will not* occur because of their limited sensitivity. Clinical trials do provide valuable information when adverse events *are* detected.
- A statistically significant increased rate in adverse events indicates that a sufficiently large number of events have occurred to allow one to conclude that the observation is unlikely due to chance alone. However, in populations and settings where no adverse event is expected, a nonsignificant trend also warrants some concern and consideration.
- Epidemiological studies that contain information on the use of dietary supplements, when available, are valuable sources of information for evaluating their safety.
- Given the state of the art in adverse event report evaluation and pharmacovigilance and risk management, and given the potential risk to the public entailed by serious adverse events, regulatory action can be justified on the basis of spontaneously reported adverse event report analysis alone or as the predominant source of information. Reports of certain adverse events warrant heightened concern because they have a known potential for significant morbidity (and in some cases, mortality).
- If spontaneously reported adverse event reports are of high quality, irrespective of number, the effect of underreporting can be somewhat mitigated. The stronger the product-adverse event relationship and the lower the incidence of (and thus rarer) the adverse event occurring *de novo*/naturalistically, the fewer the number of case reports that will be needed to perceive causality.
- Recognizing that a full range of data is unlikely to be available for many dietary supplement ingredients, historical use may be taken into account as a surrogate measure for safety in the absence of relevant scientific and experimental data. In doing so, it is important to consider the relevance of the traditional use to the current use and, as such, FDA must have information regarding both the traditional use and the current use to determine if the traditional use sheds any light on the potential risk associated with current use.
- The fact that a substance was consumed over a number of years does not indicate that it was consumed without adverse effects. Safe administration by non-oral routes of administration should not be taken as an indication of safety via oral administration. Historical information is useful only if the product in question is not so far removed from the original

substance as to constitute a distinct entity. If the current level of intake is significantly above what has been traditionally recommended, then the level of concern should be increased.

REFERENCES

Altman DG. 1998. Statistical reviewing for medical journals. *Stat Med* 17:2661–2674.

Auriche M, Loupi E. 1993. Does proof of casualty ever exist in pharmacovigilance? *Drug Safe* 9:230–235.

Bannerman RH, Burton J, Wen-Chieh C, eds. 1983. *Traditional Medicine and Health Care Coverage. A Reader for Health Administrators and Practitioners.* Geneva: World Health Organization.

Barnes J, Mills SY, Abbot NC, Willoughby M, Ernst E. 1998. Different standards for reporting ADRs to herbal remedies and conventional OTC medicines: Face-to-face interview with 515 users of herbal remedies. *Br J Clin Pharmacol* 45:496–500.

Begaud B, Moride Y, Tubert-Bitter P, Chaslerie A, Haramburu F. 1994. False-positives in spontaneous reporting: Should we worry about them? *Br J Clin Pharmacol* 38:401–404.

Blum MD, Graham DJ, McCloskey CA. 1994. Temafloxacin syndrome: Review of 95 cases. *Clin Infect Dis* 18:946–950.

CFSAN (Center for Food Safety and Applied Nutrition). 2001. *Overview of Dietary Supplements.* Online. Food and Drug Administration. Available at http://www.cfsan.fda.gov/~dms/ds-oview.html. Accessed February 22, 2002.

Chadwick DJ, Marsh J, eds. 1990. *Bioactive Compounds from Plants. Ciba Foundation Symposium 154.* New York: John Wiley and Sons.

Chen RT, Rastogi SC, Mullen JR, Hayes SW, Cochi SL, Donlon JA, Wassilak SG. 1994. The Vaccine Adverse Event Reporting System (VAERS). *Vaccine* 12:542–550.

Chyka PA, McCommon SW. 2000. Reporting of adverse drug reactions by poison control centers in the US. *Drug Safe* 23:87–93.

CIOMS (Council for International Organizations of Medical Sciences). 1990. Standardization of definitions and criteria of causality assessment of adverse drug reaction. Drug-induced liver disorders: Report of an International Consensus Meeting. *Int J Clin Pharmacol* 28:317–322.

CIOMS. 1999. *Guidelines for Preparing Core Clinical-Safety Information on Drugs, 2nd ed. Report of CIOMS Working Groups III and V.* Geneva: CIOMS.

CIOMS. 2001. *Current Challenges in Pharmacolvigilance: Pragmatic Approaches. Report of CIOMS Working Group V.* Geneva: CIOMS.

Counsell C. 1997. Formulating questions and locating primary studies for inclusion in systematic reviews. *Ann Intern Med* 127:380–387.

Dobelis IN. 1997. *Magic and Medicine of Plants. A Practical Guide to the Science, History, Folklore, and Everyday Uses of Medical Plants.* Pleasantville, NY: Reader's Digest Association.

Eisenberg DM, Davis RB, Ettner SL, Appel S, Wilkey S, Van Rompay M, Kessler RC. 1998. Trends in alternative medicine use in the United States, 1990–1997: Results of a follow-up national survey. *J Am Med Assoc* 280:1569–1575.

Faich GA. 1986. Adverse-drug-reaction monitoring. *N Engl J Med* 314:1589–1592.

Farnsworth NR. 2003. *NAPRALERT (Natural Products ALERT) Database.* Chicago: University of Chicago.

FDA (Food and Drug Administration). 2003a. Current good manufacturing practice in manufacturing, packing, or holding dietary ingredients and dietary supplements. Proposed rule. *Fed Regis* 68:12157–12263.

FDA. 2003b. *FDA News. FDA Proposes Labeling and Manufacturing Standards for All Dietary Supplements.* Online. Available at http://www.fda.gov/bbs/topics/NEWS/2003/NEW00876.html. Accessed July 2, 2003.

FDA. 2003c. Safety reporting requirements for human drug and biological products. Proposed rule. *Fed Regis* 68:12406–12497.

Finney DJ. 1971. Statistical aspects of monitoring for dangers in drug therapy. *Methods Inf Med* 10:1–8.

Fletcher AP. 1991. Spontaneous adverse drug reaction reporting vs event monitoring: A comparison. *J R Soc Med* 84:341–344.

GAO (General Accounting Office). 1992. *Cross Design Synthesis: A New Strategy for Medical Effectiveness Research.* GAO/PEMD-92-18. Washington, DC: GAO.

Gardner MJ, Machin D, Campbell MJ. 1986. Use of check lists in assessing the statistical content of medical studies. *Br Med J* 292:810–812.

Goldman SA. 1996. *The Clinical Impact of Adverse Event Reporting. A MedWatch Continuing Education Article.* Food and Drug Administration. Available at http://www.fda.gov/medwatch/articles.htm. Accessed February 25, 2003.

Goldman SA. 1998. Limitations and strengths of spontaneous reports data. *Clin Ther* 20:C40–C44.

Goldman SA, Kennedy DL, Lieberman R, eds. 1995. *Clinical Therapeutics and the Recognition of Drug-Induced Disease. A MedWatch Continuing Education Article.* Food and Drug Administration. Available at http://www.fda.gov/medwatch/articles.htm. Accessed June 4, 2003.

Griggs B. 1997. *Green Pharmacy. The History and Evolution of Western Herbal Medicine.* 2nd ed. Rochester, VT: Healing Arts Press.

Hennekens CH, Buring JE, Mayrent SL. 1987. *Epidemiology in Medicine.* Boston: Little, Brown.

Hill AB. 1971. *Principles of Medical Statistics.* 9th ed. New York: Oxford University Press.

ICH (International Conference on Harmonisation). 1995. *Guidance for Industry. E3. Structure and Content of Clinical Study Reports.* Rockville, MD: Drug Information Branch, Center for Drug Evaluation and Research, FDA.

Ioannidis JP, Lau J. 2001. Completeness of safety reporting in randomized trials: An evaluation of 7 medical areas. *J Am Med Assoc* 285:437–443.

Ioannidis JPA, Chew P, Lau J. 2002. Standardized retrieval of side effects data for meta-analysis of safety outcomes: A feasibility study in acute sinusitis. *J Clin Epidemiol* 55:619–626.

Karch FE, Smith CL, Kerzner B, Mazzullo JM, Weintraub M, Lasagna L. 1976. Adverse drug reactions—A matter of opinion. *Clin Pharmacol Ther* 19:489–492.

Kessler DA. 1993. Introducing MEDWatch: A new approach to reporting medication and device adverse effects and product problems. *J Clin Res Drug Dev* 7:183–190.

Koch-Weser J, Sellers EM, Zacest R. 1977. The ambiguity of adverse drug reactions. *Eur J Clin Pharmacol* 11:75–78.

Lewis JA. 1981. Post-marketing surveillance: How many patients? *Trends Pharmacol Sci* 2:93–94.

Moher D, Schulz KF, Altman DG. 2001. The CONSORT statement: Revised recommendations for improving the quality of reports of parallel group randomized trials. *BMC Med Res Methodol* 1:2–8.

OIG (Office of Inspector General). 2001. *Adverse Event Reporting for Dietary Supplements. An Inadequate Safety Valve.* Online. Food and Drug Administration. Available at http://oig.hhs.gov/oei/reports/oei-01-00-00180.pdf. Accessed February 26, 2003.

Prance GT, Chadwick DJ, Marsh J, eds. 1994 . *Ethnobotany and the Search for New Drugs. Ciba Foundation Symposium 185.* New York: John Wiley and Sons.

Rawlins MD. 1995. Pharmacovigilance: Paradise lost, regained or postponed? *J R Coll Physicians Lond* 29:41–49.

Rossi AC, Knapp DE. 1984. Discovery of new adverse drug reactions. A review of the Food and Drug Administration's spontaneous reporting system. *J Am Med Assoc* 252:1030–1033.

Rossouw JE, Anderson GL, Prentice RL, LaCroix AZ, Kooperberg C, Stefanick ML, Jackson RD, Beresford SA, Howard BV, Johnson KC, Kotchen JM, Ockene J. 2002. Risks and benefits of estrogen plus progestin in healthy postmenopausal women: Principal results from the Women's Health Initiative randomized control trial. *J Am Med Assoc* 288:321–333.

Rothman KJ, Greenland S. 1998. *Modern Epidemiology*. 2nd ed. Philadelphia, PA: Lippincott-Raven.

Sachs RM, Bortnichak EA. 1986. An evaluation of spontaneous adverse drug reaction monitoring systems. *Am J Med* 81:49–55.

Sackett DL, Haynes RB, Tugwell P. 1991. Deciding whether your treatment has done harm. In: Sackett DL, ed. *Clinical Epidemiology: A Basic Science for Clinical Medicine*. 2nd ed. Boston: Little Brown.

Scott HD, Rosenbaum SE, Waters WJ, Colt AM, Andrews LG, Juergens JP, Faich GA. 1987. Rhode Island physicians' recognition and reporting of adverse drug reactions. *R I Med J* 70:311–316.

Skjeldestad FE, Amundsen T, Hoibraaten E. 2000. Reporting of adverse drug reactions to the Norwegian Medicines Control Agency—A discipline with few participants. *Tidsskr Nor Laegeforen* 120:336–338.

Stolley PD. 1990. How to interpret studies of adverse drug reactions. *Clin Pharmacol Ther* 48:337–339.

Strom BL, Tugwell P. 1990. Pharmacoepidemiology: Current status, prospects, and problems. *Ann Intern Med* 113:179–181.

Tegtmeier M, Harnischfeger G. 1994. Methods for the reduction of thujone content in pharmaceutical preparations of Artemisia, Salvia and Thuja. *Eur J Pharm Biopharm* 40:337–340.

Temple R. 1999. Meta-analysis and epidemiologic studies in drug development and postmarketing surveillance. *J Am Med Assoc* 281:841–844.

Temple RJ, Jones JK, Crout JR. 1979. Adverse effects of newly marketed drugs. *N Engl J Med* 300:1046–1047.

Walker A. 2000. *The Relation between Voluntary Notification and Material Risk in Dietary Supplement Safety*. FDA Commissioned Paper. FDA Docket 00N-1200(41).

Wurglics M, Westerhoff K, Kaunzinger A, Wilke A, Baumeister A, Dressman J, Schubert-Zsilavecz M. 2001. Comparison of German St. John's wort products according to hyperforin and total hypericin content. *J Am Pharm Assoc* 41:560–566.

5

Categories of Scientific Evidence— Animal Data

GUIDING PRINCIPLE: *Even in the absence of information on adverse events in humans, evidence of harm from animal studies is often indicative of potential harm to humans. This indication assumes greatest importance when the route of exposure is oral, the formulation tested is identical or highly similar to that consumed by humans, and more than one species show the same or similar toxicity.*

Information about animal exposure to dietary supplement ingredients may be in the form of formal studies such as traditional toxicity studies, safety pharmacology data, or observations from clinical veterinary medicine. Because dietary supplements are not required to undergo formal animal toxicity testing before marketing, extensive toxicity studies common to drugs and other substances are not likely to exist, but limited amounts of animal data are available in the scientific literature for a number of dietary supplement ingredients. Despite the challenges of dealing with incomplete data, the animal data that are available warrant attention when assessing risk of dietary supplement ingredients.

The first section of this chapter describes types of animal data that may be available. Subsequent sections describe the rationale for using animal data, including its power and relevance to human health. Also described is the appropriate consideration of negative data, and how the seriousness of harm, strength of evidence, and dose administered to animals factor into assessing animal data, along with general guidelines for integrating these factors. Animal data that raise a higher level of concern warrant immediate attention to evaluate the potential of the ingredient to cause harm. For data classified as lower to moderate concern, it is important to consider whether other animal data or other types of data (e.g., human data, *in vitro* data, or data on related substances) add to the level of concern.

POWER AND RELEVANCE OF ANIMAL DATA

Animal testing provides invaluable information about the potential for ingested substances to cause harm in humans. Studies in animals are regularly used as an important step in attempting to predict untoward effects of substances in humans (see, for example, the Food and Drug Administration's [FDA's] *Redbook* [OFAS, 2001, 2003] or guidance documents for new drugs [CDER, 2002]).

Animal studies are powerful because controlled studies can be conducted to predict effects that might not be detected from customary use by humans until they result in overt harmful effects. Animal studies are especially useful in detecting effects of chronic exposures and effects on reproductive and developmental processes because epidemiological methods of studying humans are especially problematic in these areas. The ability to administer agents to animals during their entire lifespan, if necessary, enables scientists to ascertain the potential toxic effects that may arise from long-term (chronic) exposure. Animal studies thus serve as important hypothesis generators and may be sufficient to indicate potentially unreasonable risk to human health, which justifies their use in evaluating the risks dietary supplement ingredients may pose to humans.

In general, adverse effects observed in well-designed and well-conducted animal studies should be treated as if they would occur in at least some members of the human population, assuming humans receive a sufficiently high dose. With some notable and important exceptions, the biological factors affecting the capacity of chemical substances to cause toxicity are broadly similar across mammalian species. **Unless there is scientific evidence that raises significant doubt regarding the relevance of specific toxicity findings to humans, it is prudent and scientifically appropriate to consider animal studies relevant in evaluating potential human toxicity, especially in the many cases of dietary supplement ingredients where sufficient human data are not available.** Similar positions on the relevance of animal data to human health have been supported by other committees of the National Academies, as well as by other organizations in the United States and internationally (NRC, 1994, 2001; NTP, 2002; WHO, 1999).

GENERAL TYPES OF ANIMAL DATA

Different categories of animal studies (e.g., acute, subacute/subchronic [often used interchangeably], chronic, carcinogenicity) provide different information relevant to considering the potential toxic properties of a dietary supplement ingredient and can be classified as either traditional toxicology studies or as safety pharmacology studies.

Traditional Toxicology Studies

FDA's *Redbook* describes several toxicology studies that are typically conducted in assessing the safety of food additives and other ingested substances (OFAS, 2001, 2003). These studies are applicable to evaluating most ingested substances, including dietary supplement ingredients, irrespective of what is known about their biological activities. It is highly probable that animal data from each type of toxicity study will not be available for every dietary supplement ingredient. However, consideration of the typical study protocols enables the animal data that are available on the dietary supplement ingredient in question to be placed in perspective regarding what type of information and conclusions about safety are appropriate to glean from the different study designs and endpoints. Perspective can also be gained by comparing the information available about a dietary supplement ingredient with the types of data that are often available about other ingested substances before they are considered safe.

In acute (single dose), subacute/subchronic (repeated doses), and chronic toxicity testing, groups of animals are treated with increasing amounts of the test substance to determine the dose that induces overt toxic effects. The resulting toxicities might be within organs (detected by gross examination or by observing behavioral changes), cells (detected by histological examination, such as light or electron microscopic analysis of fixed tissue samples), or subcellular structures (detected in biochemical studies, such as enzyme assays or protein analysis). In chronic toxicity testing (and in subchronic toxicity testing, which is not as lengthy as chronic toxicity testing), the test substance is typically administered to animals on a daily basis for 3 to 24 months (depending on the species) to characterize possible longer-term toxicity.

When conducting animal studies, blood concentrations of the test substance and its active metabolites are often determined. These blood levels are used to provide evidence that the test substance was absorbed, to describe the blood concentration–response curve, and to determine whether the metabolites formed in the test animal are qualitatively and quantitatively similar to those formed in humans. If the metabolites, especially active metabolites formed in the animal species studied, are not the same as those formed in humans, the results are less meaningful and testing in species with metabolism similar to humans should be considered.

Genetic, reproductive, developmental, immunological, neurobiological, and behavioral toxicity studies, as well as other types of studies, provide further information regarding the toxicity of the test substance.

Safety Pharmacology Studies

Safety pharmacology studies are conducted in various animal species to detect alterations in physiological functions at dosages lower than those used to elicit overt toxic effects detected in animal toxicity protocols. Guidance for conducting safety pharmacology studies for human pharmaceuticals is provided by FDA, which defines them as "those studies that investigate the potential undesirable pharmacodynamic effects of a substance on physiological functions in relation to exposure in the therapeutic range and above" (ICH/FDA, 2001). Safety pharmacology testing generally focuses on endpoints that differ from those examined in classic toxicity testing. The studies may be *in vivo* or *in vitro* and are designed to detect harmful effects in a core battery of vital organ systems, which include the cardiovascular, central nervous, and respiratory systems.

Observations from Veterinary Medicine

Veterinary toxicological observations may also prove useful in predicting the potential effect of dietary supplement ingredients on humans. The discipline of veterinary medicine/toxicology encompasses the entire spectrum of effects of natural and synthetic toxins, including drugs, pesticides, herbicides, and fungal and plant metabolites, on wildlife, livestock, and domestic animals (i.e., pets). The specific subdiscipline best described as plant-associated veterinary toxicology is likely to correlate most closely with adverse effects of botanical-derived dietary supplement ingredients. It is distinguished from toxicological studies in that it is primarily observational information or is based on studies not designed to predict effects on human health. Nevertheless, there are numerous examples of incidents of animal poisoning that have subsequently led to epidemiological studies and ultimately controlled experiments that resulted in identification of specific toxins and their mode of action. The well-known cases of aflatoxin-induced poultry toxicity led to the controlled animal and epidemiological studies that resulted in the classification of this important fungal metabolite as a human carcinogen (Mishra and Das, 2003).

An advantage of considering plant-associated animal toxicity observations in livestock is that episodes of poisoning often occur on a large scale, affecting tens or even hundreds of animals, so that there is little doubt as to the significance of the information. Livestock poisoning also tends to be worldwide in distribution, with numerous episodes reported in North America, Australia, and South Africa, where there have been significant efforts on the part of national and state governments to control losses. More recently, efforts to confront these problems, and consequently the amount and quality of information, have increased in areas such as China and parts of South America. With domestic animals, reports may only occur on an individual basis, but the close owner-pet relationship leads to more episodes being reported and carefully analyzed, cumulating in large numbers of documented cases in aggregate.

However, the types of toxicological information obtained can differ significantly between livestock and domestic animals. Livestock producers, because of their economic interests, are often more likely to be aware of both acute toxicity and chronic effects, such as lack of weight gain, birth defects, infertility, and abortion. Owners of domestic animals, which are not only restricted to cats and dogs but may also include individual cattle, sheep, goats, and horses, frequently report only acute toxicity, typically resulting from poisoning by a house or garden plant.

Serious adverse events reported in animals, such as livestock, may also provide helpful information. Reported effects of animal intoxications, similar to spontaneous human adverse event reports, tend to be scattered, with the only nationwide tracking system being the Animal Poison Control Center operated by the American Society for the Prevention of Cruelty to Animals, although this is generally more focused on pets than livestock (ASPCA, 2003). State veterinary diagnostic laboratories, usually located in close association with university veterinary schools, receive many reports of animal poisonings, but this information may not be routinely compiled for general use. However, a comprehensive database of poisonous plants with numerous links to other compilations is maintained by the Department of Animal Science at Cornell University (Cornell University, 2002). The U.S. Department of Agriculture (USDA)/Agricultural Research Service Poisonous Plant Research Laboratory (PPRL) in Logan, Utah, is the only laboratory in the world specifically conducting research entirely devoted to poisonous plants affecting livestock (USDA/ARS, 2003). This program was initiated over a century ago and data acquired since that time are voluminous. Staff at the PPRL, consisting of animal and range scientists, veterinarians, and natural products chemists, have access to most of this historical information and are aware of the most recent episodes of plant-livestock interactions.

The veterinary literature provides anecdotal observational information, but there is no single source. There are compendia on effects of poisonous plants on livestock for North America, Australia, and Southern Africa (Cheeke, 1998; Everist, 1981; Keeler and Tu, 1983, 1991; Kellerman et al.,

1988; Kingsbury, 1964). In addition, there are five volumes of proceedings of international symposia on poisonous plants, with particular emphasis on livestock poisonings (Colegate and Dorling, 1994; Garland and Barr, 1998; James et al., 1992; Keeler et al., 1978; Seawright et al., 1985).

Most of the available veterinary toxicology reports are observational and not experimental, and the relevance of various species of livestock to human toxicity is not well established. Nevertheless, **veterinary toxicology information may be quite useful when it corroborates concerns raised by other types of data. Independent of other types of data, evidence of harm in livestock and other veterinary toxicology information is appropriate to consider as a signal prompting an initial review of an ingredient.** In addition, the veterinary toxicology literature is also useful for generating hypotheses in need of testing in well-established animal models. A careful mechanism for ensuring continuing awareness by FDA of this important data source is suggested.

CONSIDERATIONS FOR ASSESSING ANIMAL DATA

Human Versus Animal Dose

The degree of potential human risk is a function of the nature and seriousness of the observed toxicity and the dose at which it occurs in animals relative to the expected human intake of the substance. One of the unique and powerful approaches of animal testing is the administration of high amounts of a substance over a short time period. This allows the detection of effects with small groups of animals, the prediction of possible effects following prolonged human exposure, and the prediction of possible effects on particularly sensitive human subpopulations. Many animal studies focused on toxicity evaluate increasing dosages until signs of toxicity are seen. While the amount administered may not appear relevant to the nonscientist, organ toxicities at elevated intake in acute or subchronic studies can be indicative of toxicities that may develop at lower doses during chronic use of the ingredient and should therefore not be disregarded simply because the dose administered is higher than that taken by humans. On the other hand, in certain instances, data will indicate that positive animal studies conducted at high doses may falsely predict human outcomes because the excessive doses used in animals overwhelm normal detoxification mechanisms that would protect against toxicity at actual levels of human exposure.

While the assumption should be that any effects observed in animals are relevant to humans, under some circumstances known differences between humans and animals with respect to the pharmacokinetics and metabolism of a substance, interspecies differences in pharmacodynamics, or

other well-characterized biological differences may lessen or eliminate concerns about human toxicity. Clues to such differences may arise when findings in one species of animal are not observed, under similar dosing conditions, in a second species. Such an observation is, however, only a clue, and cannot be taken by itself as evidence of irrelevance to humans. Rather, data that can be used to explain species differences are necessary to draw strong inferences regarding relevance or lack thereof.

Bioavailability, Pharmacokinetics and Knowledge of Absorption, Metabolism, Excretion, and Distribution Processes

When comparing the quantified ingested dose resulting in animal adverse effects with information about a human ingested dose, it is useful to consider the relationship between the amount ingested and the amount of the substance or its metabolites that reach the active site[1] (usually indicated by the concentration of unbound compound in the blood, and described in terms of bioavailability [see Chapter 3]). Pharmacokinetic processes, such as absorption, metabolism, excretion, and distribution, affect how much of the ingested substance actually reaches sites of action in the body. Differences in the pharmacokinetic processes of humans and experimental animals can lead to differences in the plasma concentration of active constituents that result from a given intake amount. Evaluating possible pharmacokinetic differences between experimental animals and humans requires some knowledge of the comparative absorption, distribution, metabolism, and excretion of the test substance in animals and in humans (Klaassen, 2001) and a judgment regarding the degree to which any observed differences in these measures are sufficient to discount animal test findings. The reality is that quantitative information about how these pharmacokinetic variables should appropriately impact the extrapolation of safety information from animals to humans is not available for many substances, especially dietary supplement ingredients. Thus this type of evaluation should be undertaken by experts on a case-by-case basis. **When detailed understanding of absorption, distribution, biotransformation, or excretion in experimental animals or humans is not available to make a comparison possible, it is appropriate to assume the most sensitive experimental animal studies are relevant to humans.**

Linear Versus Nonlinear Dose-Response Assumption

Mechanistic or mode-of-action information may be used to improve the risk assessment by providing information about the relationship be-

---

[1]See also discussion in Chapter 8.

tween dose and response. The default assumption, in the absence of any mechanistic or mode-of-action information, should be that a threshold or low-dose nonlinear dose-response relationship exists for health effects other than cancer; that is, that for noncancer health effects, there is a dose below which concern is not warranted. **The default assumption for cancer is a linear low-dose extrapolation.** This principle is important in considering the relevance of the dose of dietary supplements causing harm, as a linear dose extrapolation leads to the conclusion that any amount of the substance is a risk. The rationale for a linear or nonlinear assumption is not without its detractors, but it is an established principle used in risk assessment of other ingested substances (Rodricks et al., 2001) that should be applied to dietary supplements as well.

Pharmacodynamic Differences

In addition to the pharmacokinetic differences described above, there are several well-described examples of pharmacodynamic differences between animals and humans, that is, differences in how a chemical affects the body (Klaassen, 2001). For example, while rodent carcinogenicity studies are often predictive for human carcinogenesis from chemicals (Huff, 1999; Rodricks et al., 2001; Tomatis, 2001), some target sites in rats and mice have been questioned as relevant endpoints for human risk assessment (Capen et al., 1999; Rodricks et al., 2001). Examples include kidney toxicity/carcinogenicity in male rats related to the production of alpha-2-globulin (Rodricks et al., 2001), liver toxicity/carcinogenicity in rodents related to peroxisome proliferation (Rodricks et al., 2001), thyroid toxicity/carcinogenicity in rats (Capen et al., 1999), and bladder tumors in rats caused by terephthalate acid or cyclamate (IARC, 1999). When these specific endpoints are observed, they raise significant questions regarding relevance to humans. Such findings, or others that suggest irrelevance of the particular animal study evidence to humans, should be used to reach conclusions about possible human toxicity only after careful review. **In the absence of specific evidence that certain animal study findings are irrelevant to humans, animal evidence should be used to evaluate potential human risk.**

Variable Sensitivity of Humans to Adverse Effects

When interpreting a substance's effects or lack of effect in animal studies, it is important to remember the variability among humans in their sensitivity to toxic effects from ingested substances. Some members of the human population are more sensitive than the so-called average (Hayes, 2001), an issue best captured under the concept of "natural variability in response," a well-documented phenomenon. Many of these differences are due to known genetic polymorphisms (i.e., differences in a gene's DNA that occur in more than 1 percent of the population) (Hayes, 2001).

In general, it can be said that the human population, because of its extremely diverse genetic, environmental, nutritional, and disease status, is far more variable in response to chemicals than are populations of experimental animals.

Lack of Adverse Effects in Animals

As with any type of scientific study in which an effect is not observed, **it is important to remember that a lack of observed or reported detrimental effects in an animal study is not adequate evidence that a particular substance is "safe" to humans.**[2] The sensitivity of animal experiments in detecting particular effects is of utmost importance when extrapolating from animal studies to humans. Use of animal data to mitigate concerns raised by other data is appropriate only if animal studies are sensitive enough to detect adverse effects if they occur. Sensitivity depends on experimental design factors, such inclusion of positive controls, study power, and whether relevant endpoints were examined in the animals. For example, if an animal study only reported how many animals died or exhibited gross toxicity following short-term administration of an ingredient, it is not acceptable to conclude that this ingredient does not cause cancer following chronic intake by humans. Even if a lack of adverse effects in an appropriate model is reported, it is not scientifically valid to use such information to mitigate other types of information suggesting risk if the study does not have the statistical power necessary, is incompletely reported, does not include positive controls, or is otherwise inadequately designed to detect a risk. In summary, it is only negative data originating from well-designed studies or other credible sources that may mitigate or eliminate a concern raised by other data.

Quality Issues

While all animal experiments may be informative, the nature of the experimental design, the quality of the methodology, and the statistical significance of the results need to be taken into consideration in weighing the evidence of toxicity. As was mentioned earlier in this chapter, recommendations for well-designed safety tests using animals are described in FDA's *Redbook* (OFAS, 2001, 2003) while general characteristics of ideal

[2]See also Chapter 10.

BOX 5-1
Characteristics of High-Quality Animal Studies

A high-quality animal study is one that:

- uses good laboratory practices;
- is specifically designed as a toxicity, safety pharmacology, or safety study and includes sufficiently large doses to detect toxicity;
- uses unanesthetized, unrestrained animals on a semipurified diet;
- includes adequate controls;
- uses fully characterized composition and formulation of the test substance;
- uses a species that has pharmacokinetics similar to humans (bioavailability, distribution, metabolism, excretion);
- tests multiple doses of test substance;
- estimates blood or other tissue levels to ensure absorption and adequate exposure to active components to increase the likelihood the response will occur in humans;
- conducts clinical chemistry, blood, and urine analysis;
- uses more than a single species;
- administers the test substance orally; and
- conducts animal necropsy and histopathology.

animal studies are given in Box 5-1. Data from animal studies not meeting these criteria may be valuable as well and should be considered if they suggest a possible risk to human health. In summary, animal evidence should be used to evaluate potential concern for harm to human health unless the evidence indicates that the results are irrelevant.

WHEN DO ANIMAL DATA WARRANT CONSIDERATION AS AN INDICATOR OF SERIOUS RISK TO HUMAN HEALTH?

Pathophysiological Effects in Animals That Raise the Most Concern

Animal toxicity outcomes with clearly definable pathological changes are more compelling with regard to their relevance to humans than are outcomes in which only physiological or biochemical abnormalities are found. Thus, the concerns about possible human toxicity rise in proportion to both the seriousness and the severity of the toxic effects observed in animals and, more closely, those effects suggest the presence of a disease or pathological condition development process.

Clearly, animal studies that predict possible serious harm or death warrant more attention than those that predict mild, self-limiting effects on humans. Certain chronic animal toxicity or adverse biological effects data should be considered as immediate cause for higher or moderate concern,

TABLE 5-1 Guidelines for Relative Seriousness for Examples of Adverse Effects Obtained from Animal Studies

Category A (most serious)
- Neoplasia (including genotoxic and nongenotoxic carcinogens), teratogenesis, mortality
- Severe target organ toxicity
  - — Necrosis, dysplasia
  - — Reproductive failure, fetotoxicity, severe developmental effects
  - — Severe neurobehavioral changes

Category B (moderately serious)
- Moderate target organ toxicity
  - — Atrophy, hyperplasia
  - — Reduced reproductive capacity, moderate developmental effects
  - — Moderate neurobehavioral changes
- Clinical chemistry changes associated with histological lesions outside reference value ranges

Category C (less serious)
- Reduced body weight gain
- Body weight/organ weight ratios
- Reduced food consumption
- Enzyme changes, other biochemical and toxicity biomarker alterations unaccompanied by histological changes
- Reversible degenerative changes

regardless of the presence of high-quality human data suggesting no acute toxicity. This is because human exposure may need to be prolonged before such toxicities would be detected. Table 5-1 contains classifications of toxicity outcomes, ranked according to the nature of the effect, and provides a perspective on which effects are of greater concern. Three broad categories of effects are described. Those in Category A represent the clearest and most serious manifestations of toxicity, and if such effects are observed in well-conducted animal studies, there is a compelling basis for significant concern about comparable human toxicity (ignoring differences that may occur in dose and metabolism). Effects in Category B, while considered adverse, are of lesser concern, and those in Category C are of concern, but the concern is less than the other categories. Depending upon the ingested dosage at which the effect has been observed in animal studies relative to the level of human intake of the substance, and assuming there is no evidence that raises significant doubts about differences in toxic effects between animals and humans, effects in Category A should raise significant concerns about human toxicity even without data from other categories of evidence (e.g., human data). Effects in Category B may need to be buttressed by other data, and effects in Category C are considered less useful in raising questions of significant human toxicity without significant additional data. In general, it would not be advisable to solely use Category B or C effects to specify the seriousness of the adverse effects expected in humans.

The level of concern appropriate for different adverse findings increases when effects have been documented in well-designed and well-conducted animal studies, when the observed effects increase in severity or incidence with increasing dose, and/or when the observed effects are otherwise clearly related to the substance. An ideal study would be appropriately controlled, define the composition of the test material, administer the test material in measured quantities by the oral route, and use standardized and validated methods to measure toxicity accompanied by appropriate statistical analysis, interpretation, and reporting (see Box 5-1). **While many studies will not meet this ideal, they will nonetheless provide useful information and should be used if they suggest possible risk to human health.**[3] The strength of the evidence for toxicity is substantially increased if the effects were observed in more than one animal species, and even more so if supported by additional experimental data (e.g., *in vitro* data) or human data.

RISK ASSESSMENT STRATEGY FOR CONSIDERING ANIMAL DATA

Evaluating Risk with Animal Data

Under current law, FDA has the burden of providing evidence that one or more uses of a dietary supplement poses some identifiable significant or unreasonable *risk* to human health. Issues confronting FDA in regulating dietary supplements are not exactly analogous to those that arise in the premarketing approvals of other substances such as food additives, for which protocols for using animal data to establish *safety* have been developed. The traditional use of animal toxicity data to establish acceptable exposures has imbedded within it an element of caution—animal toxicity findings are used without significant question regarding the predictive power of specific findings for humans, and uncertainty factors are used to ensure safety. Use of protocols for setting safe levels (as opposed to evaluating risk) are outlined in Box 5-2. In assembling evidence regarding risks to health,

[3]For example, animal data resulting from non-oral exposure may be available and indicate adverse effects. Concentration of the ingredient (or its active constituents or metabolites) in animal blood that results in adverse effect can be compared with blood levels likely to result from human ingestion, with consideration of additional uncertainty factors as discussed in the text.

BOX 5-2
Setting Safe Levels and Tolerances in Foods

Over the past half century, a large effort has been devoted to the development and validation of a wide variety of protocols to guide the study of chemical toxicity in animals. At present, such protocols are available to study a broad range of adverse health effects, including the effects of acute, subchronic, and chronic dosing, effects on reproduction and development, and effects on the nervous and immune systems (Klaassen, 2001). The premarketing approval of food additives, both direct and indirect, food-use pesticides, and the evaluation of generally recognized as safe substances all depend heavily upon results from such animal studies. Those who propose to market such substances are required to conduct such studies and to ensure compliance with Good Laboratory Practice Regulations (21 C.F.R. § 58 [1978]). Adverse effects elucidated in animal toxicology studies are used to evaluate the safety of food ingredients and pesticide residues. The following assumptions have long been applied in making those safety evaluations:

1. The most sensitive indicator of adverse effects is selected from the entire body of reported animal data, relying on quality of the data and/or weight of the evidence.[a]
2. A lowest-observed-adverse-effect level (LOAEL—the minimum toxic dose) and a no-observed-adverse-effect level (NOAEL) for that effect are identified.
3. The NOAEL is divided by a series of uncertainty factors that are designed to accommodate variability in response between animals and humans and among humans (typically, factors of 10 for each). Additional factors may sometimes be introduced to deal with uncertainties in the database or to estimate a NOAEL from a LOAEL if the former is not available from the study.

The dosage (or intake) resulting from the above is taken as a safe level of daily intake for the human population; it is assumed to satisfy the "reasonable certainty of no harm" requirements of law.

[a]In the case of ingredients that are carcinogenic in animals, direct addition to food is prohibited for substances coming within the purview of the Delaney Clause Amendment to the Food, Drug, and Cosmetic Act (and regulated by FDA/Center for Food Safety and Applied Nutrition); for other substances (regulated by Environmental Protection Agency, Consumer Product Safety Commission, FDA/Center for Drug Evaluation and Research), a quantitative estimate of risk is derived from the data and a "safe" level is established at a very low level of risk.

the questions of the predictive power of animal studies, the dosages to which humans might be expected to be exposed, and the various types of toxicity observed in animals can become meaningful and significant. The purpose of the section that follows is to offer guidance on issues of risk.

Risk is defined as the probability that a substance or situation will produce harm under specified conditions and is a combination of probabil-

TABLE 5-2 Relative Spectrum of Concern: Guidelines for Types of Evidence from Animal Studies[a]

Increasing Concern →		
At least one acceptable, quality study showing effects of Category A at Dose > 1,000× Human Intake	At least one acceptable, quality study showing effects of Category A at Dose > 100 to < 1,000× Human Intake	At least one acceptable, quality study showing effects of Category A at Dose < 100× Human Intake
OR	OR	OR
At least one acceptable, quality study showing effects of Category B at Dose > 100× Human Intake	At least one acceptable, quality study showing effects of Category B at Dose > 10 to < 100× Human Intake	At least one acceptable, quality study showing effects of Category B at Dose < 10× Human Intake
OR	OR	OR
At least one acceptable, quality study showing effects of Category C at Dose > 10× Human Intake	At least one acceptable, quality study showing effects of Category C at Dose > 1 to < 10× Human Intake	At least one acceptable, quality study showing effects of Category C at Dose ≤ 1× Human Intake
OR		
Studies showing adverse effects, but which cannot be interpreted because of deficiencies in design, conduct, or reporting		
OR		
Acceptable, quality non-oral studies indicating adverse effect from Category A, B, or C		

[a] Categories A, B, and C refer to relative seriousness of a variety of adverse effects identified in animal studies, ranging from reproductive failure (A) to reduced food consumption (C). See Table 5-1 for further examples.

ity and consequences. Risk assessment is an organized process used to describe and estimate the likelihood of adverse health outcomes from exposure to chemicals. The four steps in risk assessment are hazard identification, dose-response assessment, exposure assessment, and risk characterization (NRC, 1996). The risk assessment model proposed in this chapter for using animal data is to consider that the data are a means to integrate information about the seriousness of the observed animal toxicity (Table 5-1) with information about the human dose and the animal dose at which the toxicity occurs. The result is incorporated in the relative spectrum of concern figure for animal data (Table 5-2), providing a practical and general mechanism to estimate the relevance of animal dose when setting priorities for further evaluation.

Rationale for the Risk Assessment Strategy

Box 5-2 outlines an approach for risk assessment based on animal data. This approach starts with a dose known to cause a no-observed-adverse-effect level (NOAEL) and/or the lowest dose known to cause any effect (lowest-observed-adverse-effect level, or LOAEL) to derive a dosage that is considered safe. These concepts are generally accepted by the toxicology community to provide some general guidance when determining how much of a substance can safely be consumed. In the case of the postmarketing situation that currently exists for dietary supplements where limited resources may necessitate a focus primarily on serious adverse effects, **it is appropriate to apply some of the scientifically accepted concepts to determine which serious adverse effects observed in animals warrant further investigation or suggest an unreasonable risk may exist.**

In developing safe limits, uncertainty factors have been applied to animal toxicity threshold values (NOAELs) to reach estimates of human dosages that are likely to represent thresholds for the most sensitive members of the human population (see Box 5-2). These uncertainty factors are a scientifically accepted framework for setting priorities when complete data are not available. Uncertainty "default" values of 10 are used for each significant source of variability, such as cross-species differences and interindividual differences between and among humans.

A series of studies provides evidence that the factors of 10 are generally adequate to deal with these sources of variability and, in most cases, are more than is necessary (Dourson and Stara, 1983; Dourson et al., 1996; NRC, 1994). The factors of 10 are widely used as default values in the United States and internationally. There is wide recognition that, in specific cases, pharmacokinetic data, if available, provide better estimates of variability. As comparative pharmacokinetic data that allow the development of models for quantitative interspecies extrapolation (physiologically based pharmacokinetic models) become available, they may be used to replace at least a fraction of the interspecies default uncertainty factor.

Guidelines for Considering Seriousness of Effect and Dose Using a Risk Assessment Model

The following guidelines relate the human intake level of the dietary supplement ingredient under review to the minimum experimental dose required to cause toxicity (LOAEL). For toxic effects that fall into the most serious category, **Category A** (see Table 5-1), **human intakes that exceed**

one-one hundredth (0.01) of the test animal dose for that effect (and not for any lower dose effects that may fall into Categories B or C) should be considered to represent a significant risk to human health. Such a recommendation, which does not include several of the cautious (public health protective) assumptions that are associated with a safety assessment, nevertheless represents a balance between overinterpretation of animal findings and the need to consider population variability in response. **For toxic effects falling into Category B, human intakes that exceed one-tenth (0.10) of the test animal dose for that effect (and not for any lower dose that may fall into Category C) should be considered to represent a significant risk to human health.**

These are offered as general guidelines, but they should not be interpreted as inflexible rules. The general guidelines offered here should be seen as useful for relatively rapid decision-making to set priorities for utilization of limited resources, with more thorough evaluation of all relevant data necessary to confirm the strength of the evidence. Thus, FDA should evaluate evidence of toxicity and make some general findings regarding the strength of the evidence. For example, for effects falling into Category A and exhibiting clear dose-response relationships, similar findings in multiple species/strains/sexes of animals, supporting *in vitro* data or information about related substances, and/or evidence from human studies, there can be justification for considering human intakes at levels less than 0.01 of the animal effect dose as representing a potentially serious health risk. While studies of acceptable quality are most useful, combined evidence from other studies may also be useful depending upon the limitations of the studies. **Carcinogenicity findings, particularly those that are accompanied by evidence of genotoxicity[4] and within the 100× expected human exposure, are of particular concern.** Any dietary supplement ingredient having such activity presents the highest degree of potential seriousness (Category A).

The guidelines described above for relating the type of effect observed to the dose are summarized in Table 5-2. Situations described in the right-hand column of Table 5-2 signal the highest degree of concern for human risks and suggest a significant risk to human health, even in the absence of any human information regarding adverse effects. Situations described in the middle column are of less concern, and ingredients with this level of evidence may not represent a significant health risk unless such risk is confirmed with human or other types of data. Situations described in the left-hand column are of lower concern and thus by themselves present a relatively minor public health concern.

---

[4]Genotoxicity is discussed in Chapter 7.

SUMMARY

The guiding principle related to animal data is as follows: "Even in the absence of information on adverse events in humans, evidence of harm from animal studies is often indicative of potential harm to humans. This indication assumes greatest importance when the route of exposure is oral, the formulation tested is identical or highly similar to that consumed by humans in an ingredient, and more than one species shows the same or similar toxicity."

The rationale and importance of this principle have been presented, and the following corollaries, along with their rationales and limitations:

- In the absence of specific evidence that certain animal study findings are irrelevant to humans, animal evidence should be used to evaluate potential human risk.
- A lack of observed or reported detrimental effects in an animal study is not evidence that a particular substance is "safe."
- Veterinary toxicology information may be useful when it corroborates concerns raised by other types of data. Independent of other types of data, evidence of harm in livestock and other veterinary toxicology information is appropriate to consider as a signal prompting an initial review of an ingredient. In addition, the veterinary toxicology literature is also useful for generating hypotheses in need of testing in well-established animal models.
- When there is no detailed understanding of pharmacokinetics to make a comparison between animals or humans possible, it is appropriate to assume that the most sensitive experimental animal studies are relevant to human health.
- Much of the animal study data available for dietary supplement ingredients will not have the characteristics of ideal studies, but these studies should nonetheless be considered if they suggest possible human health risk.
- Animal studies that predict possible serious harm or death warrant more attention than those that predict mild, self-limiting effects in humans.
- Certain chronic animal toxicity or adverse biological effects data should be considered as immediate cause for higher or moderate concern, regardless of the presence of high-quality human data suggesting no acute toxicity (see Category A in Table 5-1).
- The default assumption for cancer is a linear low-dose extrapolation. Carcinogenicity findings, particularly those that are accompanied by evidence of genotoxicity and observed in animals at ingested amounts within 100× of expected human exposure, are of particular concern.

- As a general guideline, human intakes that exceed one-one hundredth (0.01) of animal doses that produce Category A effects (see Table 5-1) should be considered to represent a significant risk to human health. Human intakes that exceed one-tenth (0.1) of the animal doses that produce Category B effects should be considered to represent a significant risk to human health.

REFERENCES

ASPCA (American Society for the Prevention of Cruelty to Animals). 2003. *Animal Poison Control Center*. Online. Available at http://www.napcc.aspca.org. Accessed July 8, 2003.

Capen CC, Dybing E, Rice JM, Wilbourn JD, eds. 1999. *Species Differences in Thyroid, Kidney and Urinary Bladder Carcinogenesis. International Agency for Research on Cancer (IARC) Scientific Publication No. 147*. Lyon, France: IARC.

CDER (Center for Drug Evaluation and Research). 2002. *Guidance Documents*. Online. Food and Drug Administration. Available at http://www.fda.gov/cder/guidance/index.htm. Accessed May 2, 2002.

Cheeke PR. 1998. *Natural Toxicants in Feeds, Forages, and Poisonous Plants*. 2nd ed. Danville, IL: Interstate Publishers.

Colegate SM, Dorling PR, eds. 1994. *Plant-Associated Toxins: Agricultural, Phytochemical and Ecological Aspects*. Wallingford, UK: CAB International.

Cornell University. 2002. *Poisonous Plants Informational Database*. Online. Available at http://www.ansci.cornell.edu/plants/index.html. Accessed July 8, 2003.

Dourson ML, Stara JF. 1983. Regulatory history and experimental support of uncertainty (safety) factors. *Regul Toxicol Pharmacol* 3:224–238.

Dourson ML, Felter SP, Robinson D. 1996. Evolution of science-based uncertainty factors in noncancer risk assessment. *Regul Toxicol Pharmacol* 24:108–120.

Everist SL. 1981. *Poisonous Plants of Australia*. London: Angus & Robertson Publishers.

Garland T, Barr AC, eds. 1998. *Toxic Plants and Other Natural Toxicants*. Wallingford, UK: CAB International.

Hayes W. 2001. *Principles and Methods of Toxicology*. 4th ed. Philadelphia: Taylor and Francis.

Huff J. 1999. Long-term chemical carcinogenesis bioassays predict human cancer hazards. Issues, controversies, and uncertainties. *Ann NY Acad Sci* 895:56–79.

IARC (International Agency for Research on Cancer). 1999. Cyclamates. *IARC Monogr Eval Carcinog Risks Hum* 73:195–222.

ICH/FDA (International Conference on Harmonisation/Food and Drug Administration). 2001. *Guidance for Industry: S7A Safety Pharmacology Studies for Human Pharmaceuticals*. Rockville, MD: FDA.

James LF, Keeler RF, Cheeke PR, Bailey EM Jr, Hegarty MP, eds. 1992. *Poisonous Plants*. Ames, IA: Iowa State University Press.

Keeler RF, Tu AT, eds. 1983. *Handbook of Natural Toxins. Volume 1. Plant and Fungal Toxins*. New York: Marcel Dekker.

Keeler RF, Tu AT. 1991. *Handbook of Natural Toxins, Volume 6. Toxicology of Plant and Fungal Compounds*. New York: Marcel Dekker.

Keeler RF, Van Kampen KR, James LF, eds. 1978. *Effects of Poisonous Plants on Livestock*. New York: Academic Press.

Kellerman TS, Coetzer JAW, Naudé TW. 1988. *Plant Poisonings and Mycotoxicoses of Livestock in Southern Africa*. Cape Town, South Africa: Oxford University Press.

Kingsbury JM. 1964. *Poisonous Plants of the United States and Canada.* Englewood Cliffs, NJ: Prentice-Hall.

Klaassen CD, ed. 2001. *Casarett and Doull's Toxicology: The Basic Science of Poisons.* New York: McGraw-Hill.

Mishra HN, Das C. 2003. A review on biological control and metabolism of Aflatoxin. *Crit Rev Food Sci Nutr* 43:245–264.

NRC (National Research Council). 1994. *Science and Judgment in Risk Assessment.* Washington, DC: National Academy Press.

NRC. 1996. *Understanding Risk: Informing Decisions in a Democratic Society.* Washington, DC: National Academy Press.

NRC. 2001. *Evaluating Chemical and Other Agent Exposures for Reproductive and Developmental Toxicity.* Washington, DC: National Academy Press.

NTP (National Toxicology Program). 2002. *Report on Carcinogens.* 10th ed. Research Triangle Park, NC: NTP.

OFAS (Office of Food Additive Safety). 2001. *Toxicological Principles for the Safety Assessment of Direct Food Additives and Color Additives Used in Food. Redbook II-Draft.* Washington, DC: OFAS, Food and Drug Administration.

OFAS. 2003. *Redbook 2000. Toxicological Principles for the Safety of Food Ingredients.* Online. CFSAN Food and Drug Administration. Available at http://www.cfsan.fda.gov/~redbook/red-toca.html. Accessed June 19, 2003.

Rodricks JV, Gaylor DW, Turnbull D. 2001. Quantitative extrapolations in toxicology. In: Hayes AW, ed. *Principles and Methods of Toxicology.* 4th ed. Philadelphia: Taylor and Francis.

Seawright AE, Hegarty MP, Keeler RF, James LF, eds. 1985. *Plant Toxicology.* Brisbane: Queensland Poisonous Plants Committee.

Tomatis L. 2001. The identification of human carcinogens and primary prevention of cancer. *Mutat Res* 462:407–421.

USDA/ARS (United States Department of Agriculture/Agricultural Research Service). 2003. *Poisonous Plant Research Laboratory (PPRL).* Online. Available at http://www.pprl.usu.edu. Accessed July 8, 2003.

WHO (World Health Organization). 1999. *Principles for the Assessment of Risk to Human Health from Exposure to Chemicals.* Geneva: WHO.

6
Categories of Scientific Evidence—Information About Related Substances

It is scientifically acceptable and appropriate to use information about safety concerns of related substances to inform a decision about the risk associated with a dietary supplement ingredient, especially in the absence of information about the activity of the ingredient in question in humans, animals, or *in vitro* experiments.[1] Information about substances related to the dietary supplement ingredient of interest may be helpful when predicting risk in one of the following ways:

- Chemical relatedness—similarity to known toxic chemicals or presence of constituents similar in structure to known toxicophores. Chemical structures associated with potential adverse effects;
- Taxonomic relatedness—similarity to known toxic plant species, genus, or family; and
- Functional relatedness—the dietary supplement ingredient of interest is related to another substance because they share a common biological target or mechanism of action that is clearly tied to a toxic effect. This includes endogenous substances and mimetics of endogenous substances when the effect of increasing the amount of an endogenous substance is linked to an adverse health effect.

[1]Note that this chapter describes the application of information on risk and safety concerns of related substances to the dietary supplement ingredient in question, not the converse (using information suggesting safety to mitigate concerns about the dietary supplement ingredient).

The value and utility of these types of information, taken together, to predict risk depends on the type of dietary supplement ingredient that is being considered. Cause for concern with a botanical dietary supplement may be derived from information about risk associated with known chemical constituents, as well as information about risk associated with related toxic plants. Similarly, information about the potential risk of dietary supplements that are pure single chemical compounds may be derived by reviewing a list of known risk-associated chemical compounds and chemical moieties (toxicophores) that raise concern of safety. However, for information about what might occur following ingestion of substances that are normally present in the human body (endogenous substances), it is helpful to understand what the substances do in the body at normal concentrations and to understand their mechanisms of action well enough to shed light on what might occur if the normal concentrations are exceeded. Certainly, for particular dietary supplement ingredients, such information could be more useful than reviewing a list of unrelated toxic chemical structures or substances that are not endogenous. Finally, especially when dietary supplements have undefined chemical composition[2] but information about biological activity is available, it may be helpful and it is appropriate to consider whether the exhibited biological activity is the basis for safety concerns of other substances that are considered potentially harmful. Provided below are guiding principles and further descriptions of the different types of "relatedness" information, including discussion of when and why it is appropriate to use this type of information and specific questions that may help in extrapolating the most useful information.

CONSIDERING INFORMATION ABOUT CHEMICAL COMPONENTS AND RELATED BOTANICALS AS SIGNALS OF POTENTIAL RISK OF BOTANICAL DIETARY SUPPLEMENT INGREDIENTS

GUIDING PRINCIPLE: *Consumption of any botanical ingredient carries a certain degree of inherent risk to at least some segments of the human population, even for those plants used as foods or with a history of use for medicinal purposes. In the absence of comprehensive human trials establishing safety, scientific evidence for risk can be obtained by considering whether the plant constituents are*

[2]An example of a nonbotanical dietary supplement with undefined chemical composition might be a preparation from a living organism or otherwise complex substance—shark cartilage is an example.

compounds with established toxicity or closely related in structure to compounds with established toxicity, or whether the plant source of the botanical dietary supplement is itself a toxic plant or is taxonomically related to a known toxic plant.

It is well known that plants produce secondary metabolites with biological activities in mammals, and that plant toxicities are due to chemical constituents in plants. Indeed, the rationale for the use of botanical dietary supplements is that they are likely to affect human function. The challenge in assessing risk in the use of dietary supplements is to establish whether the plant compounds present a hazard to humans and, if so, whether the conditions of use suggest risk.

Risk is always considered a function of two factors: hazard and exposure. In the case of botanical ingredients, hazard relates to the presence of biologically active metabolites produced naturally by biosynthetic processes within the plant. In contrast, exposure may be a consequence of the amount of any particular substance produced by the plant, its concentration or dilution during manufacture, and user intake level and bioavailability (see Chapter 3). Thus consumption of a botanical containing a high level of potentially dangerous bioactive substances, consumed at high dosages or for prolonged periods, will significantly increase risk.

It is possible to make educated estimates of the potential hazard of any given botanical through consideration of the types of biologically active compounds that may be present in the plant (constituents of concern) and the nature of the plant (taxonomic relationships). The goal is to consider two likely scenarios that could provide some guidance regarding the possible toxicity of a botanical dietary supplement ingredient (1) where a known constituent of the plant is, or is structurally similar to, a known toxic compound; and (2) where a plant genus or species is, or is closely related to, a plant known to be toxic. When there is evidence that a botanical is taxonomically related to known poisonous plants and that particular constituents are established as having deleterious effects, the convergence of these factors compels detailed consideration of the potential risks associated with the use of the ingredient.

Information about the potential biological activity of a plant-derived dietary supplement ingredient is obtained by reviewing information about the plant's individual chemical components to determine if any of the constituents raise concerns. **Given that related plants have related chemical composition, with more closely related plants generally having more similar chemical constituents, it is therefore also appropriate to consider the activity of other plants in the same plant family or genus to predict composition and potential toxicity.**

This approach of considering the taxonomic relatives of the dietary supplement ingredient has its limitations, however. That is, not all genera of a given family will contain similar toxic components. Furthermore, the concentration of potentially dangerous compounds in the final product will be affected by the plant part being utilized and the manner of preparation, processing, and formulation, as well as by growth conditions that can produce variation in chemical constituents (e.g., climate, season, soil conditions).

Chemical Constituents of Concern

Secondary metabolites of plants are generally low-molecular-weight compounds (~ < 1000 Daltons), originally thought to be biosynthesized by the plant primarily for purposes other than basic nutritional and metabolic requirements for normal growth and reproduction (Harborne, 1993). When produced, these metabolites confer "fitness" on the plant, enabling it to respond to and counteract external influences, such as competition for resources, environmental stresses, herbivory, and microbiological or viral attack. The biosynthetic mechanisms by which certain of these compounds (phytoalexins) are produced may essentially shut down unless there is an external stimulus that triggers their production for defensive purposes (Fong, 2002; Harborne, 1993). Other compounds may always be present because evolutionary pressures have established their necessity.

Known Constituents of Concern

Known chemicals and classes of chemicals that are botanical constituents and warrant concern for safety are listed in Box 6-1, a list generated largely from consideration of plant genera of concern identified in the next section of this chapter. Some of the mechanisms of these compounds, as well as information about plants containing them, are described in the discussion of plant families in Appendix C. (Other compounds or classes of compounds act through mechanisms that are only theoretical or are not understood.) Appendix C describes how some of these compounds are ingested in conventional foods where the amounts ingested are limited or are in different forms due to processing (e.g., cooking). This list is not intended to be all inclusive, but rather to highlight some of the compounds that may result in adverse effects from ingesting plants. Some of these compounds cause more serious deleterious effects than others and some compounds are more potent than others. It is suggested that this list be taken as a general guideline helpful to the Food and Drug Administration (FDA) in determining which botanical substances may warrant higher priority attention. Evidence that one or more of these chemical constituents is present in a botanical dietary supplement should be considered as an indicator of increased concern for potential toxicity of the specific botanical product, except when consumed as constituents of conventional foods, unless additional information mitigates concern. Further investigation may result in mitigated concern if it is found that circulating concentrations of constituents resulting in adverse effects are substantially lower than circulating concentrations reached with dietary supplement ingestion or if quality animal toxicity studies suggest that the effects are unlikely to occur from the amounts or preparations ingested as dietary supplements. As indicated, some of the substances listed are classes of compounds rather than individual chemical constituents. In this case, some members of a given class may be of less or no concern (see also Appendix C), as will be uncovered by a search of the available literature. For example, a literature search may reveal conclusive evidence that specific structural features required for toxicity are not present for some members of a given class.

Of all classes of botanical toxic compounds, those classified as alkaloids predominate in causing concern because a large proportion have been associated with biological activities and/or toxic effects in mammals (Harborne, 1993; Seawright et al., 1985). Thus particular attention is warranted for dietary supplement ingredients containing alkaloids. Although most chemists recognize and agree on whether a particular compound is an alkaloid, there has been considerable discussion as to how to define such compounds simply because they do not conform to a single structural type. The most workable definition is probably that of Pelletier (1983), which states that "an alkaloid is a cyclic organic compound containing nitrogen in a negative oxidation state which is of limited distribution among living organisms."[3] This definition excludes simple amines, amino acids, peptides, proteins, nucleic acids, and nucleotides, which are ubiquitous, as well as nitro compounds such as aristolochic acid, in which the nitrogen is not in a negative oxidation state. It is particularly noteworthy that the definition does not carry a requirement for pharmacological activity. This is appropriate because many newly isolated alkaloids may not have been tested, and even those of long standing will not have been evaluated for each and every type of activity. Nevertheless, **alkaloid-containing plants should always be suspected of being capable of pharmacological activity and should be considered as risk factors.**

---

[3]Many other definitions often include a statement that alkaloids usually are biologically active (Cordell et al., 2001).

BOX 6-1
Specific Botanical Chemical Constituents of Concern and General Classes of Constituents of Concern

Constituents

3-hydroxy-4(1*H*)-pyridone
4'-demethylpodophyllotoxin
abrin[a]
aconitine and pseudoaconitine
anemonin
amygdalin
arecoline
atractyloside
australine
beta-phenethylamine
canavanine
carboxyatractyloside
castanospermine
colchicine[1]
convallatoxin
coriamyrtin
cycasin
cyclopamine
cytosine
dicoumarol
digitoxin
digoxin
fagopyrine
galanthamine
helenalin, hymenovin
hydrogen cyanide
hyoscyamine
hypoglycin A
indospicine
isocupressic acid
isoperoxisomicine A-1
lantadene A and B
lycoctonine
lyoniatoxin
macrozamin
mandelonitrile
methyllycaconitine
mimosine
monocrotaline
nicotine
β-nitropropionic acid
nordihydroguaiaretic acid
norephedrine (phenylpropanolamine)
α-peltatin
peroxisomicine A-1

Classes of Constituents

agroclavine alkaloids[a,b]
alkenyl catechols (urushiols)
amino-butyric and -propionic acids and nitriles
anthracene dimers
aristolochic acids[a]
bufadienolides[a]
cardenolides,[a]
cardiac glycosides
coumarins
cyanogenic glycosides (phaseolunatin) and other cyanogenic compounds[a]
cyclopropane amino acids
dibenzofurans
diterpene acids
diterpenoid alkaloids[a]
ephedrine and related alkaloids
ergot alkaloids[a,b]
furanoeremophilanes
glucosinolates[c]
grayanotoxins
indole alkaloids[a]
indolizidine alkaloids[a]
isoquinoline alkaloids[a]
labdane diterpene acids
methylazoxymethanol glycosides
morphinan alkaloids
nicotine alkaloids[a]
nitrates, nitrites
nitrophenathrenes[a]
nitrosamines[a]
nojirimycin and derivatives
oxalates
penitrem alkaloids[a,b]
phenalenones
phenylpropanolamine
phorbol esters[a]
piperidine alkaloids[a]
podophyllotoxin-type lignans
polyacetylenes
polyhydroxy alkaloids (swainsonine, calystegines)[a]
polyhydroxy nortropanes
pressor amines

Constituents	Classes of Constituents
phenylpropanolamine	pyrrolizidine alkaloids[a]
physostigmine (eserine)	quinolizidine alkaloids[a]
picrotoxin	rotenoids
podophyllotoxin	steroidal alkaloids[a]
protoanemonin	taxoids
N-propyl disulfide	thiooxazolidones
prunasin	tremetone and derivatives
ptaquiloside	trichothecenes
ranunculin	tropane alkaloids[a]
ricin[a]	
safrole	
sanguinarine	
scopolamine	
senecionine	
seneciphylline	
solanine	
solasonine	
sparteine	
strychnine	
tetradymol	
tomatine	
trichodesmine	
tutin	
tyramine	
zearalenone	
zygacine	
zygadenine	

NOTE: The chemical constituents and general classes of constituents listed in this table were largely derived from the list of botanicals in Table 6-1 by committee members knowledgeable in botanicals and phytochemicals and who consulted the references listed at the end of the chapter as needed. A review of each chemical on this list was not practical within the constraints of this report. The list should thus be considered as a general guideline for determining which chemical constituents and classes of constituents warrant attention, not as an authoritative statement on any chemical constituent or class in particular. When consumed as minor constituents of conventional foods prepared via conventional methods, these constituents are of little concern.

---

[a]Particularly hazardous, would probably be considered as "A" toxicity as defined in toxicity descriptions in Table 6-1 (A: Reports of adverse effects to the heart, liver, lungs, kidney, immune system, and reproductive system, teratogenicity, carcinogenesis, central nervous system [convulsant], or death in animals or humans).

[b]Depending on dose, alkaloids could be considered as exhibiting A, B, or C level of potential toxicities.

[c]And isothiocyanates, the toxic hydrolytic products of the naturally occurring glucosinolates (glycosides).

Identifying Other Chemical Constituents in Botanicals That May Be of Concern

In addition to known chemicals highlighted in Box 6-1, other structurally related chemical constituents should also be of concern, unless there is convincing information suggesting that particular structural features are required for toxicity and these are not present. It is important to note that if a botanical is known to contain a chemical constituent that is structurally related to a chemical that is regulated (e.g., as a drug), this is a reason for concern and should be investigated. It is not possible to specifically define all the ways that different chemicals may be related, but this concept can be illustrated with an example. Substances with similar chemical structures, such as ephedrine and amphetamine, are structurally related, and substances that stimulate or inhibit activity at the same cellular receptors or other biological targets are "functionally" related (see discussion later in this chapter). Similarity of dietary supplement ingredients to biologically active metabolic intermediates, such as cytokines or hormones, may also be important if the actions of metabolic intermediates provide clues about the activity of a dietary supplement ingredient; this concept is discussed in the "endogenous substances" section.

Taxonomic Relationships and Genera of Concern

GUIDING PRINCIPLE: *If a botanical dietary supplement was derived from a plant that belongs to a genus known to contain toxic compounds, it is scientifically reasonable to presume that the same compounds will be present in the dietary supplement and thus may pose a risk from ingestion of the ingredient, unless there is reason to believe that the plant or plant part being used does not cause the effect or contain the toxic substances.*

Frequently, information about the chemical constituents or the distribution of chemical constituents throughout a plant used to make a dietary supplement will not be complete. In this case, it will be helpful and appropriate to consider whether a botanical is related to plants that are of concern.[4] The system of naming, ranking, and classifying plants and other

---

[4]It is also appropriate to consider information about related plants even when information about the chemical constituents of the botanical in question is available.

organisms based on morphology is now being guided by analysis of metabolites and molecular genetics. There is no doubt that, as progression is made to an increasing degree of specialization through the hierarchy sequence of family, genus, species, subspecies/variety/cultivar, and plant organ, there will be a corresponding increase in congruence, not only in physical appearance, but also in the nature of secondary metabolites produced and sequestered by the plant. Therefore, as any group of plant species becomes more closely related, the compounds biosynthesized will become more similar in both structural types and specific constituents. Thus, in summary, evidence that a botanical bears a close taxonomic relationship to known toxic plants should be used to evaluate potential human risk in the absence of scientific information that such data are not relevant. (See Box 6-2 for a summary of questions to be asked and Box 6-3 for notes on botanical nomenclature.)

Plants in the same genera will not necessarily produce compounds with exactly the same structure, but they are likely to produce the same structural classes of compounds. For example, different species of the genus *Senecio* (Asteraceae), in spite of being widely distributed in many parts of the world and growing under vastly different climatic conditions, are invariably found to contain pyrrolizidine alkaloids on phytochemical examination (Hartmann and Witte, 1995). Since chemical structure and biological activity are intimately related, novel pyrrolizidine alkaloids should be assumed to possess at least some degree of the hepatotoxic activity established for the most common members of this class (Hartmann and Witte, 1995) if information to prove otherwise is not available. (In this case, data suggest that hepatotoxicity of pyrrolizidine alkaloids depends on unsaturated 1,2 bonds in one of the rings [Hartmann and Witte, 1995].) For the purposes of this framework, taxonomic classification helps in identifying plants that are likely to have similar chemical components. Therefore, much information can be gained by reviewing what is known about plants that are taxonomically related to the dietary supplement ingredient under consideration.

The chemical composition of a given plant species can vary depending on the conditions under which it was grown. However, it is rare for a chemical compound to be observed in one specimen of a species, but not in another specimen of the same species, except due to artifactual differences in analysis techniques. It is more likely that differences in the levels of particular compounds will be observed (Fong, 2002; Harborne, 1993). This is because the array of phytochemicals that a given species may contain is under genetic control; thus each plant has the potential to create the same range of phytochemicals. While the environment and growth conditions may impact phytochemicals found in a given plant, plants of a species known to contain harmful phytochemicals under some conditions should

BOX 6-2
Questions to Be Asked Regarding Taxonomic Relationships of Botanicals

- Is the supplement formulated from a plant that is in a known toxic plant *family*?
- Is the supplement classified in a *genus* known to contain toxins or suspected of being unsafe?
- Is the supplement classified in a *species/subspecies/variety/cultivar* known to contain toxins?
- Does the supplement contain a particular *plant part* known to contain toxins in a dangerous level?

BOX 6-3
Notes About Botanical Nomenclature

When searching for chemical or pharmacological information, it should be kept in mind that plant synonymy is often encountered at both the family and genus level. Although several nomenclature systems have been used over the years and changes by taxonomists are encountered, the dual names are found primarily in a few plant families, namely:

Compositae	=	Asteraceae
Cruciferae	=	Brassicaceae
Graminae	=	Poaceae
Guttiferae	=	Clusiaceae
Labiatae	=	Lamiaceae
Leguminosae	=	Fabaceae
Palmae	=	Arecaceae
Umbelliferae	=	Apiaceae

Nomenclature changes were made in those plant families ending in -ae so that all plant families would have the conventional -aceae ending.

At the genus level nomenclature is constantly being changed or corrected. For example, one can find chemical and pharmacological information in the literature for the plant *Catharanthus roseus* under the binomials *Vinca rosea, Lochnera rosea*, and *Ammocallis roseus*, which are all the same plant. At the beginning of a literature search it is essential to know the specific parameters to be used with regard to botanical terminology. It is suggested that the *Index Kewensis* (online) can be used, but botanical expertise is necessary to interpret the data (IPNI, 2004). A less complicated reference source to ascertain correct Latin binomials and family classification for a given plant or group of plants is Mabberley (1997). One can obtain the following information from this reference:

Search	*Find*
a. Common Name	Latin Binomial
b. Genus Name	Possible synonymy and common uses, including (some) toxicity

be assumed to have them even if grown under different conditions. Analyses that suggest specimens of a given plant species do not contain a hazardous phytochemical usually associated with the plant should be carefully considered to ensure that the analysis techniques are appropriately sensitive.

The presence of toxic compounds has been traditionally associated with a number of plant genera and families (e.g., Liliaceae are known to contain cardiac glycosides, Euphorbiaceae are known to contain phorbol esters and toxic diterpenes). The ability to anticipate the presence of specific classes of compounds based on plant family and genus knowledge may be helpful in predicting potential toxicity. Table 6-1[5] highlights some of the plant genera to which FDA may want to give attention. Also important are the nuances of information about each plant family, which are discussed in Appendix C. It is important to note that this table is not intended to provide a complete reference or to be inclusive, but it serves to provide FDA with a starting point of plant genera that warrant concern. The primary difficulty in using information about related plants to infer information about the toxicity of a particular plant arises when the family encompasses both valuable food plants and species capable of producing toxic compounds (see discussion of traditional use as a food plant below and specific examples in Appendix C).

Considerations Regarding Concerns Raised by Taxonomic Relationships or Chemical Constituents of Concern

There are a number of considerations that may mitigate or exacerbate concerns raised by the taxonomic relationship of a dietary supplement ingredient to a hazardous botanical or knowledge that a botanical contains chemical constituents of concern. These are described here, followed by discussion of how these and other factors should impact the use of historical consumption information as a mitigator of concern.

Plant Parts

Chemical compounds are differentially distributed in various parts of plants. When secondary metabolites are biosynthesized for the purpose of

---

[5]Note that association of these plants with toxic effects may well be a reflection of the degree of phytochemical examination to which they have been subjected, given that there is more reason to investigate plants that are cultivated for specific purposes. Other plant families may be relatively neglected (phytochemically), especially those that are of limited distribution or occur in remote areas.

TABLE 6-1 Genera of Concern

Primary Genera of Concern	Family	Compounds and Compound Classes Implicated in Toxicity
Abrus	Fabaceae	Abrin
Aconitum	Ranunculaceae	Diterpenoid alkaloids
Actaea	Ranunculaceae	Quinolizidine alkaloids
Adenostyles	Asteraceae	Pyrrolizidine alkaloids
Agave	Agavaceae	Saponins
Agrostemma	Caryopyhllaceae	Saponins
Aleurites	Euphorbiaceae	Unknown
Allium[b]	Liliaceae	N-propyl disulfide
Amsinckia	Boraginaceae	Pyrrolizidine alkaloids
Anamirta	Menispermaceae	Picrotoxin
Anchusa	Boraginaceae	Pyrrolizidine alkaloids
Anemone	Ranunculaceae	Protoanemonin
Apium[b]	Apiaceae	Coumarins
Apocynum	Apocynaceae	Cardiac glycosides
Areca	Arecaceae	Arecoline
Argemone	Papaveraceae	Isoquinoline alkaloids
Arisaema	Araceae	Oxalates
Aristolochia	Aristolochiaceae	Aristolochic acids
Armoracia	Brassicaceae	Isothiocyanates, Thiooxazolidones
Arnica	Asteraceae	Sesquiterpenes
Asclepias	Asclepidaceae	Cardiac glycosides
Astragalus	Fabaceae	Polyhydroxy alkaloids (swainsonine) Nitro-alcohols and -acids, Selenium accumulation
Atractylis	Asteraceae	Atractyloside and related compounds
Atropa	Solanaceae	Tropane alkaloids
Avena[b]	Poaceae	Nitrate accumulation
Baccharis	Asteraceae	Trichothecenes[c]
Baileya	Asteraceae	Oxalates and nitrates
Baptisia	Fabaceae	Quinolizidine alkaloids

Observed or Predicted Toxicity	Class[a]	Other Comments
Hemorrhagic	A	Only seeds are toxic
Muscle and respiratory failure, death	A	
Gastrointestinal, circulatory	B	Fruits and roots are toxic *A. racemosa* syn. *Cimcifuga racemosa* (black cohosh)
Hepatotoxic, carcinogenicity	A	
Photosensitization, hepatotoxic	B	
Gastroenteritis, coma, death	A	
Hemorrhagic	B	
Gastritis, vomiting, diarrhea	C	
Hepatotoxic, carcinogenic	A	
Convulsant	A	
Hepatotoxic, carcinogenic	A	
Gastroenteritis, death	B	
Coagulapathy, photosensitization	C	
Cardiotoxic, death	A	
Carcinogenic	A	Usually mixed with other plants
Dropsy, glaucoma, death	A	
Numbness of mouth and throat	B	Common household plant
Nephrotoxicity, carcinogenic	A	All species
Goitrogenic, death	B	Only in exceptionally large amounts
Gastrointestinal, coma	C	
Cardiotoxic, coma	A	
Abortifacient, neurotoxic; teratogenic	A	Variable toxicity depending on species
Respiratory failure, death		
Anorexia, emaciation, neurotoxicity, death		
Hepatotoxic, nephrotoxic	A	
Anticholinergic	A	
Anoxia	A	
Gastrointestinal	B	Variable toxicity based on species
Hepatotoxic, nephrotoxic	C	Large amounts in livestock
Teratogenic, respiratory failure, death	A	

continued

TABLE 6-1 Continued

Primary Genera of Concern	Family	Compounds and Compound Classes Implicated in Toxicity
Beta[b]	Polygonaceae	Oxalates Nitrates
Blighia	Sapindaceae	Cyclopropane amino acids
Borago	Boraginaceae	Pyrrolizidine alkaloids
Brassica[b]	Brassicaceae	Isothiocyanates Glucosinolates Thiooxazolidones
Brugmansia	Solanaceae	Tropane alkaloids
Buxus	Buxaceae	Steroidal alkaloids
Cacalia	Asteraceae	Pyrrolizidine alkaloids, Triterpene
Calystegia	Convolvulaceae	Polyhydroxy nortropane and indolizidine alkaloids
Canavalia	Fabaceae	Canavinine Hydrogen cyanide Indospicine β-nitropropionic acid Nitrites
Castanospermum	Fabaceae	Polyhydroxy alkaloids (castanospermine)
Castilleja	Scrophulariaceae	Pyrrolizidine alkaloids
Centaurea	Asteraceae	Sesquiterpene lactones
Chelidonium	Papaveraceae	Isoquinoline alkaloids
Cicuta	Apiaceae	Polyacetylenes
Colchicum	Liliaceae	Colchicine
Colocasia	Araceae	Oxalates
Conium	Apiaceae	Piperidine alkaloids
Convallaria	Liliaceae	Cardiac glycosides
Convolvulus	Convolvulaceae	Polyhydroxy nortropane and indolizidine alkaloids (calystegines and swainsonine)
Coriaria	Coriariaceae	Picrotoxin-like terpenes
Corydalis	Papaveraceae	Isoquinoline alkaloids, bicuculline
Crotalaria	Fabaceae	Pyrrolizidine alkaloids
Croton	Euphorbiaceae	Phorbol esters
Cupressus	Cupressaceae	Labdane diterpene acids

Observed or Predicted Toxicity	Class[a]	Other Comments
Gastrointestinal, depression, death	C	Only seeds are toxic
Hypoglycemia, convulsions, death	A	Unripe fruits are toxic
Hepatotoxic, carcinogenic	A	
Irritant to mucus membranes, death	C	Only toxic at very high levels
Anticholinergic		Atropine related compounds
Convulsant	A	All plant parts
Hepatotoxic, carcinogenic	A	
Neurotoxicity	A	
Nephrotoxic, respiratory failure	A	Only in very large amounts
Neurotoxic, gastroenteritis	A	
Hepatotoxic, carcinogenic	A	Toxins acquired from other plants through parasitism
Neurotoxicity	A	
Dropsy, glaucoma, death	A	
Convulsant, respiratory failure	A	
Antimitotic	A	
Numbness of mouth and throat	B	
Teratogenic, respiratory failure, death	A	
Cardiotoxic	A	
Neurotoxic	B	Some species are not toxic
Analeptic	A	
Convulsant	A	
Carcinogenic, pulmonary, hypertension	A	
Gastroenteritis, cocarcinogen	A	
Abortifacient	A	Mainly in livestock

continued

TABLE 6-1 Continued

Primary Genera of Concern	Family	Compounds and Compound Classes Implicated in Toxicity
Cycas	Cycadaceae	Methylazoxymethanol glycosides
Cynodon	Poaceae	Cyanogenic glycosides
		Agroclavine alkaloids[c]
Cynoglossum	Boraginaceae	Pyrrolizidine alkaloids
Cytisus	Fabaceae	Quinolizidine alkaloids
Daphne	Thymelaeaceae	Phorbol esters
Datura	Solanaceae	Tropane alkaloids
Daucus[b]	Apiaceae	Polyacetylenes
Delphinium	Ranunculaceae	Diterpenoid alkaloids
Descurainia	Brassicaceae	*Iso*thiocyanates Thiooxazolidones
Dicentra	Papaveraeae	Isoquinoline alkaloids, Bicuculline
Dieffenbachia	Araceae	Oxalates
Digitalis	Scrophulariaceae	Cardiac glycosides
Dolichos	Fabaceae	Cyanogenic compounds
Drymaria	Caryophllaceae	Saponins
Duboisia	Solanaceae	Tropane alkaloids
Echium	Boraginaceae	Pyrrolizidine alkaloids
Ephedra	Ephedraceae	Ephedrine, Norephedrine and related alkaloids
Euonymus	Celastraceae	Cardiac glycosides
Eupatorium	Asteraceae	Pyrrolizidine alkaloids Tremetol/tremetones
Euphorbia	Euphorbiaceae	Phorbol esters
Fagopyrum	Polygonaceae	Fagopyrine
Farfugium	Asteraceae	Pyrrolizidine alkaloids
Ferula	Apiaceae	Coumarins
Festuca	Poaceae	Ergot alkaloids[c]
		Penitrem alkaloids[c] Selenium accumulation
Flourensia	Asteraceae	Tremetone derivatives, Benzofurans, Polyacetylenes
Gloriosa	Liliaceae	Colchicine

Observed or Predicted Toxicity	Class[a]	Other Comments
Carcinogenic, neurotoxic, hepatotoxic	A	
Respiratory failure	A[d]	
Neurotoxic		
Hepatotoxic, carcinogenic	A	
Respiratory failure, coma, death teratogenic	A	
Cocarcinogen, allergenic	A	
Anticholinergic	A	Atropine-like compounds
Gastroenteritis	C	
Muscle and respiratory failure, cardiotoxic, death	A	
Goitrogenic	B	
Convulsant	A	All parts are toxic
Numbness of mouth and throat	B	Common household plant
Cardiotoxic	A	
Cardiotoxic respiratory failure, death	A	Mainly seeds are toxic
Gastroenteritis, coma, death	A	
Anticholinergic	A	Atropine-like compounds
Hepatotoxic, carcinogenic	A	
Hypertension, death	B	Many species do not contain alkaloids. Toxicity is dependant on amount
Cardiotoxic, coma, death	A	Fruits and leaves are toxic
Hepatotoxic, carcinogenic	A	
Gastroenteritis		
Vesicant, cocarcinogenic	A	
Photosensitization, allergenic	C	
Hepatotoxic, carcinogenic	A	
Photosensitization, coagulapathy	C	
Vasoconstriction, gangrene, tremors (See *Lolium*)	A/B[d]	Caused by fungal contamination
Anorexia, emaciation, neurotoxicity, death		
Death	B	
Antimitotic	A	

continued

TABLE 6-1 Continued

Primary Genera of Concern	Family	Compounds and Compound Classes Implicated in Toxicity
Gutierrezia	Asteraceae	Diterpene acids (?)
Halogeton	Polygonaceae	Oxalates Nitrates
Haplopappus	Asteraceae	Tremetol/tremetone derivatives
Hedera	Araliaceae	Saponins
Helenium	Asteraceae	Sesquiterpene lactones (helenalin, hymenovin)
Heliotropium	Boraginaceae	Pyrrolizidine alkaloids
Helleborus	Ranunculaceae	Cardiac glycosides
Hippomane	Euphorbiaceae	Phorbol esters
Hyacinthus	Liliaceae	Unknown
Hymenoxys	Asteraceae	Sesquiterpene lactones (helenalin, hymenovin)
Hyoscyamus	Solanaceae	Tropane alkaloids
Illicium	Illiciaceae	Sesquiterpenes
Indigofera	Fabaceae	Canavanine Hydrogen cyanide Indospicine β-nitropropionic acid Nitrite
Ipomoea[b]	Convolvulaceae	Polyhydroxy nortropane and indolizidine alkaloids
Jatropha	Euphorbiaceae	Diterpenes
Juniperus	Cupressaceae	Labdane diterpene acids
Kalmia	Ericaceae	Grayanotoxins
Karwinskia	Rhamnaceae	Quinones, peroxisomicine A-1 (anthracene dimers)
Laburnum	Fabaceae	Quinolizidine alkaloids
Lantana	Verbenaceae	Triterpenes (lantadene A and B)
Larrea	Zygophyllaceae	Nordihydroguaiaretic acid
Lathyrus	Fabaceae	Aminobutyric and amino-propionic acids and nitriles
Leucaena	Fabaceae	Mimosine
Liatris	Asteraceae	Pyrrolizidine alkaloids

Observed or Predicted Toxicity	Class[a]	Other Comments
Abortifacient	A	Mainly in livestock
Indigestion Depression, death	A	Large amounts in livestock
Hepatotoxic, gastrointestinal	A	
Respiratory failure, coma, death	B	Only one species implicated of many
Gastrointestinal, hepatotoxic, nephrotoxic, death	A	
Hepatotoxic, carcinogenic	A	
Convulsant, cardiotoxic	A	
Cocarcinogen	A	
Gastrointestinal	B	Mainly bulbs are implicated
Gastrointestinal, hepatotoxic, nephrotoxic	A	
Anticholinergic	A	Atropine derivatives
Convulsant	A	All parts of plants
Abortifacient, gastroenteritis, nephrotoxic, hepatotoxic	A	See Canavalia
Neurotoxicity	B	Many species are not toxic
Neurotoxicity	B	Mainly seeds
Abortifacient	A	Mainly in livestock
Cardiotoxic	A	
Neurotoxic, nephrotoxic	A	Mainly fruits are implicated
Respiratory failure, coma, death teratogenicity	A	
Hepatotoxic, anithrombin, possible anticholinergic	A	
Hepatotoxic, nephrotoxic	A	
Neurotoxic, neurolathyrism (skeletal deformity)	A	
Hair loss, cytotoxic, goitrogenic	A	Mimosine is metabolized to 3-hydroxy-4(1*H*)-pyridone
Hepatotoxic, carcinogenic	A	

continued

TABLE 6-1 Continued

Primary Genera of Concern	Family	Compounds and Compound Classes Implicated in Toxicity
Ligustrum	Oleaceae	Unknown
Lobelia	Campanulaceae	Piperidine alkaloids
Lolium	Poaceae	Ergot alkaloids[c] Penitrem alkaloids[c] Selenium accumulation (Selenium is acquired from Seleniferous soils, not funga)
Lupinus	Fabaceae	Quinolizidine alkaloids
Lycopersicon[b]	Solanaceae	Steroidal alkaloids Polyhydroxy alkaloids (calystegines)
Lyonia	Ericaceae	Lyoniatoxin
Macrozamia	Zamiaceae	Methyl azoxymethanol glycosides (i.e., macrozamin)
Manihot[b]	Euphorbiaceae	Cyanogenic glycosides
Melilotus[b]	Fabaceae	Dicoumarol
Myristica[b]	Myristicaceae	Safrole
Narcissus	Amaryllidaceae	Isoquinoline alkaloids
Nerium	Apocynaceae	Cardiac glycosides
Nicotiana	Solanaceae	Nicotine alkaloids
Nolina	Liliaceae	Unknown
Ornithogalum	Liliaceae	Colchicine
Oxytropis	Fabaceae	Polyhydroxy alkaloids (swainsonine)
Pachyrhizus[b]	Fabaceae	Unknown
Packera	Asteraceae	Pyrrolizidine alkaloids
Papaver	Papaveraceae	Isoquinoline alkaloids Morphinan alkaloids
Pedicularis	Scrophulariaceae	Pyrrolizidine alkaloids
Petasites	Asteraceae	Pyrrolizidine alkaloids
Phaseolus[b]	Fabaceae	Cyanogenic glycoside (phaseolunatin)

Observed or Predicted Toxicity	Class[a]	Other Comments
Gastroenteritis, death	A	Mainly fruits and leaves
Respiratory failure, coma, death	B	Mainly large doses in livestock
Vasoconstriction, gangrene Tremors Anorexia, emaciation, neurotoxicity, death	A/B[d]	Caused by fungal contamination
Respiratory failure, coma, death teratogenic	B	Many species ("sweet lupines") are not toxic
Gastroenteritis, teratogenic Gastroenteritis, neurotoxicity (i.e., same as *Solanum*)	B	Restricted occurrence of toxic substances
Convulsant	A	All parts of the plant
Hepatotoxic, neurotoxic, carcinogenic	A	
Respiratory failure, death	A	Cyanogenic toxins are removed by boiling or heating when prepared as food
Hemorrhagic	B	Dicoumarol is formed by microbial transformation (fermentation)
Carcinogenic	A	
Cardiotoxic, external irritant, emetic death	A	
Cardiotoxic, gastrointestinal, death	A	
Cholinergic toxicity	A	
Hepatoxic, gastroenteritis	A	
Animitotic	A	
Neurotoxic, teratogenic, abortifacient, gastroenteritis	A	
Convulsant	A	Mainly seeds, root edible (jicama)
Hepatotoxic, carcinogenic	A	
CNS effects	A	
Hepatotoxic, carcinogenic	A	
Hepatotoxic, carcinogenic	A	
Respiratory failure, coma, death	B	Mainly in large amounts in livestock

continued

TABLE 6-1 Continued

Primary Genera of Concern	Family	Compounds and Compound Classes Implicated in Toxicity
Phoradendron	Loranthaceae	Pressor amines
Physostigma	Fabaceae	Physostigmine (eserine)
Phytolacca	Phytolaccaceae	Saponins
Pilocarpus	Rutaceae	Pilocarpine
Pinus	Pinaceae	Labdane diterpene acids
Podophyllum	Berberidaceae	Podophyllotoxin-type lignans
Polygonatum	Liliaceae	Steroidal saponins
Prosopsis	Fabaceae	Indouizidine alkaloids, β-nitropropionic acid, tyramine
Prunus[b]	Rosaceae	Cyanogenic glycosides
Psilostrophe	Asteraceae	Unknown
Pteridium	Polypodiaceae	Ptaquiloside
Ranunculus	Ranunculaceae	Protoanemonin
Rheum[b]	Polygonaceae	Oxalates, nitrates, anthraquinones
Rhododendron	Ericaceae	Grayanotoxins
Rhodomyrtus	Myrtaceae	Dibenzofurans
Ricinus	Euphorbiaceae	Ricin
Robinia	Fabaceae	Abrin
Rudbeckia	Asteraceae	Unknown
Rumex	Polygonaceae	Oxalates, nitrates
Sambucus	Caprifoliaceae	Cyanogenic
Sanguinaria	Papaveraceae	Sanguinarine
Saponaria	Caryophyllyaceae	Unknown
Sarcobatus	Polygonaceae	Oxalates, nitrates
Sarothamnus	Fabaceae	Sparteine
Sassafras	Lauraceae	Safrole
Scilla	Liliaceae	Cardiac glycosides

Observed or Predicted Toxicity	Class[a]	Other Comments
Gastritis, vasoconstriction, death	B	Large amounts in livestock
Cholinesterase inhibition, death	A	
Extreme irritation on inhalation of root powder	B	
Cholinomimetic	A	
Abortifacient	B	Mainly in livestock
Gastroenteritis, catharsis, conjunctivitis	A	
Cardiotoxic	A	
Gastroenteritis, death	A	
Cardiac and respiratory failure, death	A	
Nephrotoxic	A	
Carcinogenic	A	The fronds (fiddle heads) are processed (salting) and are safely eaten. All toxicities reported in livestock are from unprocessed fronds
Gastroenteritis, death	A	Mainly in large doses in livestock
Indigestion, depression, death	B	Mainly in livestock
Convulsant	A	All parts
Blindness	A	Mainly in livestock
Hemorrhagic, circulatory system	A	Only seeds are toxic
Hemorrhagic, circulatory system	A	
Incoordination, gastroenteritis	C	Large amounts in livestock
Indigestion, Depression, death	C	Mainly in livestock
Cardiac and respiratory failure, death	A	
Coma	A	Rhizomes
Gastroenteritis, coma, death	B	
Indigestion, depression, death	B	Mainly in large amounts in livestock
Hypotension	B	Seeds and leaves
Carcinogenic	A	Bark, essential oils
Cardiotoxic, death	A	

continued

TABLE 6-1 Continued

Primary Genera of Concern	Family	Compounds and Compound Classes Implicated in Toxicity
Secale[b]	Poaceae	Nitrate accumulation, ergot alkaloids[c]
Senecio	Asteraceae	Pyrrolizidine alkaloids
Sesbania	Fabaceae	Quinolizidine alkaloids
Solanum[b]	Solanaceae	Steroidal alkaloids Polyhydroxyalkaloids (calystegines)
Solidago	Asteraceae	Unknown
Sophora	Fabaceae	Quinolizidine alkaloids
Sorghum[b]	Poaceae	Cyanogenic glycosides, nitrate
Spartium	Fabaceae	Sparteine
Strelitzia	Musaceae	Phenalenones
Strychnos	Loganiaceae	Strychnine
Symphytum	Boraginaceae	Pyrrolizidine alkaloids
Tanacetum	Asteraceae	Unknown
Taxus	Taxaceae	Taxoids
Tetradymia	Asteraceae	Furanoeremophilanes
Teucrium	Lamiaceae	Diterpenes (?)
Thevetia	Apocynaceae	Cardiac glycosides
Toxicodendron	Anacardiaceae	Urushiols
Trichodesma	Asteraceae	Pyrrolizidine alkaloids
Trifolium[b]	Fabaceae	Coumestrol Isoflavones
Triglochin	Juncaginaceae	Cyanogenic glycosides
Tripterygium	Celastraceae	Diterpenes
Tussilago	Asteraceae	Pyrrolizidine alkaloids
Urginea	Liliaceae	Cardiac glycosides
Veratrum	Liliaceae	Steroidal alkaloids
Vicia	Fabaceae	Aminobutyric and aminopropionic acids and nitriles
Wisteria	Fabaceae	Canavanine
Xanthium	Asteraceae	Carboxyatractyloside
Zamia	Zamiaceae	

Observed or Predicted Toxicity	Class[a]	Other Comments
Anoxia, vasoconstriction, abortifacient, neurotoxic	A/B[d]	Contamination with fungi
Hepatotoxic, carcinogenic	A	
Hemorrhagic, circulatory system, collapse	A	
Gastroenteritis, teratogenic	A	
Gastroenteritis, neurotoxicity		
Abortifacient, gastroenteritis	A	Large amounts in livestock
Respiratory failure, coma, death teratogenic	A	
Respiratory failure	B	
Abortifacient	A	
Gastroenteritis, vertigo	B	Seeds and pods
Convulsant	A	
Hepatotoxic, carcinogenic	A	All parts
Abortifacient, gastroenteritis, teratogenic	A	
Convulsant and coma	A	
Photosensitization	B	Large amounts in livestock
Nephrotoxic	A	Teucrium chamaedrys of major concern
Cardiotoxic, death	A	
Dermatitis, gastroenteritis	A	Poison ivy, poison sumac, Poison oak
Hepatotoxic, carcinogenic	A	
Photosensitization	C	
Estrogenic		
Respiratory depression	B	
Immune suppressant, antispermatogenic	A	
Hepatotoxic, carcinogenic	A	
Cardiotoxic, death	A	
Cyclopia, holoprosencephaly, limb defects	A	
Neurotoxicity, teratogenic	A	
Gastroenteritis	B	
Heptotoxic, neurotoxic, death	A	
Carcinogenic, neurotoxic, hepatoxic	A	

continued

TABLE 6-1 Continued

Primary Genera of Concern	Family	Compounds and Compound Classes Implicated in Toxicity
Zea[b]	Poaceae	Zearalenone
Zephyranthes	Amaryllidaceae	Isoquinoline alkaloids
Zygadenus	Liliaceae	Steroidal alkaloids

NOTE: The information in this table was developed by committee members knowledgeable in botanicals and phytochemicals who consulted the references listed at the end of the chapter as needed. A review of each of the genera and families on this list was not practical within the constraints of this report. The list should thus be considered as a general guideline for determining which warrant attention, not as an authoritative statement on any in particular.

[a] A = reports of adverse effects to the heart, liver, lungs, kidney, immune system, reproductive system, teratogenicity, carcinogenesis, central nervous system (convulsant), or death in animals or humans, or where well-known constituents with adverse effects on these same organs, that is, pyrrolizidine alkaloids (liver), cardiac glycosides (heart), methylazoxymethanol glycosides (cancer) are reported for the genus. B = reports of nonpotentially lethal effects in humans or animals, such as severe irritation, gastric upset, emesis, photosensitization, or

providing a protective function within the plant, they tend to be concentrated in young, tender leaves, shoots, and roots, or in reproductive structures (e.g., flowers and seeds). For example, livestock poisoning episodes have shown that there is often a bimodal distribution of toxic hazard with very young plants and plants at the reproductive stage being toxic, whereas at other growth stages no problems occur. (For a more complete discussion, see Appendix C and resources listed.) Frequently, compounds are continuously biosynthesized in a particular part of the plant, such as mature leaves where photosynthesis is at a maximum, but then they are transported and accumulated in other organs where the protective function conferred by such substances is required (Harborne, 1993).

Although it is possible for plants to contain completely different chemical entities in different parts, it is generally more likely that they will contain the same compounds or compounds that have undergone relatively minor structural transformations. The situation with respect to structural types of constituents is often under a state of continuous flux in response to environmental conditions and ecological factors. It is therefore appropriate to assume, in the absence of other information to the contrary, that a plant part marketed as a dietary supplement ingredient contains toxins that are found in other parts of the plant. That is, if a toxic chemical is present in one part of the plant, it will generally be present in the other parts of the plants, even if at lower concentrations. Indeed, **concentrations of toxins**

Observed or Predicted Toxicity	Class[a]	Other Comments
Vulvovaginitis in livestock	C	Caused by fungal contamination
Cholineesterase Inhibition	A	
Gastritis, vasomotor collapse, coma, death	A	

allergenicity. C = reports of effects that cannot be explained on the basis of known chemistry of the genus or where exceptional amounts, especially in livestock, were required to elicit the effect.

[b] Several species of these genera are common conventional food and/or condiment plants and are of little concern when consumed.

[c] Produced by endophytic fungi in some, but not all, cases.

[d] Class A concerns for *Festuca* stem from concerns about penitrem alkaloids and ergot alkaloids produced by fungal contamination, which can occur fairly frequently depending on weather conditions. Even if fungal contamination is not present, there are concerns when the plants grow in high-selenium soils, warranting at least a class B classification.

may vary and thus be less problematic in some plant parts, but the assumption should be that all parts of a plant containing toxins pose a risk unless there is credible evidence suggesting that dangerous levels of toxins are not present in the part marketed as a dietary supplement. In this case, selection of plant material at a specific growth stage to avoid incorporation of potentially toxic plant parts is desirable.

Cultivation and Other Conditions

In addition to concentration of toxic compounds in particular plant parts, levels of toxins in plants may also be influenced by growth stage, time of collection, environmental stress, herbivory, and a multitude of other factors (Fong, 2002). Blending of plant material from a number of locations will tend to dilute toxin levels that are higher in some plants if other plants are lower in toxin levels. However, in the absence of comprehensive studies, it is not possible to delineate precisely the overall influence of such conditions on constituent levels, although their role must be recognized in evaluating the safety of dietary supplements. When sporadic adverse incidents occur in association with a botanical supplement ingredient with no previous indication of risk, it may well be possible that environmental changes have resulted in an increase in levels of toxic constituents. **If a plant's content of a hazardous phytochemical varies significantly with environ-**

mental and growth conditions, then it is appropriate to consider the plant's use in dietary supplements as a risk unless quality control or other actions are implemented to ensure that levels of compounds associated with risk are not reached in raw materials or finished products.

Preparation Methods

When considering the risk associated with a dietary supplement, it is important to consider whether the method of preparation is likely to concentrate toxic constituents or otherwise increase the consumption or bioavailability of toxic compounds. Toxic plant constituents that are normally present below a given threshold of toxicity can be concentrated by a variety of processing methods. **Some methods of preparation may make specific toxins more readily available or even concentrate them** (see also discussion of relevance of historical use in Chapter 4). **An additional risk is that there may be a tendency to consume more of the plant material in an encapsulated form than if it were consumed in its "native" form.**

Some methods of extract preparation can raise levels of toxic constituents to levels of greater concern. Whereas preparation of teas (i.e., aqueous infusions) is a method designed to concentrate specific constituents, many low-molecular-weight phytochemicals[6] are not particularly water-soluble,[7] and exceptionally high levels are not likely to be attained. Furthermore, hydrolytic changes may occur that can detoxify or reduce the levels of toxic compounds. It is also difficult to consume large volumes of teas. In contrast to aqueous extracts, extraction of plant material with alcohol or aqueous alcohol in which low-molecular-weight compounds are generally very soluble will likely concentrate toxic components many fold. Thus, such extraction of botanicals that may contain hazardous constituents should be a cause for concern unless there is credible evidence to the contrary. Such procedures underlie the process by which natural products chemists isolate specific bioactive substances from plant material for further purification and identification. **Given the potential for extraction to impact the constituents consumed, it is not appropriate to assume that safety of an aqueous extract of a botanical indicates that alcoholic extracts (or other organic solvent extracts) of the same botanical are not of concern.**

[6]Although most of the toxins are small molecules (< 1,000 Daltons), there are a number of high-molecular-weight proteins, particularly lectins, that are extremely toxic. For example, ricin, occurring in the castor bean (*Ricinus communis*), is one of the most toxic substances known with a minimal lethal dose intraperitoneal injection of 1 ng/g body weight in mice (O'Neil et al., 2001).

[7]This statement must be tempered by the fact that many alkaloids occur in plants as water-soluble salts and others have high levels of hydroxylation that confer water solubility on them.

Historical/Traditional Use

Certain plant families, while being major sources of food plants, also contain some of the most toxic plant species (see discussion in Appendix C). Species of Fabaceae and Solanaceae that are toxic have been established (probably a reflection of extensive investigations of the secondary metabolite compositions of these families because they are primary food sources), but even some species that contain toxins are used as food plants. For example, plants in the following families are used as foods: Liliaceae (e.g., onion, garlic, asparagus), Apiaceae (e.g., carrots, celery, parsnips), Brassicaceae (e.g., green leafy vegetables), Fabaceae (e.g., peas and beans), and Solanaceae (e.g., potatoes, tomatoes, eggplant). In most cases, the toxin tends to be concentrated in specific plant parts (e.g., potato sprouts) that are not consumed as conventional foods (Drager et al., 1995). Levels in plant parts conventionally eaten as foods are generally known and, in some cases, regulated (e.g., steroidal alkaloids in potatoes); when present, the levels are sufficiently low that they can be metabolized and excreted without adverse effects.

Some general principles apply when considering the relevance of historical or traditional use of a plant. It is important to consider the points outlined in the previous section, particularly the importance of plant part and whether the dietary supplement ingredient preparation will allow excessive amounts to be consumed or will concentrate toxins (in capsules vs. teas, or alcoholic vs. aqueous extracts, for example). A dissimilar amount of ingested toxin could result from changes, such as a switch from cooked to raw consumption, inclusion of plant parts not traditionally consumed, excessive use of one particular vegetable foodstuff, preparation of infusions or extracts, or ingestion of plant preparations historically only applied externally. For example, plant foods are typically consumed after cooking by either dry heat or boiling in water, a process that often destroys toxins because they are thermally labile, hydrolyzed, or extracted.

That particular concern should arise when nontraditional or excessive levels of plant parts are consumed can be illustrated by several examples. Increased consumption of potato skins without the flesh, because nutrients are generally considered more concentrated in this part, may lead to ingestion of high levels of glycoalkaloids and glycosidase-inhibitory calystegines known to be concentrated in the skin, which can seriously affect digestive processes (Asano et al., 1997). Similarly, excessive use of vegetables of the family Brassicaceae can result in toxic effects due to isothiocyanates and other hydrolytic products from glucosinolates, which can cause goiter and a general inhibition of iodine uptake by the thyroid. Internal consumption of plants historically used externally, as with comfrey (*Symphytum spp.*), a pyrrolizidine alkaloid-containing plant, is especially relevant. Medieval herbalists prescribed the use of comfrey as a poultice, but more recent use as a salad vegetable or tea has resulted in evidence of liver damage (Coulombe, 2003).

In summary, plant foods and spices, when consumed in a conventional manner, can generally be assumed to be safe if the same plant part is consumed, but caution should be applied to restrict higher than conventional ingestion of those known to have some degree of toxicity. Similarly, the assumption of safety may or may not apply to plants prepared differently. Of course, not all foods are safe for all persons. If adverse events are reported, then the level of concern should be higher. Most plant species containing overtly toxic compounds are not generally consumed, and consequently there will be no normal food intake data available. For plants that are not commonly consumed by humans, the best data as to adverse effects will come from observations and/or studies with herbivorous animals (see Chapter 5).

Summary of Chemical Components and Related Botanicals

When considering the safety of a botanical dietary supplement ingredient, information about its chemical constituents may provide important clues as to the potential toxicities of the substance. Similarly, consideration of related plant species, especially those in the genera listed in Table 6-1, can provide information about chemical constituents that may be present in the ingredient, as well as toxicities associated with these chemicals. Some information about the potencies is also provided in Appendix C. The concept that it is important to consider chemical constituents and related plants of possible concern is summarized in the guiding principle at the beginning of this section: it is appropriate to consider risk by considering ". . . whether the plant source of the botanical dietary supplement is itself a toxic plant or is taxonomically related to a known toxic plant." Several corollary guiding principles are important to remember as individual supplements are considered:

- Plant foods and spices consumed in a conventional manner can generally be assumed to be safe if the same plant part is consumed, but caution applies to higher than conventional ingestion of those known to have some degree of toxicity.
- Alkaloid-containing plants should always be suspected of possibly being pharmacologically active and should be considered as a risk factor.
- Unless there is evidence to the contrary, the assumption should be that all parts of a plant containing toxins pose a risk unless there is credible evidence suggesting that dangerous levels of toxins are not present in the part marketed as a dietary supplement.

- If production of a hazardous phytochemical in a botanical appears to be particularly sensitive to environmental and growth conditions, then it may be appropriate to consider its use in dietary supplements as a risk unless quality control or other actions are implemented to assure that toxic levels of compounds are not reached in raw materials or finished products.
- Preparation affects toxicity. Materials that are traditionally consumed in cooked form may not have the same safety profile as in uncooked form, compounds that are concentrated or otherwise altered by the method of preparation will present a hazard that is of greater concern than for unprocessed material, and knowledge about the safety of one plant preparation should not be applied *prima facie* to different preparations of the same plant.
- Particular concern should arise when nontraditional or excessive levels of plant parts are consumed. There may be a tendency to consume more of the plant material in an encapsulated form than if it were used in its "native" form.
- Extraction of plant material with alcohol or aqueous alcohol, in which low-molecular-weight compounds are generally very soluble, will likely concentrate toxic components several fold. Thus, for botanicals containing toxic compounds, a shift from aqueous to alcoholic extracts should be a cause for concern unless there is credible evidence to mitigate this concern.

OTHER APPROACHES FOR CONSIDERING STRUCTURAL SIMILARITY TO KNOWN CLASSES OF TOXIC COMPOUNDS

GUIDING PRINCIPLE: *Compounds that are similar in structure may have similar biological functions. If the chemical structure of a dietary supplement is known, but additional insight into the biological activity is needed, then it is scientifically appropriate to consider the information about the biological activity of structurally related substances and the general knowledge about adverse effects associated with toxicophores.*

The physical–chemical properties and biological effects of a substance are derived from its chemical structure. If the chemical structure of a dietary supplement is known, but additional insight into the biological activity is needed, then it is scientifically appropriate to consider the information about the biological activity of structurally related substances. It is assumed that the biological effects of chemicals, including toxic effects, are implicit in their molecular structures (referred to as toxicophores when they are associated with toxic effects). This concept is most clearly illustrated with the example of ephedra, which is considered by some scientists to have similar physiological actions, although less potent, to the chemically related substance amphetamine, as well as the recently banned pharmaceutical agent phenylpropanolamine (FDA, 2004; Furuya and Watanabe, 1993; Lake and Quirk, 1984).

Along these lines, FDA and other agencies have developed chemical structure classes of concern to describe well-known toxicophores. The structure of regulated chemicals (e.g., pesticides or food additives) is compared with structural classes of concern to predict which may cause adverse effects. For ingredients regulated by premarket approval, structures of higher concern classes lead to a requirement for particular studies to provide additional information about the likelihood of adverse effects occurring in humans. The structural class approach is discussed in Box 6-4 and in the FDA *Redbook II* (OFAS, 2001). **When the structure of a dietary supplement ingredient or its constituents belongs in one of the higher classes of concern identified via the Structure Category Assignment, it should be considered as a potential risk if mitigating information suggesting other-**

BOX 6-4
Chemical Relatedness (Structure Category Assignment)

In the United States, the Food and Drug Administration, Office of Food Additive Safety, has detailed the value of considering chemical relatedness in the process of assessing the potential of an unknown agent to cause undesirable adverse effects upon consumption in sufficient dosages (see *Redbook II*). This document proposes that it is reasonable to expect that the structure and associated physiochemical properties of a compound play an important role in its toxicity. Four variables for consideration in structure activity relationship (SAR) modeling are as follows:

- Topological parameters
- Geometric parameters
- Electronic parameters
- Physiochemical parameters

Thus chemicals with unknown toxicological properties may be assigned to a chemical structure category based on the presence or absence of chemical groups that have been associated with certain types of toxicity. Moreover, the guidelines provided in *Redbook II* allow for the assignment of an unknown chemical to an initial Concern Level for potential adverse toxic effects (OFAS, 2001). These SAR indicators should be utilized when evaluating dietary supplement ingredients.

wise does not exist. The rationale behind this recommendation is that the dietary supplements with structures of concern are no less likely to produce adverse effects than other ingested substances. Ideally, the use of information about the structural classes of concern will provide guidelines for manufacturers or other scientists to study the ingredient's safety in more depth.

Based on the understanding that biological effects are implicit to molecular structures, computational programs have been developed to predict the biological activity of less-characterized chemicals by comparing their chemical structures with other well-characterized compounds. Computer programs designed to assist in predictive toxicology are useful in predicting the potential propensity for a chemical to cause particular effects. For example, *The Open Practical Knowledge Acquisition Toolkit* program (AIAI, 2003) uses chemical structures and a variety of models to estimate carcinogenicity and teratogenicity, among other toxicological endpoints, and is used by the Cosmetic Industry Review in setting priorities for review. An endorsement or comparative evaluation of individual programs is beyond the scope of this report, but these types of programs in general are believed to have value in providing insight into the potential for a dietary supplement ingredient to demonstrate toxicological outcomes, especially if there is a paucity of experimental or other data relevant to the ingredient's safety.

Computational prediction is most useful for predicting biological activities of pure compounds because it is possible to circumvent the multitude of variables that influence toxicological endpoints, such as the presence of unknown chemicals, the animal species, strains, experimental conditions, and other factors. Even then, however, care must be exercised in selecting data that may be considered valid. Additional complexities, even vagaries, such as metabolic transformation and the multitude of modulating factors that determine a biological outcome under prescribed conditions, may obviate any meaningful predictive conclusion.

Moreover, other confounding factors are the often unique susceptibilities of individuals in animal and human populations that are dependent on complex genetic, environmental, and lifestyle factors. Even more difficult is the reliability of predictions of toxic response where there are effects of simultaneous exposures to a variety of compounds. Even the common example in humans of combining alcohol and tobacco smoke can exercise a striking influence on the toxic manifestations of another (test) material (Izzotti et al., 1998).

In summary, the understanding that toxic effects result from molecular structures that act on biological targets provides a good rationale for comparing chemical structures of a dietary supplement ingredient with other chemical structures to predict possible toxicities. Nonetheless, the practicalities of how to make such comparisons in a systematic way and the limitations inherent in systematic prediction software may limit the usefulness of this approach, as may the important fact that small changes in chemical structure can result in major changes in physiological activity.

CONSIDERATION OF SUBSTANCES RELATED TO ENDOGENOUS SUBSTANCES

GUIDING PRINCIPLE: *Dietary supplement ingredients that are endogenous substances or may be structurally or functionally related to endogenous substances should be evaluated to determine if their activities are likely to lead to serious effects. Considerations should include the ingredient's ability to raise the steady-state concentration of biologically active metabolites in tissues and whether the effect of such increases is linked to a serious health effect.*

A number of dietary supplement ingredients may be structurally or functionally related to endogenous substances. Such substances include hormones, metabolites and their precursors, and ingredients created as mimetics of these substances (see Table 6-2 for examples). Any safety issues of ingredients related to endogenous substances are based on the extent to which the ingredient's similarity to an endogenous substance alters homeostasis. Concern about one of these ingredients is warranted when certain characteristics or qualities are present, as discussed below.

Relevant Characteristics

Physiologically relevant amount of ingredient ingested: It is important to consider whether the ingredient is delivered to potential sites of action at a concentration that is physiologically relevant. For example, a supplement ingredient ingested at an amount that is clearly a small fraction of the amount typically provided in the diet is less likely to pose a risk because the likelihood of physiological impact is low.

Concentration at the site of action that can cause harm: The next consideration is whether the substance reaches the site of action at a concentration that can cause harm, which is largely determined by the substance's bioavailability, rate of metabolism, and excretion. For example, dietary supplement ingredients for which evidence suggests negligible uptake from the gastrointestinal tract would be unlikely to pose a risk beyond local effects, such as gastrointestinal upset. In contrast, ingredients that may result in concentrations of endogenous substances above the normal

TABLE 6-2 Examples of Dietary Supplement Ingredients Related to Endogenous Substances

Hormones and Ingredients Containing Hormones or Precursors	Lipids and Related Ingredients	Metabolites and Cofactors	Others[a]
Androstenediol	Conjugated linoleic acid	S-Adenosyl-L-methionine	Chondroitin sulfate
Androstenedione	Docoshexaenoic acid		Collagen
Dehydroepiandrosterone (DHEA)	(DHA)	Creatine	Enzymes
Glandulars	Eicosapentaenoic acid	α-Lipoic acid	Glucosamine
Human growth hormone	(EPA)	NADH	Indole-3-carbinol
Melatonin	Inositol hexaphosphate	Pyruvate	Probiotics
Pregnenolone	Phosphatidyl choline Phosphatidyl serine	Nucleic acids	

[a] In addition to this list, there are also many other plant and animal constituents known to convert to biologically active substances similar to endogenous substances.

range at the site of action are worthy of further consideration, because of the potential for their activities to be adverse.

Having determined whether an ingredient is likely to be absorbed from the gut at a concentration that could alter cellular, biochemical, or biological activities, the next issue to consider is whether the compound is readily metabolized or degraded to an inactive metabolite. For example, effects on endpoint cells and tissues are unlikely if there are efficient mechanisms for metabolizing these compounds into inactive compounds.

Sensitivity of the target system to variation in the endogenous substance: An important question to ask about endogenous substances is whether a homeostatic regulatory system would attenuate biological effects that could otherwise occur. If the target system is one that is not tightly regulated by feedback or other mechanisms to maintain homeostasis, then there is greater likelihood of potential risk.

Example

Hormones are an illustrative example for how some ingredients related to endogenous substances can be evaluated. Exogenous hormones can be potent substances often used clinically as pharmaceuticals to treat specific deficiency states (e.g., insulin to treat diabetes, thyroid stimulating hormone to treat hypothyroidism, human growth hormone to treat dwarfism) in order to achieve physiological homeostasis. **Use of dietary supplements containing hormones, hormone precursors, or hormone mimetics known to be highly potent raises the possibility of significant and substantial harm unless there is demonstrated hormonal insufficiency.**

CONSTITUENTS FUNCTIONALLY RELATED TO KNOWN CLASSES OF TOXIC COMPOUNDS

> **GUIDING PRINCIPLE:** *When data (i.e.,* in vitro *or animal data) suggest that a dietary supplement constituent targets a receptor, enzyme, or other biological target in a manner similar to a compound known to be toxic, concern is warranted, especially if the dietary supplement constituent is known to reach the biological target in a relevant concentration.*

Compounds that appear to be structurally dissimilar may nonetheless affect the same biological targets or have the same mechanism of action and thus result in the same downstream adverse health effect. Thus, if data strongly suggest that similar biological activity or mechanisms of action exist between an ingredient and a substance known to be dangerous, there is scientific merit in considering whether similar adverse health effects might also occur. This is especially true if the ingredient or its relevant metabolites are bioavailable at the target site.

Although the actual data for such consideration will fall into the categories of data described in the previous chapters (*in vitro,* animal, or human data), the consideration of functional relatedness is described here rather than in the other chapters because (1) the concept applies to all types of data and (2) because the concept is similar to the concept of considering substances related in other ways (either structurally or, for botanicals, taxonomically). That is, a safety evaluation should consider the relationship between the dietary supplement ingredient in question and compounds known to be toxic. This type of information may be most useful in assessing the safety of a dietary supplement ingredient for which chemical constituents are not known or, for botanicals, when not much is known about the plant genus.

Functionally related substances may have similar actions *in vitro*, such as genetic effects or effects on cellular processes (e.g., enzymatic effects, effects on intracellular cell signaling). One example of such functional relatedness illustrated in Chapter 11 is saw palmetto and the drug finasteride. Finasteride is considered unsafe for consumption during pregnancy because of effects on male genitalia development (Bowman et al., 2003; Clark et al., 1990, 1993; Kurzrock et al., 2000). This effect is due to inhibition of the 5-α-reductase enzyme, which is important in testosterone production (Anderson and Clark, 1990; Prahalada et al., 1997). Saw palmetto also inhibits 5-α-reductase, as shown in *in vitro* experiments (Bayne et al., 1999), and thus would be considered as functionally related to finasteride. Thus, in the absence of mitigating data suggesting that saw palmetto does not also lead to male genitalia development problems, it would be scientifically appropriate to consider saw palmetto as a risk for consumption by pregnant women.

When considering which substances a given dietary supplement may be functionally related to, the purported mechanism of action of the ingredient should be considered. For example, shark cartilage has been referred to as an angiogenesis inhibitor. If angiogenesis inhibition is considered as dangerous, or angiogenesis inhibiting drugs are only used with caution by pregnant women because of this mechanism, then it would be appropriate to consider whether shark cartilage is indeed a risk for the same reason.

When evaluating whether functional relatedness to other chemicals provides helpful information about the safety of a dietary supplement ingredient, it is very important to consider that overt expression of toxicity is dependent on exposure (i.e., amount ingested or dose). When animal or human data do not exhibit the toxic effects predicted based on functional relatedness, then it is necessary to consider whether the possible effects would not have been detectable, even if they did occur (such as would be expected for genetic effects or latent effects) (see also see "lack of effects" discussion in Chapter 10). Similarly, the amount of dietary supplement ingredient necessary to produce the effect in humans should be compared to the amount actually consumed.

In summary, if there is information about the mechanism of action of a substance suggesting that it exerts action similar to other classes of substances that are either considered dangerous or restricted in their use, then it may be appropriate to extrapolate such information to the dietary supplement ingredient, especially if little other information about the action of the supplement ingredient is available.

SUMMARY

This chapter emphasizes the importance and scientific appropriateness of including information about related substances when considering the safety of a particular dietary supplement ingredient. For botanicals, the taxonomic and chemical relationships questions can be considered in parallel. Although evidence from one relationship alone may be sufficient to cause an awareness of significant risk, a higher level of concern arising from consideration of both relationships will amount to compelling evidence that the risk has to be seriously examined.

When a dietary supplement contains a known toxic substance, the hazard of ingestion must be assumed to be high unless mitigated by information about dose. Similarly, if the complete toxicity information about a given compound is not known, but it falls into a structural class of known toxins, then that compound is also likely to be a risk unless there is mitigating information about bioavailability or exposure levels.

Table 6-3, the relative spectrum of concern for relatedness information, provides general guidelines about the relative amount of concern for example scenarios using the different types of relatedness information. The information in the right-hand column suggests a significant risk to public health even in the absence of direct human data documenting adverse effects caused by the dietary supplement ingredient. In many situations like those described in the left-hand column, a conclusion of imminent risk may require corroboration with other types of information.

TABLE 6-3 Relative Spectrum of Concern for Relatedness Information

Type of Information	Increasing Concern →		
Botanical chemical constituents of concern	Plant contains constituents that are known to be toxic to humans, but the constituents are commonly consumed in similar amounts in conventional food products	Plant contains constituents that are known to be toxic to humans at low concentrations, but the concentration of these substances in the plant part used for the supplement is *not* characterized OR Plant *part* used for the supplement contains constituents that are toxic to humans, but there is credible reason to believe that the constituent may not cause serious adverse effects at the amount typically ingested	Plant contains constituents that are known to be toxic to humans at low concentrations and the concentration of substances found in the plant *part* used for formulating the supplement has been characterized
Taxonomic relationship to other botanicals of concern	In a plant family that contains known toxic genera, but the supplement is not in a genus known to be toxic AND It has a history of use as a food in a preparation and method similar to its current use	Same genus known to be toxic to humans or animals OR In a plant family that is known to contain toxic plants but not in a genus known as a food plant OR	Same species as a known toxic plant that is not ingested as a food

continued

TABLE 6-3 Continued

Type of Information	Increasing Concern →		
		In a plant family that is known to contain toxic plants,and in a genus that may have a history of food use, but supplement is either a concentrated extract or from a different plant part than is ingested as a food	
Chemical structure	Structurally similar to, or likely contains, a chemical compound known to be toxic to humans or animals when ingested in high doses	Supplement contains chemical constituent known to be toxic to humans or animals	Supplement contains chemical constituent known to be toxic at very low doses to humans
Endogenous substances or mimetics of endogenous substances	*May result* in tissue concentrations that would be expected to cause biological effects (either because homeostasis is disrupted or because the substance has potent biological activities), but the seriousness of the biological effect is not definite	Results seen in tissue concentrations that would be expected to cause biological effects (either because homeostasis is disrupted or because the substance has potent biological activities), but the seriousness of the biological effect is not definite	Results seen in tissue concentrations that would be expected to cause biological effects (either because homeostasis is disrupted or because the substance has potent biological activities) that are considered serious

REFERENCES

AIAI (Artificial Intelligence Applications Institute). 2003. *TOPKAT—The Open Practical Knowledge Acquisition Toolkit*. Online. University of Edinburgh. Available at http://www.aiai.ed.ac.uk/~jkk/topkat.html. Accessed July 9, 2003.

Anderson CA, Clark RL. 1990. External genitalia of the rat: Normal development and the histogenesis of 5 alpha-reductase inhibitor-induced abnormalities. *Teratology 42*:483–496.

Asano N, Kato A, Matsui K, Watson AA, Nash RJ, Molyneux RJ, Hackett L, Topping J, Winchester B. 1997. The effects of calystegines isolated from edible fruits and vegetables on mammalian liver glycosidases. *Glycobiology* 7:1085–1088.

Bayne CW, Donnelly F, Ross M, Habib FK. 1999. *Serenoa repens* (Permixon): A 5 alpha-reductase types I and II inhibitor–A new evidence in coculture model of BPH. *Prostate* 40:232–241.

Bowman CJ, Barlow NJ, Turner KJ, Wallace DG, Foster PMD. 2003. Effects of in utero exposure to finasteride on androgen-dependent reproductive development in the male rat. *Toxicol Sci* 74:393–406.

Clark RL, Antonello JM, Grossman SJ, Wise LD, Anderson C, Bagdon WJ, Prahalada S, MacDonald JS, Robertson RT. 1990. External genitalia abnormalities in male rats exposed in utero to finasteride, a 5 alpha-reductase inhibitor. *Teratology* 42:91–100.

Clark RL, Anderson CA, Prahalada S, Robertson RT, Lochry EA, Leonard YM, Stevens JL, Hoberman AM. 1993. Critical developmental periods for effects on male rat genitalia induced by finasteride, a 5 alpha-reductase inhibitor. *Toxicol Appl Pharmacol* 119:34–40.

Cordell GA, Quinn-Beattie ML, Farnsworth NR. 2001. The potential of alkaloids in drug discovery. *Phytother Res* 15:183–205.

Coulombe RA. 2003. Pyrrolizidine alkaloids in foods. In: Taylor SL, ed. *Advances in Food and Nutrition Research*. Vol 45. Amsterdam: Academic Press. Pp. 61–99.

Drager B, van Almsick A, Mrachtz G. 1995. Distribution of calystegines in several *Solanaceae*. *Planta Med* 61:577–579.

FDA (Food and Drug Administration). 2004. Final rule declaring dietary supplements containing ephedrine alkaloids adulterated because they present an unreasonable risk; Final rule. *Fed Regis* 69:6787–6854.

Fong HHS. 2002. Integration of herbal medicine into modern medical practices: Issues and prospects. *Intergr Cancer Ther* 1:287–293.

Furuya I, Watanabe S. 1993. Discriminative stimulus properties of ephedra herb (*Ephedra sinica*) in rats. *Yakubutsu Seishin Kodo* 13:33–38.

Harborne JB. 1993. *Introduction to Ecological Biochemistry*. 4th ed. London: Academic Press.

Hartmann T, Witte L. 1995. Chemistry, biology and chemoecology of pyrrolizidine alkaloids. In: Pelletier SW, ed. *Alkaloids: Chemical and Biological Perspectives*. Vol 9. Oxford, UK: Levier Science.

IPNI (International Plant Names Index). 2004. *About Index Kewensis*. Online. Available at http://www.ipni.org/ik_blurb.html. Accessed March 22, 2004.

Izzotti A, Balansky RM, Blagoeva PM, Mircheva ZI, Tulimiero L, Cartiglia C, De Flora S. 1998. DNA alterations in rat organs after chronic exposure to cigarette smoke and/or ethanol ingestion. *FASEB J* 12:753–758.

Kurzrock EA, Jegatheesan P, Cunha GR, Baskin LS. 2000. Urethral development in the fetal rabbit and induction of hypospadias: A model for human development. *J Urol* 164:1786–1792.

Lake CR, Quirk RS. 1984. CNS stimulants and the look-alike drugs. *Psychiatr Clin North Am* 7:689–701.

Mabberley DJ. 1997. *The Plant Book*. 2nd ed. Cambridge, UK: Cambridge University Press.

OFAS (Office of Food Additives Safety). 2001. *Toxicological Principles for the Safety Assessment of Direct Food Additives and Color Additives Used in Food. Redbook II-Draft*. Washington, DC: OFAS, Food and Drug Administration.

O'Neil MJ, Smith A, Heckelman PE, eds. 2001. *The Merck Index: An Encylopedia of Chemicals, Drugs, and Biologics*. 13th ed. Whitehouse Station, NJ: Merck and Co.

Pelletier SW. 1983. The nature and definition of an alkaloid. In: Pelliter SW, ed. *Alkaloids: Chemical and Biological Perspectives*. New York: Wiley. Pp. 1–31.

Prahalada S, Tarantal AF, Harris GS, Ellsworth KP, Clarke AP, Skiles GL, MacKenzie KI, Kruk LF, Ablin DS, Cukierski MA, Peter CP, VanZwieten MJ, Hendrickx AG. 1997. Effects of finasteride, a type 2 5-alpha reductase inhibitor, on fetal development in the rhesus monkey (*Macaca mulatta*). *Teratology* 55:119–131.

Seawright AE, Hegarty MP, Keeler RF, James LF, eds. 1985. *Plant Toxicology*. Brisbane, Australia: Queensland Poisonous Plants Committee.

7

Categories of Scientific Evidence—*In Vitro* Data

Guiding Principle: In vitro *studies can serve as signals of potential harmful effects in humans. Validated*[1] in vitro *studies can stand alone as independent indicators of risk to human health if a comparable exposure is attained in humans and the* in vitro *effects correlate with a specific adverse health effect in humans or animals. Alone,* in vitro *data from nonvalidated assays serve as hypothesis generators and as indicators of possible mechanisms of harm.*

Numerous publications have described *in vitro* experiments on dietary supplement ingredients. Some experiments are specifically designed to examine safety endpoints, while others provide less specific information about an ingredient's biological activity. Because no battery of tests is required on dietary supplement ingredients, results from safety tests common to other chemicals are not widespread, although they are available for some ingredients.

The first section of this chapter describes the unique power of in vitro studies and considerations for interpreting them. The next section describes various types of *in vitro* data that may be available, with descriptions of

[1]In this report, *in vitro* assays are considered validated when their results have been proven to predict a specific effect in animals and/or humans with reasonable certainty (not necessarily universally accepted or without detractors).

both the types of endpoints examined and the model systems used. Next is a description of validated *in vitro* assays—assays that are accepted for use in predicting effects on whole organisms. The seriousness of harm predicted by a given assay is then pointed out as an important consideration. Several annexes present information on genetic toxicology experiments, examples of validated *in vitro* assays, and a description of new *in vitro* methods that are evolving in toxicology. Finally, a spectrum of concern figure is presented to integrate the considerations discussed.

CONSIDERATIONS AND RELEVANCE TO HUMANS

A range of *in vitro* experimental systems is used to gain insight into the risk of adverse effects of compounds. These systems include isolated organs, isolated cells, microorganisms, subcellular organelles, and molecular entities such as enzymes, receptors, transport proteins, isolated membranes, and genes or gene fragments. A primary advantage of conducting *in vitro* studies is that their reductionist approach allows insight into a compound's mechanisms of action that might be more difficult to obtain in a "whole-animal study." The control possible with *in vitro* experiments enables examination of effect on the target process or structure in isolation from confounding factors. For example, control over the concentration of the chemical of interest or of one or more of its metabolites enables the interactions among chemicals or metabolites to be studied. *In vitro* experiments are also generally more rapid and less expensive to conduct than *in vivo* studies, thus *in vitro* studies are more likely than *in vivo* studies to be available for assessment of dietary supplement safety.

While the reductionist approach of *in vitro* studies makes them powerful and inexpensive methods useful for learning about effects and mechanisms of actions of compounds, the reductionist approach also requires careful consideration of limitations. It is important to consider the degree to which the particular *in vitro* system replicates the biology of the human target cells and their responses to toxic substances, as discussed below.

Another consideration is that *in vitro* procedures may be less informative if performed with substrate concentrations that are not comparable with those reached *in vivo* or if the substrate is not metabolized similarly *in vitro* and *in vivo*. It is important, for example, to consider the relationship between the compound applied directly to the *in vitro* system and the identity and concentration of the compound that reaches the target (e.g., tissue, receptor, subcellular component) following human ingestion of the dietary supplement ingredient. After a substance is ingested, the metabolic fate of the compound and the amount of the biologically active compound that actually reaches the target site is dependent on a multitude of processes, including absorption, distribution, metabolism, and excretion in what are often complex pathways. The various processes that influence what compound reaches the active site, and at what concentration, are collectively referred to as pharmacokinetics information. Knowledge of a dietary supplement ingredient's pharmacokinetics and *in vivo* metabolism, if available from animal or human studies, will allow the most appropriate interpretation of the relevance of compound concentrations used in *in vitro* experiments to amounts ingested by humans.

GENERAL TYPES OF *IN VITRO* ASSAYS

As described above, *in vitro* assays are valuable because they allow scientists to answer questions that otherwise may not be answerable due to various constraints with whole-animal and human studies. It is not possible to describe the complete realm of *in vitro* assays in this report, but consideration of the value provided by those described here gives perspective to the value of *in vitro* assays as a scientific tool for predicting risk.

Assay Types by Effect Observed

Effects on Cellular Receptors

A number of different assays focus on examining effects of supplement ingredients on cellular receptors. Knowledge of which receptors are activated or inhibited, combined with general knowledge about what physiological processes are stimulated by different types of receptors, will increase understanding of how dietary supplement ingredients will affect humans. General types of assays for examining receptor activity are:

- *Receptor binding assays*—used to measure how strongly a substance (such as a dietary supplement ingredient or its constituent) binds to various receptor types to determine if the substance is likely to activate or inhibit cellular receptor activity.
- *Cell function assays*—used to measure agonism or antagonism of receptor activity in the intact cell by examining effects that are downstream of the receptor itself.

Receptor activation is often a critical event in biological pathways that leads to a functional effect, hence many manufactured pharmacological agents are selected for intentional receptor targeting. Strong agonist or antagonist action does not generally warrant particular attention in and of itself, but it may warrant attention when combined with general knowledge about the receptor. Many receptors are characterized well enough to know whether sufficient activation or inhibition in target tissues is associated with a pharmacological or toxicological process that presents a health risk. Thus whether cellular receptor effects should be considered as indicative of a risk depends on what is known about downstream effects of receptor activation and whether the agent in question reaches the receptor (the site of action) in a sufficient concentration (see Chapter 3 for a discussion about concentration at site of action).

When activity at receptors is not associated with detrimental effects *per se*, understanding how the ingredient may affect the receptors may still prove valuable in providing a biological mechanism that can be used to understand adverse effects observed in intact (whole) and component biological systems (e.g., human, animal).

Effects on Ion Channel Activity and Electrophysiology

A number of assays can predict possible effects on the electrophysiology of the cells, either by directly measuring the membrane potential of the cells or by using other methods to examine effects on ion channels, the cellular proteins that control the cell's ion distribution. For example, certain substances inhibit or block ion transport through particular types of ion channels, which, depending on the channel and the cells involved, can have a detrimental effect.

Effects on some ion channels are associated with specific adverse physiological outcomes. For example, some drugs can induce what is called "long QT syndrome," a rare, but potentially fatal heart disorder that may trigger arrhythmias including "torsades de pointes." This syndrome results when drugs interact with potassium channels (usually with human ether-a-go-go-related gene (HERG) channels specifically), changing the action potential duration in cardiac cells. In the pharmaceutical world, concern about drugs that may induce this syndrome has led to the development of well-accepted *in vitro* assays to identify drugs that may exert this adverse effect on potassium channels (Roche et al., 2002). Such assays are a good example of validated assays (see discussion of validated assays below) and will also be helpful for identifying dietary supplement ingredients of concern.

Effects on Enzyme Activity

At the molecular level, enzyme activity assays measure substances' abilities to inhibit or induce enzyme activity, either by directly affecting the enzyme's activity or by affecting the amount of enzyme in the cell (e.g., affecting translation or enzyme stability). Whether the results of these assays in and of themselves warrant concern about risk depends on what is known about the enzyme and the resultant physiological impact if its function is altered, as well the extent of the effect. For example, effects on cytochrome P450 enzymes important in metabolism of xenobiotics may suggest risk for pharmacokinetic interaction with other ingested substances (see Chapter 8).

Effects on Genes and Nucleic Acids

A number of techniques are capable of identifying genetic alterations that may be responsible for disease processes, alterations such as nucleic acid mutations, or effects on chromosomes. These assays are of growing importance for risk assessment because they measure events that could lead to delayed or latent adverse health effects. Annex 7-1 provides an expanded description of genetic toxicology information, and Annex 7-2 describes several specific types of validated genetic toxicity tests. The current challenge is to demonstrate a connection between changes in specific genes or combinations of genes and the underlying mechanism responsible for a given disease. New technology that may eventually aid in assessing risk of toxicity of compounds, including dietary supplement ingredients, is described in Annex 7-3.

Assay Types by Experimental System

The previous paragraphs organized *in vitro* assays by the effects assessed: effects on enzymes, ion channels, and nucleic acids. These and other *in vitro* tests may be conducted in a variety of experimental systems, such as isolated tissues or in isolated cells, each of which has its own considerations.

Isolated Tissues

In some experiments, animal tissues are isolated and then treated with test substances (e.g., dietary supplement ingredient). Tissues in many ways resemble an intact *in vivo* system because they contain a variety of cell types organized in their native structure and, because they are usually recently isolated from an animal, the protein expression is relatively similar to that *in vivo*. Detrimental effects observed in tissue or isolated organ assays may be predictive of effects *in vivo*. Nevertheless, the toxicological value of these effects can be limited by the inability of an isolated tissue to react with other reciprocating organ-body systems.

For example, there are limitations inherent in excluding the gastrointestinal system in an experiment using isolated tissue. Botanical extracts provide an example of how important it is to consider how absorption of the ingested substance may affect which compounds reach the target tissue.

Botanical extracts often contain polyphenolic compounds (e.g., tannin) that can reversibly or irreversibly bind to subcellular components, such as enzymes, signal transduction factors, and receptors. When administered orally to humans, however, these compounds may bind to food components or gastrointestinal cells, or they can be metabolized by gastrointestinal mucosal or bacteria enzymes and therefore not exert the same effects *in vivo* as seen in isolated tissue (Bravo, 1998; Yang et al., 2001).

In summary, if the impact of excluding effects of other organ systems is considered or compensated for, isolated tissue can be a valuable tool for studying physiological effects of dietary supplement ingredients.

Isolated Cells

Suspensions of isolated cells or cultures of cells derived from animal tissue or from continuously replicating cell lines offer numerous advantages for studying chemical toxicity. The test substance can be examined in direct contact with the cell type of interest, the concentration of the test substance can be rigorously controlled, and the secondary effects of such extracellular influences as metabolic factors, matrix, and cell-to-cell contact can be excluded or controlled for. However, substances that are insoluble in culture media may not adequately reach the target cell *in vitro*, leading to misleading negative results. In addition, adaptation of cells to culture generally results in spontaneous alterations of gene expression so that caution must be exercised in extrapolating to whole organisms the results of chemical effects in culture.

It is also important that the appropriate cell model is used. All cell types do not respond similarly to a single substance, even when the cells originate from the same organ. One cell type may exclude or excrete a compound, whereas another cell will not, and another may behave differently due to its unique biochemical pathways. Cell lines may have different activities than the parent tissue. For example, a problematic interpretation can be made using certain hepatocyte cultures that, unlike the liver, do not always support expression of metabolizing enzymes, causing some data generated in these assays to be misleading. A better choice for some tests might be cell cultures established specifically to evaluate metabolism of substances. Another approach is to add substrates to cell cultures that replace and/or activate metabolic enzymes, thus producing reactive metabolites that simulate *in vivo* metabolism of a given chemical/dietary supplement.

VALIDATED *IN VITRO* ASSAYS

In vitro studies vary in their value as predictors of harm. An *in vitro* assay will have the most direct predictive value when the measured effects are known to correspond to a specific functional change characteristic of an adverse health effect. It may often be appropriate to use *in vitro* data as hypothesis generators, as potential indicators of harmful health effects, or as information about biological plausibility or mechanism, rather than as standalone demonstrated indicators that in themselves indicate risk. However, some types of *in vitro* assays should be considered validated as predictors of possible harm, and thus when carefully conducted and interpreted, will provide valuable information beyond simply reinforcing observations from other categories of data or generating hypotheses. *In vitro* assays warrant attention and are appropriate to use as standalone indicators of risk to human health when the relationship between the results of an *in vitro* assay and actual clinical or animal outcomes has been demonstrated, thus validating the predictive value of the assay.

A number of validated *in vitro* tests are in standard use for regulated materials and are often required for premarket approval by a regulatory authority. These form an important established battery of tests that are useful in predicting possible adverse effects. Although the regulatory situation is such that completion of these or other *in vitro* tests is not required for dietary supplement ingredients, the scientific value of these assays in predicting adverse effects in humans is as valuable in assessing the safety of dietary supplements as it is in assessing the safety of other substances. For example, specific types of *in vitro* tests are used by the Environmental Protection Agency (EPA) and the Food and Drug Administration (FDA) to identify potential pesticides and food additives that may lead to adverse effects (see Annex 7-2). In summary, it is recommended that *in vitro* assays—such as those contained in the *Redbook* (OFAS, 2001, 2003); Protection of Environment (40 C.F.R. § 150–189 [1998]); and the Consumer Product Safety Commission and its subacts, the Federal Hazardous Substances Act (15 U.S.C. § 1261–1278 [1960]) and the Labeling of Hazardous Art Materials Act (15 U.S.C. § 1277 [1988])—all be considered, among others, as important validated assays in the prediction of possible adverse effects in humans.

Assays used by regulatory bodies are by no means the only assays or *in vitro* observations that should be considered as validated and thus independent predictors of risk. Other specific assays, such as certain receptors or ion channel assays, should also be considered validated. The important concept is that for an assay to stand alone as a predictor of risk, a connection between the observed biological effect and an adverse effect needs to have been made. (In Chapter 10, this concept is illustrated by the need for linkages between observed biological effects and adverse health effects.)

In addition to the types of *in vitro* effects considered validated, other *in vitro* information is also valuable for assessing biological plausibility of concerns raised by other observations, such as observations of adverse effects in animals or humans. The assessment of biological plausibility becomes an issue when interpreting data and trying to predict the likelihood of causal relationships (see Chapter 10). While it is not necessary to establish a rational mechanism of harm to conclude that an ingredient poses an unreasonable risk, it is nonetheless valuable to identify possible mechanisms that explain the totality of the data. Many *in vitro* studies can be useful for this purpose.

SERIOUSNESS OF HARM PREDICTED BY THE ASSAY

In addition to considering the correlation of the particular *in vitro* assay with a particular adverse health outcome, it is of utmost importance to consider the *seriousness* of the outcome when evaluating the level of concern warranted by results of *in vitro* studies. Assays that warrant the most attention are those that predict biological effects/outcomes associated with toxicological manifestations, pathologies, or effects that could reasonably be hypothesized to lead to *serious* risks. This concept is analogous to Table 5-1, which categorizes the relative seriousness of various types of effects observed in animals.

SUMMARY

There is no quantitative method of assigning a weight to the outcome of each *in vitro* experiment and imputing an appropriate level of concern for public health risk from such data. Instead, it is important for experts to reach a judgment about the *in vitro* results based on the seriousness of the effect predicted, the validity of the assay in identifying substances that cause a particular adverse effect, the quality of the individual studies, and the consistency among the collection of studies. Considerations on study quality discussed in the human and the animal chapters (Chapters 4 and 5) apply to *in vitro* systems as well. Considerations include the strength of the association, its reproducibility in the same and corresponding systems, the specificity of the findings for both cause and effect, and the coherence of the evidence—all of which give more confidence that the findings are meaningful.

When considering the information, it will be helpful to answer the following questions to decide how much concern for public health is warranted by the *in vitro* evidence:

- Is the *in vitro* test validated or commonly used to predict a serious adverse effect? For example, assays used in regulatory situations to predict possible carcinogenic effects are considered as such.
- Is the assay considered predictive of a particular adverse effect?

• How serious is the adverse effect that might be predicted? Mutagenicity in many assays, DNA damage in human cells, cell transformation, and production of DNA adducts *in vitro* are evidence of higher levels of concern, especially for potential carcinogenesis. Evidence of enzyme induction without DNA damage or mutagenesis is of lesser concern.

• Does the evidence provide mechanistic or mode of action information which lends biological plausibility to effects observed in humans or animals?

• Is the mechanism or mode of action consistent with the type of effect, caused by similar substances, such as plants in the same family?

• Is there information suggesting that the concentrations used *in vitro* are relevant or irrelevant? Concern should increase if the active ingredient and/or metabolite of concern reach relevant concentrations in blood or tissue (see Chapter 3).

• Is there consistency in more than one assay?

The answers to these questions determine the appropriate level of concern, as described in Table 7-1. Information such as that in the right column warrants higher levels of concern about public safety and risk of consumption. *In vitro* information such as that described in the left column warrants lower levels of concern, while information described in the middle column warrants concern, but additional information may be required to warrant conclusion that a risk exists.

ANNEX 7-1
USE OF GENETIC TOXICOLOGY INFORMATION

Genetic toxicology is the study of the ability of substances to cause selective damage to the DNA of living organisms (or RNA in the case of RNA viruses). In addition to providing the raw materials for evolution, genetic alterations are associated with a large proportion of human diseases, including cancer. Chromosomal aberrations, such as deletions, inversions, and translocations, have been associated with leukemia, lymphoma, and some solid tumors.

The term genotoxic is applied to substances (or physical agents like ultraviolet light or X-rays) that have an intrinsic ability to damage DNA (not simply due to gross toxicity that may secondarily result in damage to DNA). Different genotoxicants interact with DNA in different ways, cause different types of DNA alterations, and can be detected using different assay systems (Preston and Hoffmann, 2001).

For example, substances that cause heritable changes in DNA sequence are called mutagens. A mutation may result from an alteration in a single DNA base or addition or deletion of one or more DNA bases (point muta-

TABLE 7-1 Relative Spectrum of Concern for *In Vitro* Data

Increasing Concern →		
Standardized[a] subcellular and cellular assays validated for the purpose of establishing *in vivo* toxic effect AND Multiple different assays suggesting the same pathological condition or endpoint AND Poor consistency/ reproducibility in response AND No knowledge about concentration of toxicant in blood or tissue	Standardized subcellular and cellular assays validated for the purpose of establishing *in vivo* toxic effect AND Multiple different assays suggesting the same pathological condition or endpoint AND Consistency in response AND No knowledge about concentration of toxicant in blood or tissue	Standardized subcellular and cellular assays validated for the purpose of establishing *in vivo* toxic effect AND Multiple different assays suggesting the same pathological condition or endpoint AND Knowledge of presence of toxicant in blood or tissue enhanced by knowledge of concentrations comparable with those causing toxicity *in vitro*
OR	OR	OR
Standardized assays validated for the purpose of establishing organ toxicity AND Multiple different assays suggesting the same pathological condition or endpoint	Standardized assays validated for the purpose of establishing organ toxicity AND Multiple different assays suggesting the same pathological condition or endpoint	Standardized assays validated for the purpose of establishing organ toxicity AND Multiple different assays suggesting the same pathological condition or endpoint

tions) that alters the amino acid in a protein coded for by a particular DNA triplet. This is the type of mutation that occurs in the heritable human disease sickle-cell anemia. Agents that cause these kinds of genetic effects are detected using assays that detect changes in specific genes, such as the Ames assay in *Salmonella* bacteria or the mouse lymphoma $TK^{+/-}$ assay in mammalian cells *in vitro*. Some genotoxicants cause visibly identifiable types of changes—alterations in chromosome structure or chromosome number (chromosome mutations, or clastogenicity). These types of changes can be detected by observation of cells (generally fixed and stained) with a microscope.

The ability of some substances to cause DNA damage can also be assessed by determining whether the substance increases the normal level of activity of certain DNA repair processes or whether it is more lethal to cells

TABLE 7-1 Continued

Increasing Concern →		
AND Poor consistency/ reproducibility in response AND No knowledge about concentration of toxicant in blood or tissue OR Results obtained with nonstandardized, nonvalidated assays OR Results from microarray experiments show a gene expression pattern predictive of dangerous compounds[b]	AND Consistency in response AND No knowledge about concentration of toxicant in blood or tissue	AND Knowledge of presence of toxicant in blood or tissue at concentrations comparable with those causing toxicity *in vitro*

[a] Standardized in this context means that the assay is performed consistently across laboratories and often is officially promulgated by a standardization body, such as AOAC International (formerly the Association of Official Analytical Chemists), or the protocol is specified by a regulatory agency.

[b] Toxicogenomics is a relatively new field, the impact of which is not possible to predict at this point. However, these types of data may become more important as the field progresses. If the value of genomics, proteomics, and other new technologies in identifying dangerous compounds is demonstrated in the future, then such results may warrant more concern than is indicated in this figure.

deficient in a specific DNA repair system than to otherwise identical cells that have the DNA repair system.

Because of the importance of genetic alterations in cancer development, and the observation that many carcinogens were also mutagenic, the original focus of genetic toxicology on evaluating potential hazards to the human gene pool shifted in the early 1970s to the use of genotoxicity assays as rapid screens for potential carcinogens (Ames et al., 1973, 1975; Bridges, 1976). The subsequent finding that many animal carcinogens are not genotoxic and that some chemicals show genotoxic activity in at least some assay systems, but do not show detectable carcinogenic activity in standard animal carcinogenicity studies, has somewhat lessened the attractiveness of genotoxicity assays (Tennant et al., 1987; Zeiger et al., 1990).

Regulatory agencies that require safety testing of chemicals, for example, EPA for pesticides (40 C.F.R. § 158.340 [2001]) and FDA for food additives (21 C.F.R. § 170 [2000]) and drugs (FDA, 1997), currently require testing for genotoxicity (see Annex 7-2 for specific assays). The required battery of tests varies slightly from agency to agency, but includes at least one assay for gene mutations (generally the Ames assay), and an assay for chromosome damage (*in vitro* and/or *in vivo*). Some programs require a mammalian gene mutation assay in addition to the typical Ames bacterial gene mutation assay, and the test battery may include an assay for induction of DNA repair. Also, testing in additional assays may be triggered by positive results in the initial battery.

While genotoxicity assays are no longer viewed as a quick and inexpensive way to detect chemical carcinogens, they do still have substantial utility. Under EPA's recently revised cancer risk assessment guidelines (EPA, 2003a), for example, much greater emphasis is placed on using information on the mode of action of a carcinogen to guide how the risk assessment is performed. Evidence of lack of genotoxicity, together with positive evidence of another mode of carcinogenic action, may lead to use of a risk assessment model that is not linear at low doses and predicts lesser risk at low doses than the default low-dose linear model. In this regard, EPA's approach has become more like that employed in many European countries, where nongenotoxic carcinogens have long been treated as presenting less risk at low doses than genotoxic carcinogens and are typically regulated in the same manner as noncarcinogens (identification of a no-effect level and application of an uncertainty factor to derive an allowable exposure level).

Similarly, the International Agency for Research on Cancer (IARC) sometimes uses evidence of genotoxicity to modify its ranking of a chemical. For example, ethylene oxide was recently elevated to a class 1 human carcinogen despite there being only "limited evidence" in human studies, because the available positive animal carcinogenicity and clear evidence of genotoxicity in a wide variety of assay systems *in vitro* and *in vivo* was considered by the IARC reviewers as being convincing evidence that there was a clear human cancer risk from ethylene oxide exposure (IARC, 1994).

In summary, genotoxicity data are not currently used alone in regulation of chemicals, and this is not likely to change. More commonly they are used to trigger a requirement for carcinogenicity testing. Internally, companies may use genotoxicity assays at an early point in product development as part of a screening system to identify promising leads—they may not wish to risk investing large amounts of time and money on a chemical that may turn out to be a carcinogen. This approach is consistent with Zeiger's (1998) conclusion that "if a chemical is mutagenic in Salmonella, it should be considered a potential rodent carcinogen, unless ancillary information suggests otherwise."

While it is estimated that only about 60 to 70 percent of mutagens are carcinogens depending on the system (Tennant et al., 1987), current approaches are to require follow-up testing when genotoxic data are observed for other substances. **It is consistent with these current approaches to consider genotoxic data about a dietary supplement ingredient as indicative of a possible carcinogen and a substantial risk of harm. If information suggests an ingredient is genotoxic, then responsible manufacturers will conduct additional research to determine if it is carcinogenic, which in many cases will provide mitigating information.**

ANNEX 7-2
IN VITRO TESTS VALIDATED FOR USE IN REGULATORY TOXICOLOGY CONTEXTS

It is necessary to understand if chemicals have the potential to affect the genetic components of mammalian cells because of the importance of mutations and chromosomal aberrations to cancer development and genetic disorders, whether in somatic cells or germ cells, as discussed in Annex 7-1. Despite the controversy surrounding use of genotoxic tests to predict which chemicals are carcinogenic, EPA (2003b) has selected a battery of tests "to detect, with sensitive assay methods, the capacity of a chemical to alter genetic material in cells" and "to determine the relevance of these mutagenic changes to mammals." "When mutagenic potential is demonstrated, these findings are incorporated in the assessment of heritable effect, oncogenicity, and possibly, other health effects" (EPA, 2003b). All of these tests are not universally accepted as fail-proof predictors of adverse human health effects, and the importance placed on each is not without debate (and, as indicated in the definition of "*validated*," assays should be considered validated even if their value as predictors is not universally agreed upon), but tests held in such high regard by a governmental agency do, on their own, indicate a potential for significant or unreasonable risk if results are not mitigated by other information.

In addition to mutagenicity tests, there is the opportunity to examine agents of interest in a battery of other *in vitro* tests that measure cytotoxicity, structural chromosomal aberrations, DNA damage, developmental toxicity, estrogenicity, and cell transformation (there are many other specific tests that could be used and these examples should not be viewed as inclusive):

- Cytotoxicity assays evaluate the ability of test materials to inhibit cellular proliferation in cells in culture. Often CHO-K_1-B_4 (Chinese hamster ovary) cells are used in this assay (Morita et al., 1992). For example, cytotoxicity of chromium picolinate was examined in Chinese hamster ovary cells (Stearns et al., 1995, 2002).

- The chromosomal aberration assay may also be conducted in CHO cells and detects the capacity of test agents to alter chromosomal structure (Buckton and Langlands, 1973; Gollapudi et al., 1986; Sinha et al., 1984). For example, genotoxicity assays assessing chromosomal aberrations were published for chromium picolinate (Stearns et al., 1995).
- Several methods are available for detection of developmental toxicity *in vitro*. One of these is the limb-bud micromass assay where fetal mouse limb-buds are allowed to differentiate via incubation in culture for 5 days with a test material. The test material's effect on cytotoxicity and limb-bud differentiation are compared to determine if differentiation is inhibited at concentrations that are not cytotoxic, a sign of a potentially teratogenic compound (Flint and Orton, 1984).
- A popular and standardized method for assessing DNA damage (cells may be exposed either *in vivo* or *in vitro*) is the alkaline Comet Assay. This assay has been shown to be a sensitive and simple assay in monitoring DNA strand breaks in human leukocytes (Collins et al., 1997; Rojas et al., 1999; Tice and Strauss, 1995).
- Estrogenic activity of test materials *in vitro* may be assessed relative to the activity of 17-β-estradiol. One such assay is an estrogen receptor transactivation assay usually preformed in MCF-7 cells (Charles et al., 2000a, 2000b). For example, norhydroguaiaretic acid, a constituent of prototype monograph substance chaparral, was tested for estrogen-like activity in MCF-7 cells (Sathyamoorthy et al., 1994).
- The Syrian Hamster Embryo cellular transformation assay shares similarities with multistage carcinogenesis *in vivo* (Isfort et al., 1996). The assay may be used to study underlying mechanisms of genotoxic and nongenotoxic chemical carcinogenesis (Zhang et al., 2000).

FDA also uses *in vitro* tests to identify potentially problematic chemicals of concern. In the *Redbook 2000,* it is recommended that a variety of short-term genetic toxicity tests be conducted for all chemicals that are direct food additives or color additives used in foods (OFAS, 2003). The data from genetic toxicity assays assist FDA in evaluating animal carcinogenicity data and in determining heritable effects of chemicals.

Specifically, the guidelines for specific toxicity studies suggest the following short-term tests for genetic toxicity:

- Bacterial Reverse Mutation Test,
- *In Vitro* Mammalian Chromosome Aberration Test,
- *In Vitro* Mouse Lymphoma $TK^{+/-}$ Gene Mutation Assay, and
- *In Vivo* Mammalian Erythrocyte Micronucleus Test.

FDA considers that positive results from these tests are sufficient to suggest risk unless there is further testing, in animals for example, that mitigates the concern. The value of such *in vitro* tests is no different if the test compound is a food additive or a dietary supplement. In fact, dietary supplement ingredients may sometimes be ingested in higher amounts than food additives. **If these tests, or similarly accepted tests, are positive for dietary supplement ingredients or products, then it is scientifically justifiable to consider that a risk exists unless there is mitigating information.**

ANNEX 7-3
USE OF NEW TECHNOLOGIES IN PREDICTING RISKS

Gene arrays, metabolomics, and proteomics are potential tools in the safety assessment of dietary supplements and many other materials. A number of recent publications discuss the use of these new technologies in their application to toxicology (Bartosiewicz et al., 2001; Farr and Dunn, 1999; Kuiper et al., 2001; Pennie et al., 2000; Robinson, 2001). One basic theme is that these technologies may provide a "fingerprint" of gene regulation associated with a toxic or adverse effect.

Gene arrays (also known as genomics, transcriptomics, DNA chips, or microarrays) allow quantitative comparisons of the expression levels of potentially thousands of individual genes among different biological samples, allowing comparisons of normal with treated cells or tissues. Metabolomics provides a means to systematically analyze nonpeptide small molecules, such as vitamins, sugars, hormones, fatty acids, and other biochemicals, and is distinct from traditional analyses that target individual metabolites or pathways. An organism's biochemical profile may be a better indicator of its cell physiology than a profile of its proteome or genome. Metabolomics may be able to detect differences in small molecules in cells, tissue, or fluid that are caused by chemical exposure. Such differences may eventually be used to understand mechanistic effects of substances and may provide insight into predicting potentially harmful substances. Proteomics is the analysis of many proteins and/or peptides simultaneously. Proteomics is used to identify proteins and their post-translational modifications, to quantify variation in protein content, and to study protein-protein interactions.

Several efforts are specifically focused on developing these new technologies into approaches for predicting potential toxicities based on limited *in vitro* and *in vivo* data (Castle et al., 2002; Hamadeh et al., 2002; Pennie and Kimber, 2002; Ulrich and Friend, 2002; Waring and Halbert, 2002). In the arena of prescription pharmaceutical development, such an approach might enable resources to be focused on compounds predicted to have less safety concerns. If they prove successful in predicting toxicity, there is no biological reason that the same technologies will not provide similar information in predicting risk from dietary supplement ingredients. The limitations in use of such techniques, however, are likely to be in determining the level of risk predicted by the tests and whether it is considered an "unreasonable risk" in regulatory terminology. The answers to these questions will depend on the eventual ability of these technologies to reliably identify toxic substances.

REFERENCES

Ames BN, Durston WE, Yamasaki E, Lee FD. 1973. Carcinogens are mutagens: A simple test system combining liver homogenates for activation and bacteria for detection. *Proc Natl Acad Sci USA* 70:2281–2285.

Ames BN, Mccann J, Yamasaki E. 1975. Methods for detecting carcinogens and mutagens with the Salmonella/mammalian-microsome mutagenicity test. *Mutat Res* 31:347–364.

Bartosiewicz M, Penn S, Buckpitt A. 2001. Applications of gene arrays in environmental toxicology: Fingerprints of gene regulation associated with cadmium chloride, benzo(a)pyrene, and trichloroethylene. *Environ Health Perspect* 109:71–74.

Bravo L. 1998. Polyphenols: Chemistry, dietary sources, metabolism, and nutritional significance. *Nutr Rev* 56:317–333.

Bridges BA. 1976. Short term screening tests for carcinogens. *Nature* 261:195–200.

Buckton KE, Langlands AO. 1973. The Edinburgh Thorotrast Series—Report of a cytogenetic study. *RISO Report* 294:114–125.

Castle AL, Carver MP, Mendrick DL. 2002. Toxicogenomics: A new revolution in drug safety. *Drug Discov Today* 7:728–736.

Charles GD, Bartels MJ, Zacharewski TR, Gollapudi BB, Freshour NL, Carney EW. 2000a. Activity of benzo[a]pyrene and its hydroxylated metabolites in an estrogen receptor-alpha reporter gene assay. *Toxicol Sci* 55:320–326.

Charles GD, Gennings C, Clemons J, Zacharewski TR, Gollapudi BB, Carney EW. 2000b. Optimization of an estrogen receptor-alpha transcriptional activation assay for testing a diverse spectrum of chemicals. *J Appl Toxicol* 20:449–454.

Collins AR, Dobson VL, Dusinska M, Kennedy G, Stetina R. 1997. The comet assay: What can it really tell us? *Mut Res* 375:183–193.

EPA (U.S. Environmental Protection Agency). 2003a. *Draft Final Guidelines for Carcinogen Risk Assessment.* Online. Available at http://www.epa.gov/ncea/raf/cancer2003.htm. Accessed July 7, 2003.

EPA. 2003b. *EPA Pesticides: Data Requirements.* Online. Available at http://www.epa.gov/pesticides/regulating/data.htm. Accessed December 16, 2003.

Farr S, Dunn RT 2nd. 1999. Concise review: Gene expression applied to toxicology. *Toxicol Sci* 50:1–9.

FDA (Food and Drug Administration). 1997. International conference on harmonisation. Guidance on genotoxicity: A standard battery for genotoxicity testing of pharmaceuticals. *Fed Regis* 62:62471–62475.

Flint OP, Orton TC. 1984. An in vitro assay for teratogens with cultures of rat embryo midbrain and limb bud cells. *Toxicol Appl Pharmacol* 76:383–395.

Gollapudi BB, Sutcliffe DJ, Sinha AK. 1986. Assessment of cytogenetic response to folic acid deprivation in rat lymphocytes. *In Vitro Cell Dev Biol* 22:681–684.

Hamadeh HK, Amin RP, Paules RS, Afshari CA. 2002. An overview of toxicogenomics. *Curr Issues Mol Biol* 4:45–56.

IARC (International Agency for Research on Cancer). 1994. Ethylene oxide. *IARC Monogr Eval Carcinog Risks Hum* 60:73–159.

Isfort RJ, Kerckaert GA, LeBoeuf RA. 1996. Comparison of the standard and reduced pH Syrian Hamster Embryo (SHE) cell *in vitro* transformation assays in predicting the carcinogenic potential of chemicals. *Mutat Res* 1:11–63.

Kuiper HA, Kleter GA, Noteborn HP, Kok EJ. 2001. Assessment of the food safety issues related to genetically modified foods. *Plant J* 27:503–528.

Morita T, Nagaki T, Fukuda I, Okumura K. 1992. Clastogenicity of low pH to various cultured mammalian cells. *Mutat Res* 268:297–305.

OFAS (Office of Food Additive Safety). 2001. *Toxicological Principles for the Safety Assessment of Direct Food Additives and Color Additives Used in Food. Redbook II–Draft.* Washington, DC: OFAS, Food and Drug Administration.

OFAS. 2003. *Redbook 2000 Toxicological Principles for the Safety of Food Ingredients.* Online. CSFAN, Food and Drug Administration. Available at http://www.cfsan.fda.gov/~redbook/red-toca.html. Accessed June 19, 2003.

Pennie WD, Kimber I. 2002. Toxicogenomics: Transcript profiling and potential application to chemical allergy. *Toxicol In Vitro* 16:319–326.

Pennie WD, Tugwood JD, Oliver GJ, Kimber I. 2000. The principles and practice of toxicogenomics: Applications and opportunities. *Toxicol Sci* 54:277–283.

Preston RJ, Hoffmann GR. 2001. Genetic toxicology. In: Klaassen CD, ed. *Casarett and Doull's Toxicology: The Basic Science of Poisons.* New York: McGraw-Hill. Pp. 321–350.

Robinson C. 2001. *Genetic Modification Technology and Food: Consumer Health and Safety. ILSI Europe Concise Monograph Series.* Washington, DC: ILSI Press.

Roche O, Trube G, Zuegge J, Pflimlin P, Alanine A, Schneider G. 2002. A virtual screening method for prediction of the hERG potassium channel liability of compound libraries. *Chembiochem* 3:455–459.

Rojas E, Lopez MC, Valverde M. 1999. Single cell gel electrophoresis assay: Methodology and applications. *J Chromatogr B* 722:225–254.

Sathyamoorthy N, Wang TT, Phang JM. 1994. Stimulation of pS2 expression by diet-derived compounds. *Cancer Res* 54:957–961.

Sinha AK, Linscombe VA, Gollapudi BB, McClintock ML, Flake RE, Bodner KM. 1984. The incidence of spontaneous cytogenetic aberrations in lymphocytes cultured from normal humans for 48 and 72 H. *Can J Genet Cytol* 26:528–531.

Stearns DM, Wise JP, Patierno SR, Wetterhahn KE. 1995. Chromium (III) picolinate produces chromosome damage in Chinese hamster ovary cells. *FASEB J* 9:1643–1648.

Stearns DM, Silveira SM, Wolf KK, Luke AM. 2002. Chromium (III) tris (picolinate) is mutagenic at the hypoxanthine (guanine) phosphoribosyltransferase locus in Chinese hamster ovary cells. *Mut Res* 513:135–142.

Tennant RW, Margolin BH, Shelby MD, Zeiger E, Haseman JK, Spalding J, Caspary W, Resnick M, Stasiewicz S, Anderson B, Minor R. 1987. Prediction of chemical carcinogenicity in rodents from *in vitro* genetic toxicity assays. *Science* 236:933–941.

Tice RR, Strauss GHS. 1995. The single cell gel electrophoresis/comet assay: A potential tool for detecting radiation-induced DNA damage in humans. *Stem Cells* 13:207S–214S.

Ulrich R, Friend SH. 2002. Toxicogenomics and drug discovery: Will new technologies help us produce better drugs? *Nat Rev Drug Discov* 1:84–88.

Waring JF, Halbert DN. 2002. The promise of toxicogenomics. *Curr Opin Mol Ther* 4:229–235.

Yang CS, Landau JM, Huang MT, Newmark HL. 2001. Inhibition of carcinogenesis by dietary polyphenolic compounds. *Annu Rev Nutr* 21:381–406.

Zeiger E. 1998. Identification of rodent carcinogens and noncarcinogens using genetic toxicity tests: Premises, promises, and performance. *Regul Toxicol Pharmacol* 28:85–95.

Zeiger E, Haseman JK, Shelby MD, Margolin BH, Tennant RW. 1990. Evaluation of four *in vitro* genetic toxicity tests for predicting rodent carcinogenicity: Confirming of earlier results with 41 additional chemicals. *Environ Mol Mutagen* 16:1S–14S.

Zhang H, Xu Y, Kamendulis LM, Klaunig JE. 2000. Morphological transformation by 8-hydroxy-2'-deoxyguanosine in Syrian hamster embryo (SHE) cells. *Toxicol Sci* 56:303–312.

8

Interactions

GUIDING PRINCIPLE: *The principles used in identifying drug-food and drug-drug interactions should be applied to identifying possible dietary supplement-induced interactions with other bioactive compounds, including drugs, foods, and other dietary supplement ingredients.*

One of the major concerns about the safety of dietary supplement ingredients is that interactions between a supplement and other ingested substances (e.g., drugs, other dietary supplements,[1] conventional foods) will result in adverse clinical outcomes due to an increase or decrease in the level of the dietary supplement in the organism, an increase or decrease in the level of other xenobiotics,[2] or combined toxicities. Potential adverse clinical outcomes may result if a dietary supplement lowers a drug's effective concentration. Such a drop in active drug concentration can have serious consequences, especially for persons whose health depends on the therapeutic effects of a drug. As examples, AIDS patients must maintain a therapeutic

---

[1]Many dietary supplement products are mixtures of two or more substances, some of unknown structure, making an evaluation of interactions more complex, but also more likely to be of clinical concern as they are consumed simultaneously.

[2]A chemical substance or compound that is foreign to the human body or to other living organisms.

level of antiviral activity, cancer patients must maintain an effective concentration of chemotherapeutic agents, those with organ transplants must maintain a therapeutic level of immunosuppressant, and those with hypertension must maintain effective levels of antihypertensive drugs. Conversely, interactions can raise a drug's level (or that of the dietary supplement ingredient itself) above the therapeutic range, which may lead to toxic effects.

Interactions can be detected with human, animal, or *in vitro* studies or predicted on the basis of how related substances behave. Therefore, types of interactions are discussed in this chapter, experimental methods for identifying ingredients that may cause these types of interactions are described, and guidance on how to interpret the results from studies using these methods is provided. In addition, types of individuals most vulnerable to the various types of interactions are discussed.

TYPES OF INTERACTIONS

There are numerous mechanisms for interactions among xenobiotics, but most can be categorized as direct chemical-chemical, pharmacodynamic, or pharmacokinetic interactions.

Direct Chemical-Chemical Interactions

The formation of chemical-chemical complexes can modify the action of one or both chemicals. In general, these types of interactions require ingestion of both chemicals within a relatively short time of each other. An example of a direct chemical-chemical interaction occurs in the small intestine, where calcium carbonate taken as a supplement may bind to an acid substance, such as the antibiotic tetracycline, to form an insoluble product (Gugler and Allgayer, 1990). In this case, since the acid was a drug, the action of the drug would be reduced or lost. Other examples include cholestyramine, which adsorbs other drugs, thereby decreasing their availability for absorption, and antacids, which can block iron or zinc uptake. In addition to forming complexes, antacids may significantly change the rate of absorption of other chemicals by altering gastric pH or gastric emptying time, depending on the extent to which pH affects the amount of chemical in the un-ionized state (Azarnoff and Hurwitz, 1970; Hurwitz, 1971, 1977; Hurwitz and Scholzman, 1974; Hurwitz and Sheehan, 1971; Hurwitz et al., 1976).

Pharmacodynamic Interactions

Pharmacodynamic interactions are interactions that result in a change in the response to either the dietary supplement ingredient or the xenobiotic, but with no change in the plasma concentration of either. Pharmacodynamic interactions can result when two xenobiotics with similar pharmacological action produce an additive or synergistic response or when two xenobiotics with opposing pharmacological effects produce a reduced response. Predicting when a pharmacodynamic interaction may occur and the clinical results of this interaction depends on understanding the sites and mechanism of biological activity of both chemicals and predicting whether adequate levels are achieved at the sites of action.

Direct Pharmacodynamic Interactions

Direct pharmacodynamic interactions occur at the same site, such as an extracellular receptor or an enzyme where each xenobiotic exerts its pharmacological effect. The two xenobiotics may produce an additive physiological effect or, in the case of one being an antagonist or a weaker agonist, the result may be to decrease the response to the stronger agonist.

Indirect Pharmacodynamic Interactions

Indirect pharmacodynamic interactions occur when two xenobiotics act on the same physiological pathway from the receptor to the effector, but at different molecular sites of action. For example, two substances may each affect the same organ, but in different ways, and when taken together may greatly increase the propensity for organ damage, even if toxic effects are not detected independently.

Interactions with Dietary Supplements

There are examples of pharmacodynamic interactions that have been noted with dietary supplement ingredients. The antihypertensive effect of guanabenz acetate (a drug used for hypertension) is due to its central agonistic α-2-adrenoceptor activity (Grossman et al., 1993; Wenzel et al., 2001). Thus concomitant consumption of yohimbine bark, which contains an α-2-adrenoreceptor antagonist, may diminish the antihypertensive activity of guanabenz through its opposing pharmacodynamic effect. Another example is between the inotropic drug digitalis (Katzung, 2001) and hawthorne leaf or flower; data suggest that both the hawthorne leaf and the flower may also have a positive inotropic and electrophysiological effect on the heart (Schwinger et al., 2000). If digitalis and the hawthorne leaf or flower are taken together, the additive response may be excessive and lead to a serious adverse event (Schwinger et al., 2000). Another additive effect would be exhibited by the ginkgo leaf if its purported antagonism of platelet-activating factor occurred; if ingested with a cyclooxygenase inhibitor, such as aspirin, an increased propensity for bleeding would occur (Braquet, 1987; Lenoir et al., 2002; Vale, 1998; Vogensen et al., 2003).

Pharmacokinetic Interactions

Pharmacokinetic interactions are interactions that occur when one substance affects the absorption, distribution, metabolism, or excretion of another substance, resulting in altered levels of one of the substances or its metabolites. These interactions include effects caused by the chemicals on xenobiotic metabolizing enzymes and transporters that affect the time course of the concentration of one or both of the chemicals in the body. These interactions commonly take place in the intestines, liver, or kidney and are further categorized based on their site of action.

Altered Metabolism

Interactions that alter metabolism warrant attention. Xenobiotics often undergo extensive metabolic alteration by enzymes, resulting in the formation of structurally modified derivatives (metabolites) that may possess different pharmacologic activities (either greater or less) when compared with that of the consumed parent compound. There are more than 30 families of xenobiotic metabolizing enzymes in humans, many of which may be limiting for biotransformation of the consumed xenobiotic. If an ingested xenobiotic increases or decreases the amount or activity of a given enzyme, its own rate of metabolism may be altered, as well as that of other consumed compounds. The clinical effect of changes in enzyme metabolism rates will depend on the xenobiotic(s) involved and their metabolites and potencies.

An important group of xenobiotic metabolizing enzymes are the cytochrome P450 (CYP) enzymes, a superfamily of hemoproteins that mediate the biotransformation of endogenous and exogenous compounds (Nelson et al., 1996) in the liver, as well as in the intestine and elsewhere. Some CYP isozymes found to be involved with significant pharmacokinetic reactions in humans are CYP1A2, 2C9, 2C19, 2D6, 2E1, and 3A4 (Health Canada, 2000; Ingelman-Sundberg, 2001). In addition, CYP2A6 and CYP2B6 are involved in metabolizing certain xenobiotics (Health Canada, 2000). Since many chemicals are substrates for the same CYP isozymes, one compound may inhibit the activity of the enzyme metabolizing another compound that is ingested concomitantly. In addition, ingestion of a chemical hours before another chemical may induce the production of more enzyme or inhibit normal enzyme synthesis, thus affecting the rate of metabolism of a second chemical metabolized by that same enzyme. While not without controversy, grapefruit juice provides one example of an interaction associated with

CYP enzymes; it is reported to suppress CYP3A4 and change the concentration of drugs metabolized by the enzyme (Fuhr, 1998). When considering dietary supplement ingredient safety, assays for xenobiotic alterations of enzyme metabolism may generate important signals of possible concern, as discussed below.

Altered Absorption, Distribution, and Excretion

Until recently, pharmacokinetic interactions were considered as primarily attributable to the effects on xenobiotic metabolizing enzymes. However, an increasing number of transporters that affect chemical absorption, distribution, and excretion now seem to also play a significant role in pharmacokinetic interactions (Evans and Relling, 1999; Meyer, 2000). Transporters regulate the flux of substances into and out of cells or perform a variety of transmembrane transport functions. Depending on their location and activity, they may have a significant effect on the concentration of a chemical at its site of action (Kim, 2002).

Important transporters are the multidrug resistance transporters, which include P-glycoproteins encoded by the MDR1 gene. P-glycoprotein functions as an efflux pump located in the cell membranes of enterocytes and hepatocytes, as well as the renal tubule epithelium (Fleisher et al., 1999; Yu, 1999).

Interactions between chemicals resulting from competition at transporters are not uncommon. Thus *in vitro* methods to evaluate the effect of chemicals on particular transporters have been developed (Cummins et al., 2001). Due to differences in human and animal transporters, the methods often employ human transporter proteins expressed in artificial *in vitro* systems, enabling the detailed study of human transporter protein functions with regard to drugs and other xenobiotic substances, including dietary supplement ingredients.

The concentration of the immunosuppressant drug cyclosporine attained in blood is controlled by the MDR1-encoded transporter and CYP. St. John's wort is an example of a dietary supplement that has been shown to affect both the MDR1-encoded transporter and the enzyme CYP3A4 (Markowitz et al., 2003; Wang et al., 2001). St. John's wort consumption by organ transplant patients requiring immunosuppressance can result in significant reductions in the concentration of cyclosporine, leading to organ rejection (Bauer et al., 2003; Karliova et al., 2000; Ruschitzka et al., 2000).

Another example is the reported interaction between St. John's wort and oral contraceptives. Circulating estrogen levels following oral contraceptive intake is regulated in part by the activity of MDR1-encoded transporters (Barnes et al., 1996). A woman who was taking oral contraceptives became pregnant after consuming St. John's wort, which may have been due to enhanced efflux leading to ineffective levels of the oral contraceptive (Schwarz et al., 2003).

Competition for Protein Binding

Another type of potential pharmacokinetic interaction is binding to plasma proteins. Competition for protein binding sites by xenobiotics can alter the amount of unbound xenobiotic (i.e., free drug or other substance) available to exert its pharmacological effect (Shoeman and Azarnoff, 1975). The concern is that displacement of a highly plasma protein-bound xenobiotic by another compound may result in increased activity of the displaced compound.

Although protein binding has long been described as a potential site of interaction, its actual importance has recently come under debate as some have provided evidence that changes in plasma protein binding are not clinically relevant (Benet and Hoener, 2002). It will be necessary to evaluate the potential for displacement from protein binding sites as an interaction on a case-by-case basis. The extent of protein binding, the protein binding site, and the concentration in blood of each substance are the main factors to consider.

Effects on Excretion

Renal or biliary excretion of xenobiotics, and thus the steady-state plasma concentration of xenobiotics, may also be affected by other xenobiotics. Changes in renal clearance of one xenobiotic can occur through effects of another substance on the urinary pH. Another mechanism for interaction is the effect of one substance on the active secretion of another substance into the renal tubule. Methods to evaluate the effects of a xenobiotic on excretion are available; they include measurement of tubular uptake, such as perfused kidney assays, or assays at the cellular level. Dietary supplement ingredients that inhibit tubular uptake or in any other way disrupt molecular mechanisms important to excretion of other xenobiotics should be considered of potential concern.

PREDICTING THE POTENTIAL OF INGREDIENTS TO CAUSE PHARMACOKINETIC INTERACTIONS

Techniques currently available allow the determination of the extent to which one substance may impact the concentration of other concomitantly ingested substances. There are numerous well-accepted *in vitro* assays designed specifically to determine if a drug may interact with other substances. There are also approaches for describing structures of chemicals likely to cause interactions. These *in vitro* studies and other approaches have focused on determining which drugs affect metabolizing enzymes and transporters and could similarly be used to determine which dietary supplements may lead to interactions. Whether an interaction predicted on the basis of *in vitro* studies actually occurs clinically will depend on whether the dietary supplement compound attains a concentration *in vivo* adequate to reproduce the effect observed *in vitro*, as discussed in more detail below.

In Vitro Prediction of Pharmacokinetic Effects

In vitro studies for determining which xenobiotics affect transporters and metabolic enzymes ideally employ human transporter proteins or human metabolic enzymes. For example, subcellular fractions of human liver tissue are commonly used, as are whole-cell models such as isolated human hepatocytes (Li, 1997; Sinz, 1999), liver slices (Ferrero and Brendel, 1997), and cell lines derived from human cancer cells (Yee and Day, 1999). Human transporters and enzymes can also effectively be studied by expressing them in other cell types (Crespi and Penman, 1997; Rodrigues, 1999). Changes in either the activity or amount of enzyme or transporter are detected with activity assays, pharmacological assays, and immunochemical or mRNA assays that detect changes in protein or transcription (Li, 1997).

In vitro assays for predicting possible interactions are a well-accepted staple of the drug development process. The limitation to using these assays to predict clinical interactions lies, like most *in vitro* assays, in relating the dose at which enzyme or transporter effects are observed with the amount of unbound xenobiotic present at the active site *in vivo*. If information about the concentration of xenobiotic reached *in vivo* is available, a comparison of a dietary supplement ingredient's inhibitory binding constants (K_i) for the CYP enzymes and the *in vivo* concentration (C_{max}) may place the *in vitro* information in the appropriate perspective.

Animal and Human *In Vivo* Data in Predicting Pharmacokinetic Effects

Given the inter- and intraspecies differences in xenobiotic metabolizing enzymes, it is ideal to study xenobiotic metabolism using human cells, subcellular fractions of human tissue, or heterologously expressed human proteins (see Health Canada, 2000), although information about effects on animal proteins may serve as a preliminary indicator of concern. The study of human proteins in transgenic animals may improve ability to relate effects observed in animals or animal cells to humans.

Humans themselves may also be studied to determine if a given xenobiotic may cause an observable interaction. Such tests are usually designed to compare the levels of a test substrate with and without the xenobiotic in question. For example, a study of St. John's wort in humans demonstrated that it increased the metabolism of CYP3A4 substrates (Markowitz et al., 2003). Even if specific interaction assays are not done, information about the *in vivo* concentrations achieved in humans is useful in placing *in vitro* information in perspective.

Databases for Predicting Interactions

Databases helpful for identifying substances likely to interact with other substances have been organized. For example, the database produced by the University of Washington is useful for locating information about potential interactions of particular dietary supplements with other substances (UW, 2003). The database also organizes information, such as drug effects on CYP enzymes, that may be useful for identifying potential interactions between particular drugs and supplements. A publicly available website at the Indiana University School of Medicine provides information about drugs metabolized by specific P450 isoforms (Indiana University, 2003).

Vulnerable Subpopulations

Some individuals are particularly sensitive to adverse effects from xenobiotic interactions because of polymorphic differences that affect the metabolism of some xenobiotics (Ingelman-Sundberg et al., 1999). There are recognized genetic polymorphisms that account for diminished or absent expression of one or more forms of xenobiotic-metabolizing enzymes. There are documented adverse effects directly resulting from the altered metabolism of certain drugs metabolized by these enzymes. A well-known example is people who exhibit little or no CYP2D6 activity in the liver because of inherited genes defective in expression of this form of CYP—a condition that affects 7 to 10 percent of Caucasians, by one estimate (Cascorbi, 2003). As a result, such individuals are found to experience toxic effects from ordinary doses of the antihypertensive agent debrisoquine, as well as many other drugs for which metabolic elimination is primarily catalyzed by CYP2D6 (Cascorbi, 2003).

It would be reasonable to expect that any dietary supplement ingredient dependent on CYP2D6 for metabolic conversion could potentially produce toxic effects in such persons. Numerous other polymorphisms in xenobiotic metabolism have been or are being identified. Such data can serve to identify people who may be particularly sensitive to dietary supplements cleared by these polymorphic xenobiotic metabolizing systems.

Practical Impact of Shared Pharmacokinetic Pathways on Predicting Interactions

A dietary supplement that affects the pharmacokinetics of one xenobiotic may be of concern when concomitantly consumed with any of a number of other xenobiotics because the pharmacokinetic pathways are shared by so many substances. This is especially true for dietary supplements that interact with the CYP enzymes. CYP3A, for example, is considered to be largely responsible for the metabolism of a large number (some have estimated 50 percent) of clinically prescribed drugs and probably a large share of other xenobiotics, including other chemicals and dietary supplements (Ingelman-Sundberg et al., 1999).

The state of scientific understanding in this field is such that it is unnecessary to test each and every combination of xenobiotics to predict potential risks. Reasonable scientific inferences can be made to anticipate risks without accumulating clinical examples of each combination. For example, there is sufficient knowledge about the catalytic functions of human CYP3A to confidently predict that if St. John's wort causes the loss of function of HIV drugs by inducing CYP3A (Piscitelli et al., 2000), the same interaction extends to some of the other known substrates of CYP3A. The same thought process and scientific reasoning would apply to the other xenobiotic metabolizing and transporting systems, as well. That is, the more general the pathway affected by the dietary supplement ingredient, the more widespread the potential for interaction.

SUMMARY

Dietary supplements have a potential to adversely affect public health by interacting with other substances. Whether this concern is addressed by labeling precautions, withdrawal of such dietary supplements from the market or requiring warning labels related to usage with other xenobiotics is a regulatory decision. Pharmacists and physicians are made aware of drugs and foods that can potentially interact with other drugs, and drug labeling warns about potential problems. There is no analogous prescribed mechanism to prevent dietary supplement-mediated interactions.

A number of pieces of information can suggest a possible interaction between a dietary supplement ingredient and other substances. The potential seriousness of these interactions varies and is placed in perspective by considering if a particular interaction leads to serious adverse events and the likelihood that the interaction will occur. This relative spectrum of concern is illustrated in Table 8-1.

TABLE 8-1 Spectrum of Concern for Interactions

Increasing Concern →		
Pharmacokinetic and/or pharmacodynamic data suggesting a supplement-drug/food/other dietary supplement interaction that might lead to a serious adverse event and/or identifying a population at risk for a serious adverse event	Pharmacokinetic and/or pharmacodynamic data documenting a supplement-drug/food/ other dietary supplement interaction that might lead to a serious adverse event and/or identifying a population at risk for a serious adverse event	Pharmacokinetic and/or pharmacodynamic data documenting a supplement-drug/food/other dietary supplement interaction that leads to a serious adverse event

REFERENCES

Azarnoff DL, Hurwitz A. 1970. Drug interactions. *Pharmacol Physicians* 4:1–7.

Barnes KM, Dickstein B, Cutler GB Jr, Fojo T, Bates SE. 1996. Steroid transport, accumulation, and antagonism of P-glycoprotein in multidrug-resistant cells. *Biochemistry* 35:4820–4827.

Bauer S, Stormer E, Johne A, Kruger H, Budde K, Neumayer HH, Roots I, Mai I. 2003. Alterations in cyclosporin A pharmacokinetics and metabolism during treatment with St John's wort in renal transplant patients. *Br J Clin Pharmacol* 55:203–211.

Benet LZ, Hoener BA. 2002. Changes in plasma protein binding have little clinical relevance. *Clin Pharmacol Ther* 71:115–121.

Braquet P. 1987. The ginkgolides: Potent platelet-activating factor antagonists isolated from *Ginko biloba* L: Chemistry, pharmacology and clinical applications. *Drugs Future* 12:643–699.

Cascorbi I. 2003. Pharmacogenetics of cytochrome P4502D6: Genetic background and clinical implications. *Eur J Clin Invest* 33:17S–22S.

Crespi CL, Penman BW. 1997. Use of cDNA-expressed human cytochrome P450 enzymes to study potential drug-drug interactions. *Adv Pharmacol* 43:171–188.

Cummins CL, Mangravite LM, Benet LZ. 2001. Characterizing the expression of CYP3A4 and efflux transporters (P-gp, MRP1, and MRP2) in CYP3A4-transfected Caco-2 cells after induction with sodium butyrate and the phorbol ester 12-O-tetradecanoylphorbol-13-acetate. *Pharm Res* 18:1102–1109.

Evans WE, Relling MV. 1999. Pharmacogenomics: Translating functional genomics into rational therapeutics. *Science* 286:487–491.

Ferrero JL, Brendel K. 1997. Liver slices as a model in drug metabolism. *Adv Pharmacol* 43:131–169.

Fleisher D, Li C, Zhou Y, Pao LH, Karim A. 1999. Drug, meal and formulation interactions influencing drug absorption after oral administration. Clinical implications. *Clin Pharmacokinet* 6:233–254.

Fuhr U. 1998. Drug interactions with grapefruit juice. Extent, probable mechanism and clinical relevance. *Drug Safe* 18:251–272.

Grossman E, Rosenthal T, Peleg E, Holmes C, Goldstein DS. 1993. Oral yohimbine increases blood pressure and sympathetic nervous outflow in hypertensive patients. *J Cardiovasc Cardiol* 22:22–26.

Gugler R, Allgayer H. 1990. Effects of antacids on the clinical pharmacokinetics of drugs. An update. *Clin Pharmacokinet* 18:210–219.

Health Canada. 2000. *Therapeutic Products Programme Guidance Document. Drug-Drug Interactions: Studies In Vitro and In Vivo*. Online. Available at http://www.hc-sc.gc.ca/hpfb-dgpsa/tpd-dpt/drug_int_e.pdf. Accessed July 7, 2003.

Hurwitz A. 1971. The effects of antacids on gastrointestinal drug absorption. II. Effect on sulfadiazine and quinine. *J Pharmacol Exp Ther* 179:485–489.

Hurwitz A. 1977. Antacid therapy and drug kinetics. *Clin Pharmacokinet* 2:269–280.

Hurwitz A, Schlozman DL. 1974. Effects of antacids on gastrointestinal absorption of isoniazid in rat and man. *Am Rev Respir Dis* 109:41–47.

Hurwitz A, Sheehan MB. 1971. The effects of antacids on the absorption of orally administered pentobarbital in the rat. *J Pharmacol Exp Ther* 179:124–131.

Hurwitz A, Robinson RG, Vats TS, Whittier FC, Herrin WF. 1976. Effect of antacids on gastric emptying. *Gastroenterology* 71:268–273.

Indiana University. 2003. *Drug Interactions. Defining Genetic Influences on Pharmacologic Responses*. Online. Available at http://medicine.iupui.edu/flockhart. Accessed March 15, 2004.

Ingelman-Sundberg M. 2001. Implications of polymorphic cytochrome P450-dependent drug metabolism for drug development. *Drug Metab Dispos* 29:570–573.

Ingelman-Sundberg M, Oscarson M, McLellan RA. 1999. Polymorphic human cytochrome P450 enzymes: An opportunity for individualized drug treatment. *Trends Pharmacol Sci* 20:342–349.

Karliova M, Treichel U, Malago M, Frilling A, Gerken G, Broelsch CE. 2000. Interaction of *Hypericum perforatum* (St. John's wort) with cyclosporin A metabolism in a patient after liver transplantation. *J Hepatol* 33:853–855.

Katzung BG. 2001. *Basic and Clinical Pharmacology*. 8th ed. New York: McGraw–Hill.

Kim RB. 2002. Transporters and xenobiotic disposition. *Toxicology* 181:291–297.

Lenoir M, Pedruzzi E, Rais S, Drieu K, Perianin A. 2002. Sensitization of human neutrophil defense activities through activation of platelet-activating factor receptors by ginkgolide B, a bioactive component of the *Ginkgo biloba* extract EGB 761. *Biochem Pharmacol* 63:1241–1249.

Li AP. 1997. Primary hepatocyte cultures as an *in vitro* experimental model for the evaluation of pharmacokinetic drug-drug interactions. *Adv Pharmacol* 43:103–130.

Markowitz JS, Donovan JL, DeVane CO, Taylor RM, Ruan Y, Wang J, Chavin KD. 2003. Effect of St. John's wort on drug metabolism by induction of cytochrome P450 3A4 enzyme. *J Am Med Assoc* 290:1500–1504.

Meyer UA. 2000. Pharmacogenetics and adverse drug reactions. *Lancet* 356:1667–1671.

Nelson DR, Koymans L, Kamataki T, Stegeman JJ, Feyereisen R, Waxman DJ, Waterman MR, Gotoh O, Coon MJ, Estabrook RW, Gunsalus IC, Nebert DW. 1996. P450 superfamily: Update on new sequences, gene mapping, accession numbers and nomenclature. *Pharmacogenetics* 6:1–42.

Piscitelli SC, Burstein AH, Chaitt D, Alfaro RM, Falloon J. 2000. Indinavir concentrations and St John's wort. *Lancet* 355:547–548.

Rodrigues AD. 1999. Applications of heterologous expressed and purified human drug-metabolizing enzymes: An industrial perspective. In: Woolf TF, ed. *Handbook of Drug Metabolism*. New York: Marcel Dekker. Pp. 279–320.

Ruschitzka F, Meier PJ, Turina M, Luscher TF, Noll G. 2000. Acute heart transplant rejection due to Saint John's wort. *Lancet* 355:548–549.

Schwarz UI, Buschel B, Kirch W. 2003. Unwanted pregnancy on self-medication with St John's wort despite hormonal contraception. *Br J Clin Pharmacol* 55:112–113.

Schwinger RH, Pietsch M, Frank K, Brixius K. 2000. Crataegus special extract Ws 1442 increases force of contraction in human myocardium CAMP-independently. *J Cardiovasc Pharmacol* 35:700–707.

Shoeman DW, Azarnoff DL. 1975. Diphenylhydantoin potency and plasma protein binding. *J Pharmacol Exper Ther* 195:84–86.

Sinz MW. 1999. *In vitro* metabolism: Hepatocytes. In: Woolf TF, ed. *Handbook of Drug Metabolism.* New York: Marcel Dekker. Pp. 401–424.

UW (University of Washington). 2003. *Metabolism and Transport Drug Interaction Database.* Online. Available at http://depts.washington.edu/didbase. Accessed September 24, 2004.

Vale S. 1998. Subarachnoid haemorrhage associated with *Ginkgo biloba. Lancet* 352:36.

Vogensen SB, Stromgaard K, Shindou H, Jaracz S, Suehiro M, Ishii S, Shimizu T, Nakanishi K. 2003. Preparation of 7-substituted ginkgolide derivatives: Potent platelet activating factor (PAF) receptor antagonists. *J Med Chem* 46:601–608.

Wang Z, Gorski JC, Hamman MA, Huang SM, Lesko LJ, Hall SD. 2001. The effects of St John's wort (*Hypericum perforatum*) on human cytochrome P450 activity. *Clin Pharmacol Ther* 70:317–326.

Wenzel RR, Bruck H, Mitchell A, Schaefers RF, Baumgart D, Erbel R, Heemann U, Philipp T. 2001. Interaction of the sympathetic nervous system with other pressor systems in antihypertensive therapy. *J Clin Basic Cardiol* 4:185–192.

Yee S, Day WW. 1999. Application of Caco-2 cells in drug discovery and development. In: Woolf TF, ed. *Handbook of Drug Metabolism.* New York: Marcel Dekker. Pp. 507–522.

Yu DK. 1999. The contribution of P-glycoprotein to pharmacokinetic drug-drug interactions. *J Clin Pharmacol* 39:1203–1211.

9

Vulnerable Groups and Prevalence of Use

The information in Chapters 4 through 8, which describe the scientific bases for evaluating safety of dietary supplement ingredients, is critical in determining which dietary supplement ingredients warrant the most immediate attention, that is, in setting risk-based priorities. However, it is also appropriate to take other information into consideration when setting priorities. For example, given *similar* degrees of concern about risk, attention from the Food and Drug Administration (FDA) is more appropriately directed towards a supplement that is being used by a greater portion of the population. It is also important to consider the safety of the most sensitive groups. This chapter describes these additional considerations.

USE BY VULNERABLE SUBPOPULATIONS

GUIDING PRINCIPLE: *When data indicate that an identifiable subpopulation may be especially sensitive to adverse effects from a specific dietary supplement ingredient, this should be taken into account when setting priorities.*

When considering the safety of dietary supplement ingredients, it is important to consider that some individuals may be particularly vulnerable to adverse effects from certain dietary supplement ingredients. Vulnerable subpopulations can be defined as groups of individuals who are more likely to experience an adverse event related to the use of a particular dietary supplement ingredient, or individuals in whom the specific adverse effects identified are more likely to be serious in comparison with the general population. Characteristics that contribute to such vulnerability may be physiological (including genetic predisposition), disease-related, or due to other aspects, such as lifestyle or therapeutic interventions that are commonly utilized by a subgroup.

Age-Related Changes

Physiological characteristics frequently result in an individual's increased susceptibility compared with the general population; an example of this is the change in the capacity to metabolize various dietary supplement ingredients across the lifespan. Changes in metabolism may lead to variable concentrations of active compounds at sites of action, resulting in different responses. For example, elderly individuals are a potential vulnerable subpopulation for some ingredients in that aging is associated with changes in the ability to digest, metabolize, or excrete some ingested substances (Munro, 1989; Rosenberg et al., 1989). Other age-related changes may involve receptors or kinetic parameters, such as the volume of distribution (Mangoni and Jackson, 2004).

Supplement ingredients that are normally excreted or altered by the kidney or liver may potentially pose a greater risk to the elderly subgroup than to a younger population. This fact should be considered for supplements specifically directed toward an older population, such as those consumed to prevent osteoporosis or Alzheimer's disease.

Children also metabolize some chemical substances differently than do adults, which for certain supplement ingredients may make children more susceptible to adverse effects (Guzelian et al., 1992). This should be taken into consideration for supplements marketed toward children or likely to be given to children. Infants have limited liver function that may make them particularly susceptible to certain hepatotoxic substances (Brown, 1968).

Pregnancy and Fetus Considerations

Pregnancy-related physiological changes may make pregnant women more susceptible to adverse effects associated with particular dietary supplement ingredients. In addition, the fetus may also be particularly vulnerable; special concerns are warranted for supplement ingredients that may have teratogenic effects. Fetuses may be harmed if they are exposed to dangerous substances *in utero*, as may infants if they are exposed to substances released into human milk. A well-known example is the teratogenicity of high doses of vitamin A in the periconceptual period (Eckhoff and Nau, 1990; Lammer et al., 1985; Rothman et al., 1995). Animal studies or chemical characteristics may provide clues that fetuses or infants are particularly susceptible to other supplement ingredients as well. Given these concerns, unless a supplement has been specifically tested for risk during pregnancy or is required for medical reasons, use of dietary supplements during pregnancy cannot be supported.

Disease Considerations

In addition to life stages that may alter responses to ingested substances, the presence of disease may also result in enhanced susceptibility to adverse effects from particular ingredients. Disease or pre-existing conditions, such as hypertension, cardiac arrhythmias, or other early stages of cardiovascular disease, can be expected to exacerbate susceptibility to substances that specifically affect the organ exhibiting the disease or condition. In conditions such as hepatitis or renal disease, xenobiotic clearance and excretion is markedly altered, allowing compounds that are normally cleared rapidly to accumulate to toxic levels. Similarly, dietary supplement ingredients that affect insulin and glucose regulation are of concern to individuals with diabetes, unless data are available that mitigate this concern.

Interactions with Other Xenobiotics

People who use prescribed medications on a chronic basis, many of which are critically important to their health, may also be at greater risk of harm from interactions of their drugs with various supplement ingredients. For example, people who have HIV/AIDS or other chronic diseases may be taking drug combinations that can interact with supplement ingredients, such as St. John's wort, that alter cytochrome P450 activity (Ernst, 1999; Piscitelli et al., 2000). (See Chapter 8 for a more detailed discussion on interactions.) Interactions between drugs and dietary supplements may be of particular concern when both are taken for the same pathology and are thus potentially taken at the same time, and possibly without the knowledge of the prescribing physician. For example, vitamin E supplements, which are often recommended to patients with atherosclerotic vascular disease, may interact with statin drugs (Brown et al., 2001).

Summary of Vulnerable Population Considerations

Certain segments of the population may be particularly susceptible to the effects of some dietary supplement ingredients for a variety of reasons. Factors such as age, disease, pre-existing conditions, ethnicity, sex, or history of specific xenobiotic exposure (such as to drugs or other chemicals, including pesticides) can alter the effects of supplement exposure, and supplement exposure can affect pharmacodynamics and clearance of drugs prescribed for health reasons.

When evaluating risk and reviewing data, it is important to ask if ingredients are more likely to cause harmful effects to particular subgroups of the population. In this Framework, vulnerability of a population subgroup is described as a modifying factor in that whether identifiable subpopulations are particularly susceptible to harm should always be taken into consideration when setting priorities. **In conclusion, greater priority should be given to dietary supplement ingredients for which there is a concern about risk to particular subpopulations, especially if those subpopulations are known to consume the particular ingredient of concern.**

PREVALENCE OF USE IN THE POPULATION

GUIDING PRINCIPLE: *Ingredients that are widely used by the general population should be given higher priority for critical safety evaluation than less widely used ingredients with similar degrees of safety concerns. This is consistent with the public health goal of producing the most impact from limited resources.*

The relative number of individuals who could be at risk for harm due to overall use of a particular dietary supplement ingredient in the United States can be roughly estimated from various sources that provide estimates of the relative popularity of different ingredients. Across the wide variety of dietary supplement ingredients that are currently available, there is a wide range of usage patterns in the population. Some ingredients are used only rarely or by a small fraction of the population, while others are used by a considerable fraction, and/or taken frequently and chronically by a subset of the population, such as the elderly or athletes. Dietary supplements that are used only rarely, or are used by few consumers, would be expected to result in a low level of exposure on a population basis.

Estimating prevalence of use allows a qualitative consideration of population exposure and therefore the relative number of individuals that may be at risk if an ingredient is harmful—a factor that is important in setting priorities to optimize the impact of a risk/safety evaluation on public health. **That is, from a public health perspective, it is more logical to first allocate resources to evaluate potentially harmful ingredients may harm many people before evaluating those ingredients that may only affect a small fraction of the population, assuming other information about risk is equivalent.**

Relative consumption and prevalence of use of various dietary supplement ingredients in the general population can be estimated from two types of data. One type is industry estimates of production or sales. Dietary supplement industry publications, such as the *Nutrition Business Journal,* provide such data. Additionally, manufacturers and distributors collect production data, unit sales data, and total sales information in dollars as a normal component of business operations. The industry may be willing to make this information available.

The second type of data about prevalence of use is that collected in surveys about supplement usage. Such surveys ask respondents about patterns of use and can provide data on prevalence of use in the general population as well as in specific population subgroups.

National surveys that have traditionally collected information from a large number of persons regarding health issues and conventional food consumption information are increasingly also collecting valuable information about specific supplement use. An example is the expanded monitoring efforts of the National Health and Nutrition Examination Survey (CDC, 2004). Although it may be 2 to 3 years before the collected information is available, the planned expanded data collection will provide more detailed and useful information than is currently available in the older national survey data sets.

There are inherent limitations to many of the older survey data sets. They are often deficient in reporting frequency of use information and brand-specific information on ingredients and concentration, and they contain limited information on the collection and interpretation of data on products or ingredients that are typically used in combination (in addition to formulation and sales of single-ingredient products).

In summary, when setting priorities for which dietary supplements warrant attention first, it is not only appropriate to consider use by subpopulations that may be at risk for adverse effects, but also the extent of use by the general population, assuming that other information about risk is equivalent or comparable. Ingredients that are widely used by the general population should be given higher priority for critical safety evaluation than less widely used ingredients with similar degrees of safety concerns. These concepts are consistent with the FDA's mission of protecting the public health.

REFERENCES

Brown AK. 1968. Bilirubin metabolism in the developing liver. In: Assali N, ed. *Biology of Gestation.* Vol 2. New York: Academic Press.

Brown BG, Zhao XQ, Chait A, Fisher LD, Cheung MC, Morse JS, Dowdy AA, Marino EK, Bolson EL, Alaupovic P, Frohlich J, Albers JJ. 2001. Simvastatin and niacin, antioxidant vitamins, or the combination for the prevention of coronary disease. *N Engl J Med* 345: 1583–1592.

CDC (Centers for Disease Control and Prevention). 2004. *National Health and Nutrition Examination Survey, 1999–2004 Survey Content.* Available at http://www.cdc.gov/nchs/data/nhanes/comp3.pdf. Accessed March 22, 2004.

Eckhoff C, Nau H. 1990. Vitamin A supplementation increases levels of retinoic acid compounds in human plasma: Possible implications for teratogenesis. *Arch Toxicol* 64:502–503.

Ernst E. 1999. Second thoughts about safety of St John's wort. *Lancet* 354:2014–2016.

Guzelian PS, Henry CJ, Olin SS, eds. 1992. *Similarities and Differences Between Children and Adults: Implications for Risk Assessment.* Washington, DC: ILSI Press.

Lammer EJ, Chen DT, Hoar RM, Agnish ND, Benke PJ, Braun JT, Curry CJ, Fernhoff PM, Grix AW Jr, Lott IT, Richard JM, Sun SC. 1985. Retinoic acid embryopathy. *N Engl J Med* 313:837–841.

Mangoni AA, Jackson SH. 2004. Age-related changes in pharmacokinetics and pharmacodynamics: Basic principles and practical applications. *Br J Clin Pharmacol* 57:6–14.

Munro HN. 1989. The challenges of research into nutrition and aging. Introduction to a multifaceted problem. In: Munro HN, Danford DE, eds. *Nutrition, Aging, and the Elderly.* New York: Plenum. Pp. 1–21.

Piscitelli SC, Burstein AH, Chaitt D, Alfaro RM, Falloon J. 2000. Indinavir concentrations and St John's wort. *Lancet* 355:547–548.

Rosenberg IH, Russell RM, Bowman BB. 1989. Aging and the digestive system. In: Munro HN, Danford DE, eds. *Nutrition, Aging, and the Elderly.* New York: Plenum. Pp. 43–60.

Rothman KJ, Moore LL, Singer MR, Nguygen UDT, Mannino S, Milunsky B. 1995. Teratogenicity of high vitamin A intake. *N Engl J Med* 333:1369–1373.

10

Scientific Principles for Integrating and Evaluating the Available Data

Chapters 4 through 8 describe principles for how to consider the different categories of information likely to be available: *in vitro* data, human data, animal data, and data about related substances. This chapter describes how to appropriately weave different pieces of information together when complete safety data are not available and individual pieces of data may not be conclusive or are inconsistent. The described approach and its emphasis on biological plausibility and consistencies across different types of data are consistent with scientifically accepted approaches for making judgments, as well as with the safety standard outlined by the Dietary Supplement Health and Education Act (DSHEA), which authorizes the Food and Drug Administration to act when there is unreasonable or significant risk that overturns the assumption of safety.

The first section of this chapter explains why it is not possible to use a formulaic or algorithmic approach to integrate and evaluate the data. The next section describes how the systematic integration of knowledge and judgment can be used to assess dietary supplements for risk in a practical, informative, and transparent manner using causal models. The second half of this chapter describes concepts for weighing evidence that may initially appear inconsistent, focusing especially on interpretation of negative data. Finally, a short but important discussion about proof of harm describes underlying principles that are important when determining if an unreasonable or significant risk exists.

A FORMULAIC APPROACH FOR INTEGRATING DATA IS NOT PRACTICAL

Under the current legal and regulatory framework, the safety of many dietary supplement ingredients is more difficult to evaluate than other substances because of a general lack of quality data in the public domain, as well as the lack of requirement for premarket safety evaluation to drive future safety studies.[1] In the absence of scientific studies specifically designed to assess the safety of dietary supplement ingredients, it is not possible to apply a specific algorithmic or formulaic approach to determining safety, and expert[2] judgment in the interpretation of data is likely to be important, as it is for other substances. The Framework outlined in this report is different than frameworks that have formulaic components or that rely largely on assumptions that apply to the particular type of product being evaluated (see Appendix A). For example, the Flavor and Extract Manufacturers Association process relies largely on the fact that flavors will not be ingested in large amounts, and the Cosmetic Ingredient Review is unique in that many of the ingredients it evaluates are not bioavailable. The framework for Dietary Reference Intakes of the Institute of Medicine's (IOM's) Food and Nutrition Board includes a model for determining tolerable upper intake levels for ingestion of vitamins and minerals (IOM, 1998). The model is based on applying an uncertainty factor to the level at which no adverse events are observed from consumption of a nutrient, or if no data are available, to the lowest level of chronic intake at which adverse events are observed.

It is also not appropriate to develop a hierarchical approach to considering the different types of data—human data, animal data, *in vitro* data, or information about related substances—for various reasons. In part, such an approach is not feasible because of limitations in the quality of the data and what different types of studies can reveal, but these limitations can be overcome with other types of data. Although a hierarchical approach is not practical, it is possible to weigh the various types of data available to make conclusions regarding risk to human health. The second part of this chapter provides guidance on comparing animal and human studies with seemingly inconsistent results, but each situation will need to be evaluated to weigh the data appropriately.

---

[1]Exceptions to this include some nutrients and dietary supplements that have been evaluated for specific medicinal use as drugs (e.g., niacin and melatonin).

[2]Note that "expert" could describe a number of different types of experts, with several persons providing different viewpoints, including a perspective on the historical use of the substance.

AMOUNT OF INFORMATION NEEDED TO DRAW A CONCLUSION

GUIDING PRINCIPLE: *In the absence of scientific studies designed specifically to test the safety of a dietary supplement, concern for public safety may be raised by the presence of even a few reports of possible safety concerns when viewed together and constituting the weight of available evidence.*

Even if there are only one or two convincing reports of safety concerns about a dietary supplement, from either *in vitro*, animal, or human data, it may not be necessary to gather much additional information to raise concern about the implications for public health. However, in other cases, it may be necessary to assemble several data reports and reach a conclusion about risk based on the totality of available evidence, overall consistency, and biological plausibility of the evidence (a "weight of evidence" approach). In the absence of data on the safety of a specific ingredient, convincing information about safety of chemically or functionally related substances may be used to judge concern.

INTEGRATING INFORMATION

GUIDING PRINCIPLE: *Integration of data across different categories of information and types of study design can enhance biological plausibility and identify consistencies, leading to conclusions regarding levels of concern for an adverse event that may be associated with use of a dietary supplement ingredient.*

Individual pieces of information from any one of the categories of information (human, *in vitro*, animal, or related substances data) may sometimes be sufficiently compelling to both exceed a threshold level of concern and to justify focused evaluation or action. In many circumstances, however, data will need to be collated within the same category or across several categories to determine the appropriate level of concern. That is, even if concern raised by one category of data—for example, human data—does not meet a threshold for action, the body of evidence available across several categories may raise the level of concern. In integrating observations across categories of data, *consistency* and evidence of biological *plausibility* should raise the level of concern. In other words, **available evidence from**

each category of data, by itself, may be insufficient to indicate concern, but when a pattern of mechanistically related adverse effects is observed across two or more categories in a consistent manner, this can establish biological plausibility and warrant heightened concern for potential harmful effects in humans.

Causal Models for Considering Consistency and Biological Plausibility

Synthesis is the concept or process of integrating safety data from different types of study designs and across different categories of data. Data synthesis can be facilitated, and conceptually illustrated, by the use of causal evidence models. A causal evidence model (see Figure 10-1) provides a structure to help interpret available data from a number of sources that address a specific safety question (Harris et al., 2001). The model can describe the relationship among a dietary supplement, potential adverse health outcomes (e.g., liver failure, death), and biological effects[3] by depicting the relationship as linkages that are illustrated with arrows. The type of arrow illustrates the type of evidence: convincing data are depicted by solid arrows and weaker or less conclusive data are depicted by dashed arrows. A "path" between the dietary supplement ingredient and an adverse health effect illustrates a relationship. When the available information is integrated, multiple links between the dietary supplement ingredient and a given health outcome are illustrated by multiple arrows, as discussed below.

A solid arrow (Arrow A, Figure 10-1) linking the ingredient to the adverse health effect illustrates that a clear association between the ingredient and the effect has been demonstrated. An arrow (Arrow B, Figure 10-1) linking the ingredient to the biological effect illustrates a situation where the ingredient is known to cause the biological effect, whether or not the biological effect has been linked directly to the adverse health effect (Arrow C, Figure 10-1). Note that Arrow B could be present without Arrow C for many situations, but that a conclusive situation occurs when the ingredient is linked to the biological effect and the biological effect is linked to the adverse health effect, illustrated by Arrows B and C together.

Figures 10-2 through 10-4 illustrate other possible scenarios where conclusive data (human, animal, or *in vitro*) exist. Figure 10-2 illustrates two possible scenarios of conclusive animal data. The first diagram illustrates a situation where the dietary supplement ingredient is known to

[3]The term "biological effects" does not necessarily mean health effects. For example, it can include mechanistic effects, such as enzyme inhibition.

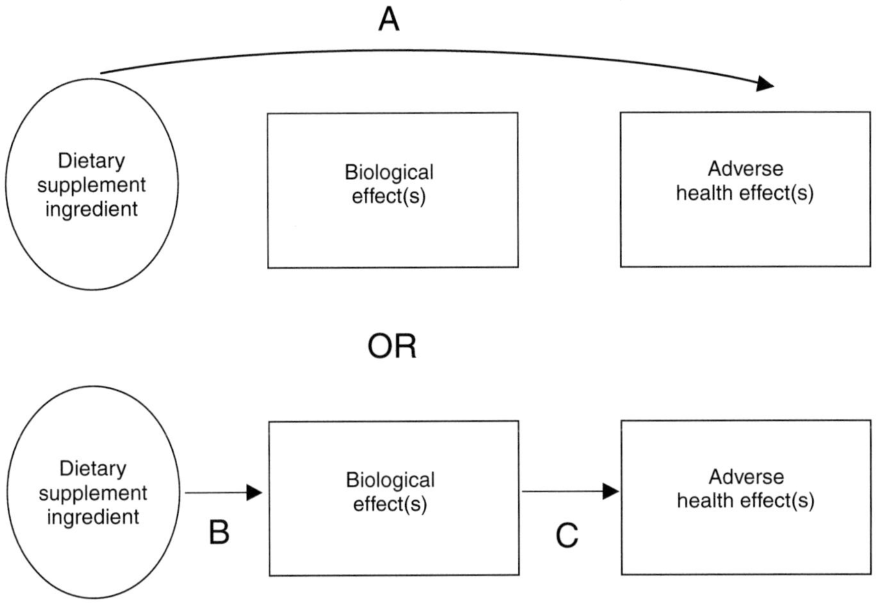

FIGURE 10-1 Illustration of causal model concept for conclusive human data. A solid arrow (A, B, or C) illustrates a clear association between the two linked items.

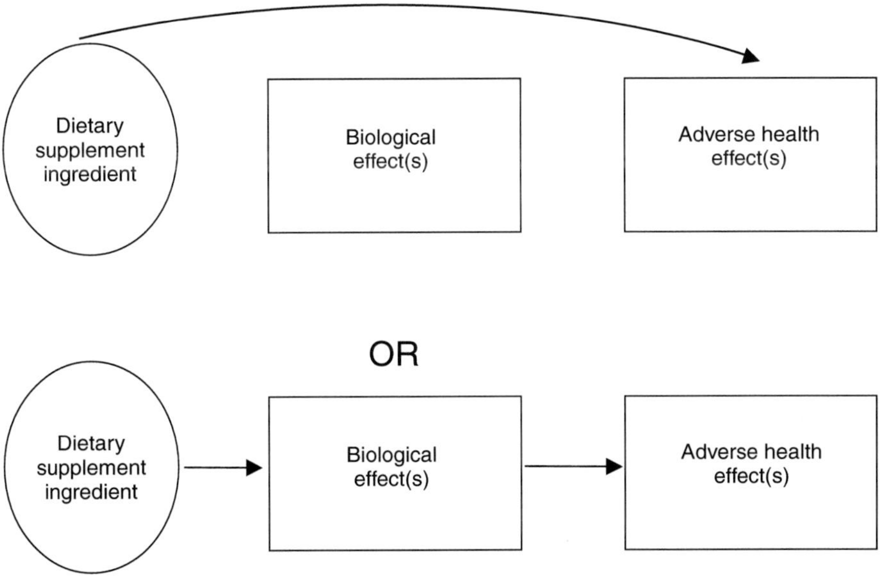

FIGURE 10-2 Illustration of causal model concept for conclusive animal data.

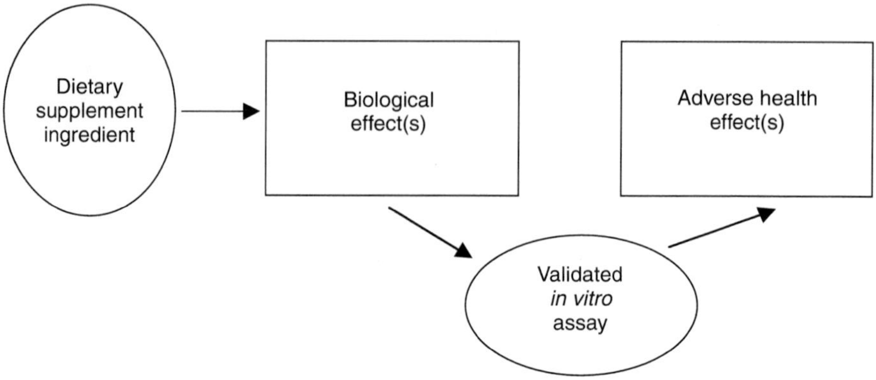

FIGURE 10-3 Illustration of causal model concept for *in vitro* data.

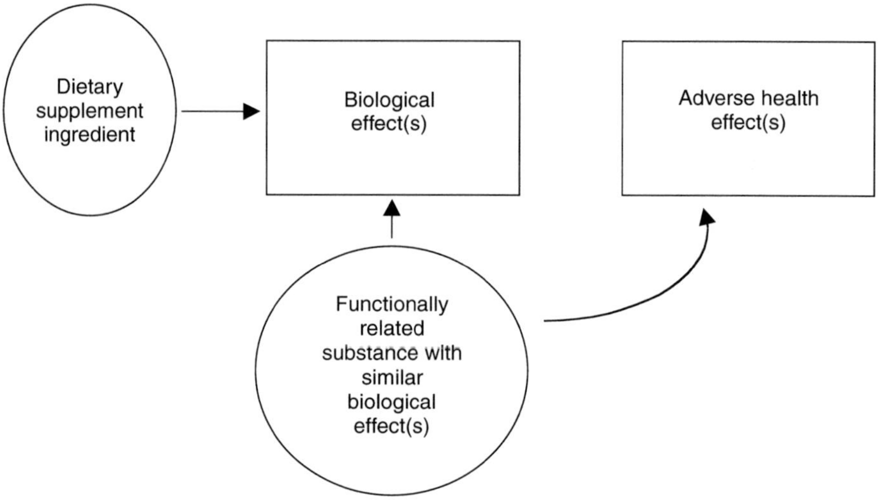

FIGURE 10-4 Illustration of causal model concept for conclusive information about "functionally related" substances. The solid arrow from the ingredient to the biological effect represents an association between the two as evidenced by human, animal, or *in vitro* data.

cause the adverse health effect in animals. The second diagram illustrates a situation where the dietary supplement ingredient is known to cause a biological effect in the animal that is related to the possible adverse health effect. Figure 10-3 illustrates conclusive *in vitro* data. The dietary supplement ingredient in 10-3 is known to cause the *in vitro* biological effect.

Validation of the *in vitro* assay for the biological effect provides a link between it and the adverse health outcomes. Figure 10-4 illustrates how information about functionally related data is used to make a link between the biological effect and the adverse health outcome. The fact that a related substance causes the adverse health effect through the biological effect provides a path of arrows between the dietary supplement ingredient and the adverse heath effect.

Evidence from all types of study designs may form linkages to aid in determining the extent of association between dietary supplement exposure and adverse health outcomes. Each causal model illustrates a specific ingredient's relationship to a particular adverse health outcome, thus separate causal models should be constructed for adverse events associated with different mechanisms (e.g., cardiotoxicity, hepatotoxicity, neurotoxicity). The same model structure should be used for different categories of data (e.g., human, animal, or *in vitro* data).

Figure 10-5 illustrates how one model integrates different types of data, demonstrating the power of the model in drawing conclusions. In Figure 10-5A, dashed lines are used to illustrate weak or incomplete data and each category of data is illustrated in a separate diagram. None of the models in Figure 10-5A are conclusive. That is, none include a path between the dietary supplement ingredient and the adverse health effect. Figure 10-5B is an integrated illustration of all that is known about a particular dietary supplement ingredient's relationship to the particular adverse effect. The weaker links are strengthened by consistent data of several types and a relationship path between the dietary supplement ingredient and the adverse health effect is apparent.

The following specific example illustrates use of the causal model diagramed in Figure 10-6. In this case, a biological effect caused by a dietary supplement ingredient may be known to occur following exposure to a different chemical that has known adverse health effects. For example, saw palmetto causes the biological effect inhibition of 5-α-reductase *in vitro* and in animal data. The drug finasteride is also known to have this biological effect, which has been linked to finasteride-induced developmental defects in male genitalia *in utero*. When the models are integrated, the relationship between saw palmetto and defects in male genitalia is illustrated; this link between the biological activity (inhibition of 5-α-reductase) of the known teratogen finasteride and saw palmetto is sufficient to raise concern about the safety of saw palmetto use in women who could become pregnant because this inhibitory effect of finasteride on 5-α-reductase is considered causative in the teratogenic effect.

Individual studies from a single category of data also form links in a causal evidence model, with multiple and consistent evidence for the same link strengthening the linkage (illustrated with multiple overlapping arrows

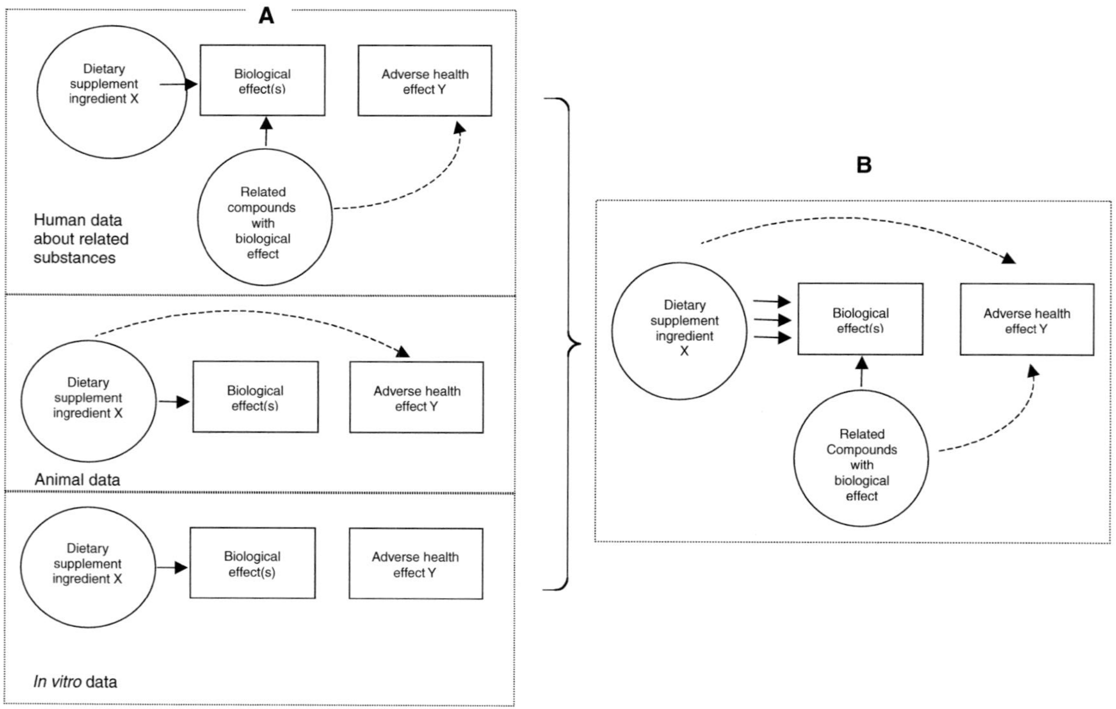

FIGURE 10-5 Illustration of a causal model used to integrate different types of data. Panel A describes categories of available data that are not independently very strong or conclusive regarding ingredient X's relationship to adverse effect Y. Panel B describes data that, when integrated across the different categories, allow for a stronger conclusion by strengthening the linkages between ingredient X and adverse effect Y. Dashed arrows indicate weak or inconclusive data.

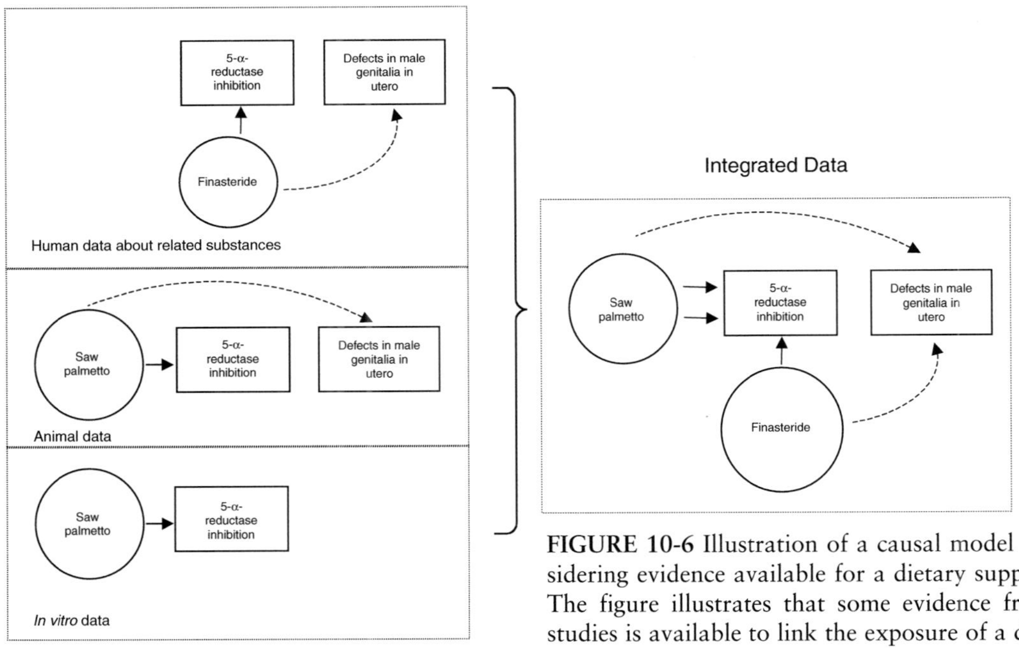

FIGURE 10-6 Illustration of a causal model in a hypothetical scenario of considering evidence available for a dietary supplement ingredient (saw palmetto). The figure illustrates that some evidence from human, animal, and *in vitro* studies is available to link the exposure of a dietary supplement ingredient with a biological effect. In the illustrated situation, there is some evidence that a dietary supplement ingredient causes the biological effect in humans. The animal data suggest that the ingredient causes some biological effect, and it directly indicates that the ingredient is linked with the adverse health outcome. There is also some *in vitro* evidence linking the ingredient with the biological effect. Finally, a related substance is known to cause the biological effect in addition to the adverse health effect. The consistency of the evidence across different types of data taken together raises the level of concern regarding risk to human health.

following integration). Thus the multiple links illustrate the *consistency* concept: consistency increases the linkage and thus increases the concern warranted. Figures 10-5 and 10-6 show that summing, or synthesizing, data addressing different linkages forms a more complete causal evidence model and can provide the biological plausibility needed to establish the association between a dietary supplement and an adverse event.

In summary, causal models are useful when individual pieces of evidence are weak and are of different types or when they do not clearly illustrate a relationship, when viewed individually, as may often be the case with dietary supplement ingredients. Frequently, in studies of dietary supplement activity, a single category of data supporting a causal evidence model is incomplete or weak, precluding firm conclusions. By linking data from more than one category, such as human and animal data, causal models create a more complete picture of the data and provide a more complete understanding of the relationship between biological effects and potential adverse health outcomes. Similarly, different types of study design (e.g., experimental and observational studies) within a category of data may also be assessed together to provide more robust conclusions.

Cross-Design Synthesis

Cross-design synthesis, a *quantitative* method that combines studies of different designs with different endpoints and different categories of data, has been proposed in the past (NRC, 1992). However, there is little current experience with this approach. As a result, the *qualitative* synthesis described here, and the weight of evidence as judged by experts, are appropriate approaches for evaluating the body of assembled evidence for safety of dietary supplements.

WEIGHING EVIDENCE THAT MAY APPEAR INCONSISTENT

Differences in Exposure or Product Formulation May Explain Inconsistencies

GUIDING PRINCIPLES: *Risk is a function of exposure. Analysis therefore needs to link risk of harm to relevant dietary supplement ingredient exposure. One formulation of an ingredient may or may not be relevant to other formulations: relevance depends on similar bioequivalence of the active ingredients.*

Some apparent inconsistencies in data may be explained by differences in the level of ingredient exposure, which in some cases may be related to differences in formulation. If different studies produce different conclusions about potential adverse effects, it is important to consider whether the exposures were comparable. Exposure at the site of action depends upon the amount ingested (amount of a constituent[4] in the product), the route of exposure,[5] and the bioavailability of the formulation. These concepts are reflected in the manner in which data were analyzed in the prototype monographs released with this report and summarized in Appendixes D through K. The amount of product ingested, route of exposure, and the processing and composition as well as the formulation of the ingredient used in each study, were all taken into consideration in determining the relevance of datasets for use in evaluating the level of concern for safety of the dietary supplement ingredients reviewed. As these prototype analyses were prepared, two underlying concepts were considered—concepts that are generally relevant and important to bear in mind when considering inconsistencies. These are (1) that the amount of active chemical constituents in products can vary, and (2) in the absence of evidence to the contrary, it is assumed that adverse effects observed at higher than ingested levels have some relevance to the safety of ingested levels of ingredient.

In studies that use controlled amounts of purified or well-characterized ingredients, it is relatively straightforward to relate a certain level of ingredient to an adverse effect. However, in many instances, the amount of a specific biologically active constituent in a dietary supplement is unknown and can be expected to vary from preparation to preparation (Feifer et al., 2002; Fong, 2002). For botanicals in particular, variation in final product can stem from inconsistent harvesting, storage, and processing, or differences in the plant genotype or growing environment (Fong, 2002). An example of preparation difference is that alcoholic extracts and dried botanicals for hot water extraction may be sold under the same name, although alcohol and water will extract a different array as well as different quantities of chemical constituents. In another example, shark cartilage is sold both as washed, ground material and as a water extract, each having different compositions. For these reasons, unless composition is confirmed by analysis, the amount of a particular chemical constituent in an ingredi-

[4]In this report, the term "ingredient" is considered to be a plant part for botanicals, therefore the term "constituent" is used to indicate a chemical compound that may be part of the ingredient in the case of a plant, or may be the ingredient itself, in the case of dietary supplements that consist of only one chemical constituent.

[5]A dietary supplement, by definition, is taken orally, but information about effects of other routes of exposure are appropriate to consider, although the relevance of such data will vary.

ent cannot be determined even when a statement on a supplement label suggests a certain volume of material contains a particular amount of active ingredient. That even different formulations containing the same amount of an active ingredient cannot be assumed to be bioequivalent is well understood; this is one reason premarketing bioequivalence studies are required for new drug formulations to be sold under generic labels. Such testing is not conducted with dietary supplements even though formulation, processing, and preparation technologies can significantly alter composition and bioavailability.

Because of these and other possible inconsistencies, direct extrapolation of evidence of *safety* from one product formulation to another is ill advised without clear evidence of bioequivalence between the preparations. **Evidence of *risk* should be treated differently, however; a general guideline to follow is that if adverse effects are observed with one product formulation, they should be assumed to occur following intake of other formulations as well, unless enough is known about the other preparations to discount the possibility that they have the potential for the same concern.**[6] For example, seemingly inconsistent results from different formulations of the same original substance might be explained by convincing evidence from animal data or chemical analysis comparing the two formulations.

In general, studies conducted using amounts of the ingredient greater than those likely to be consumed when using a product as a dietary supplement can be used in evaluating the appropriate level of concern about risk. This is because the amount of constituent ingested by humans may vary significantly, as discussed above, and because there may be consistency between the types of adverse effects observed following ingestion of these elevated amounts and lesser but similar effects observed following ingestion of lower amounts typically consumed as a dietary supplement. Alternatively, the effects seen at these higher levels may provide biological plausibility for less serious effects observed following consumption of lower amounts. For example, dose-response studies of nordihydroguaiaretic acid (NDGA, a constituent of chaparral) showing hepatotoxicity at high doses were useful in considering possible adverse effects on liver function related to reports of jaundice following ingestion of chaparral containing lower amounts of NDGA (see chaparral-focused prototype monograph, Appendix J). However, even without these elements of consistency or biological

[6]If a monograph is developed on a dietary supplement ingredient, and a manufacturer has information that its product does not demonstrate the toxic effect/hazard identified in the monograph, then it should be the manufacturer's responsibility to provide information regarding the product's lack of harm during the data gathering step of monograph development.

plausibility, the results from studies using amounts not possible to obtain through ingestion of the dietary supplement may still be useful, as explained in Chapters 4 and 5 for human data and animal data, respectively, and to indicate what types of studies should be pursued to determine the potential for harm.

Poor Data Quality May Explain Inconsistencies

GUIDING PRINCIPLE: *To evaluate the safety of an ingredient, it is best to consider all relevant data, but each study should be evaluated individually for quality.*

Another possible explanation for apparent inconsistencies in the observation of adverse effects may be differences in the quality of the reports. Important aspects of studies from each category of data, including human, animal, and *in vitro* studies, have been discussed in detail in Chapters 4 through 7. However, there are a number of overarching considerations that bear emphasizing. Decisions to consider unpublished data in addition to published data should depend on the quality and completeness of the data set. Unfortunately, publication in the scientific literature does not in itself qualify data as acceptable for evaluation, and many published articles contain insufficient detail to allow the data described to be of much use in risk evaluations. Consideration of statistical power, validation of analytical methods, analytical approaches, consistency with the published literature, peer review of the data, and bias due to conflict of interest by the authors are all important in evaluating usefulness of a dataset.

Lack of Evidence as an Apparent Inconsistency

GUIDING PRINCIPLE: *Absence of evidence of risk does not indicate that there is no risk.*

In some cases, some data will indicate a risk, while other data will not suggest the risk exists, producing what could be interpreted as an inconsistency. Inconsistencies may be explained by the inability of some systems to detect adverse effects or differences in formulation, differences in frequency or length of exposure, differences in pre-existing human physiology (e.g., sex differences or chronic illness), or many other causes. Even if a study showing lack of adverse effects is reported, if the study is not adequately designed to identify risk (e.g., not sufficiently powered, incompletely reported, does not include positive controls, or otherwise has inadequate mechanisms for detecting adverse events), it is not scientifically valid to use such information to mitigate suggested risk from other sources. Only negative data originating from well-designed studies or other credible sources may mitigate, if not fully eliminate, concerns raised by other sources of information and even well-designed, credible data are often not appropriate to use this way as discussed below. The basic principle that "absence of evidence of risk does not indicate there is no risk" leads to the question of how to weigh seemingly inconsistent data where some information suggests a risk and other information does not. How to compare this type of information is discussed here, with particular emphasis on inconsistencies between animal and human data.

Because of the relevance of human data, serious adverse events arising from randomized clinical trials, spontaneous reports with strong attribution, or case series are generally more compelling than other categories of data when they raise the level of concern. In general, if there is scientifically based evidence from human studies indicating that a concern for safety exists, then the lack of adverse events in animal studies, *in vitro* studies, or even other human studies cannot be used to overrule or disregard the evidence of harm. The absence of adverse findings in animal studies, no matter how well designed, does not prove that pathological effects will not occur in humans; thus, the absence of an effect or observation in animals cannot mitigate concern raised by human data.

Whereas animal studies cannot be used to mitigate findings of toxicity in humans, animal testing can and should be used to further investigate adverse events that have been reported in humans but for which sufficient attribution cannot be reached. For example, animal data may be used to identify problems specific to particular formulations and sources or products (e.g., in their content, contamination, bioavailability) by comparing groups of animals given the different formulations. This approach might be used, for example, to identify the presence of a contaminant due to a novel processing technology by comparing the effects of feeding the two formulations to the appropriate animal species. Appropriate positive controls would, of course, be necessary to conclude that one formulation has a different effect than another formulation. Also, animal models of human conditions and physiological states can be used to uncover particular vulnerabilities in humans in order to determine specific circumstances under which the dietary supplement ingredient may cause safety concerns in humans by modeling particular conditions (e.g., an animal model of diabetes).

Similarly, it is rarely appropriate to discard observations of adverse effects in animals simply because similar effects were not observed in humans. Evidence of risk from well-designed animal studies using appropriate models cannot be overruled by lesser-quality human data, such as a lack of spontaneously reported adverse events in current or historical use, less than adequate clinical or *in vitro* studies, or lack of structural similarities to any known poison. To justify disregarding animal observations, the event occurring in animals would need to be specifically monitored for and detectable in humans under the conditions reported. For example, a lack of cancer in humans exposed to an animal carcinogen assumes greater importance when there are data of sufficient quality and power to detect the cancer if it were to occur. Thus, even though an event such as breast cancer that occurs with some frequency in the human population would be difficult, statistically, to attribute to an ingredient used in a human study, a lack of resolving power in epidemiologic studies does not rule out a relationship between the ingredient and human cancers.

Human exposure may need to be prolonged to detect latent or chronic toxicities. Therefore, regardless of the presence of even high-quality human data suggesting no toxicity following short-term exposure, certain chronic animal toxicity or biological activity data could warrant elevated concern. In particular, animal studies that warrant special concern are those that indicate the following potential effects in humans: evidence of cancer, reproductive system effects, developmental toxicity effects including teratology, or other delayed serious toxicities (see Table 5-1).

There are only a few scientifically appropriate reasons to discount animal observations because human effects are not observed, such as the well-understood differences in pharmacokinetics and/or pharmacodynamics between humans and the experimental animal described in Chapter 5. One example is manifestation of toxic effects that depends on metabolic pathways present in animals but not in humans, thus producing animal study results that are not very applicable to human health. (A hypothetical example is an adverse effect that results because the dietary supplement ingredient blocks a pathway that humans are not dependent on.) While it is unusual in the dietary supplement field at present to have such detailed knowledge, occasionally an understanding of the pathway responsible for the toxicity can mitigate the extrapolation to humans of concerns raised in animal studies.

PROOF OF HARM

For a number of dietary supplements ingredients, decisions regarding safety must be made despite sparse data and shortcomings in the studies that are available. In making such decisions, interpretation of available data must be made by weighing it against the assumption that all dietary supplement ingredients are safe (see Chapter 1, description of DSHEA). The assumption that dietary supplement ingredients are safe is not equivalent to a scientific determination of safety, and thus the information required to overcome this assumption is not required to be absolute proof or evidence that a harm or adverse effect has occurred or will inevitably occur. Instead, the information required is something less. Rather than a quantitative, probabilistic assessment of risk, which is preferable and often possible when data about a chemical are substantial or at least include standard toxicology tests, it may be prudent or necessary to make a qualitative determination by using judgment and scientific inference to consider the limited data. In summary, **to evaluate dietary supplements under DSHEA, it is necessary to determine only if an "unreasonable or significant risk" exists, not to have complete evidence that a dietary supplement causes a serious adverse event.** That is, the standard of "unreasonable or significant risk" put forward by DSHEA is a lower standard than conclusive scientific proof, a fact that is likely to facilitate the ability to take action.

REFERENCES

Feifer AH, Fleshner NE, Klotz L. 2002. Analytical accuracy and reliability of commonly used nutritional supplements in prostate disease. *J Urol* 168:150–154.

Fong HHS. 2002. Integration of herbal medicine into modern medical practices: Issues and prospects. *Intergr Cancer Ther* 1:287–293.

Harris RP, Helfand M, Woolf SH, Lohr KN, Mulrow CD, Teutsch SM, Atkins D. 2001. Current methods of the U.S. Preventive Services Task Force: A review of the process. *Am J Prev Med* 20:21S–35S.

IOM (Institute of Medicine). 1998. *Dietary Reference Intakes: A Risk Assessment Model for Establishing Upper Intake Levels for Nutrients.* Washington, DC: National Academy Press.

NRC (National Research Council). 1992. *Combining Information: Statistical Issues and Opportunities for Research.* Washington, DC: National Academy Press.

11
Applying the Framework: Case Studies Using the Prototype Safety Monographs

The second phase of the Food and Drug Administration's (FDA's) request to the Institute of Medicine (IOM), after proposing a framework for the safety evaluation of dietary supplement ingredients and releasing it for comment, was to develop at least six prototype monographs for dietary supplement ingredients using the system outlined in the initial framework and, through this process, evaluate the proposed framework and revise it as necessary.

Based on this experience and on comments received by industry representatives and other stakeholders about the proposed process (see Appendix B for a summary of the comments received), the framework was revised to that described in Chapters 3. The prototype monographs are available on the Internet (www.iom.edu/fnb) and, for the sake of brevity, the summary and conclusions for each of the six ingredients are included in Appendixes D through I. This chapter contains a discussion of the process used to evaluate each dietary supplement ingredient, the principles derived from the process of evaluation, and a rationale for *focused* monographs, developed following review of two of the full prototype monographs (saw palmetto and chaparral).

PROTOTYPE MONOGRAPH DEVELOPMENT

The monographs developed to evaluate the proposed framework and process are referred to as "prototypes" for several reasons. Because the six monographs were simultaneously prepared within the timeline of the overall report, the information collected is not expected to be as complete as what might be collected if qualified staff at FDA or another organization were specifically charged with undertaking only monograph generation. For example, the timeline of this project required that industry and other stakeholders be given only a few weeks to a month to review the information included in the draft prototype monographs to determine if there was a need to volunteer data in their possession prior to the public meeting. In addition, the sources of information and the process for systematically collecting information were evaluated during this process and thus continually modified as subsequent monographs were developed. Thus the monographs, as well as the monograph summaries and the focused monographs in this volume, are considered prototypes and as such are not authoritative statements of the National Academies or the IOM on the safety of the specific dietary ingredients, but are put forward as examples of what might be done.

The six supplement ingredients selected to serve as the subjects of the prototype monographs were chaparral, chromium picolinate, glucosamine, melatonin, saw palmetto, and shark cartilage. Development of the prototype monographs proved to be a useful tool to assess the practicality and ability of the Framework to guide a dietary supplement ingredient safety evaluation.

Criteria Used to Select Prototype Monograph Ingredients

The six ingredients were selected to fulfill several criteria and thus test the proposed framework from a variety of perspectives. One criterion, for example, was to review a variety of types of ingredients; thus the selection of ingredients for prototype monographs included at least one botanical, one well-characterized vitamin or mineral, one animal product, one hormonal product, and one "new" (post-October 1994) product. Another criterion was that the selected ingredients include substances for which a range in the types and quality of available information were anticipated. Finally, it was decided that selected ingredients should not be undergoing safety research by committee members. The range of ingredient types, available data sources, and resulting level of concern allowed the evaluation of various aspects of the proposed framework and provided an opportunity to improve the recommended approach.

Signal Detection

It is worth noting that the reasons substances were flagged initially as described in the *proposed* framework (the report previously released for comment) would have also brought them to FDA's attention according to the Framework presented in this final report. In the case studies that follow, additional reasons that might have generated a signal for FDA to examine the dietary supplement ingredient are also noted. Using the Framework, FDA would have considered the *nature of the evidence* readily available as a result of the signal detected and decided, based on initial review, that a level of concern existed. A decision whether to continue monitoring or to move into the integrative evaluation of the dietary supplement ingredient would then have been made.

Integrative Evaluation

An IOM staff monographer developed a search strategy for each ingredient based on recommendations from the committee and began collecting and collating the data available. In order to simulate the initial evaluation in which an internal scientific review would determine which aspects were relevant to include in a comprehensive evaluation, a working group was assembled that included some committee members plus consultants who were chosen based on specific expertise relevant to the dietary supplement ingredient. An initial meeting was held of each prototype working group with the monographer to give direction to the literature search and additional relevant data to be included; at this point, the main activity was to complete the monograph outline.

The working groups reviewed and revised the developing draft monographs as new information was provided and consulted with the monographer via conference calls. Following the procedures outlined in the proposed framework, draft prototype monographs without recommendations or conclusions were released for comment and additional input. Stakeholders were notified of their existence and how to provide comment and feedback.

External Advisory Committee

The role of the working group next changed to become a prototype of an external advisory committee in which participants reviewed and analyzed the data and developed statements regarding concerns about safety. A second meeting was held of each working group in which the group served in the capacity of an external advisory committee. At the second meeting, they received oral comments from stakeholders and reviewed additional information received. They subsequently drafted recommendations and conclusions (see summary analyses, Appendixes D through I).

USE OF THE FRAMEWORK IN EVALUATING PROTOTYPE INGREDIENTS

The goal of the monograph development phase was to test the proposed process and learn from it to improve the overall framework. Below, each prototype is described as a case study to illustrate how principles and concepts from the Framework were used to meet the objectives of each step. The triggering signals are indicated as *presumed* in this illustration as it is not possible to know whether FDA would have initially detected them as signals or not.

Chaparral

Presumed Signals

Concerns expressed about the safety of chaparral by several authoritative sources signaled that chaparral's safety should be investigated, as did several SN/AEMS[1] reports of serious adverse events associated with chaparral use (coma, severe hepatic injury, hepatitis, and kidney failure).[2] Authoritative sources included FDA itself which, before the Dietary Supplement and Health Education Act, issued a press release warning of a potential relationship between chaparral use and liver toxicity (FDA, 1992), and the American Herbal Products Association's *Botanical Safety Handbook* (McGuffin et al., 1997) notation that Health Canada did not allow chaparral as an orally administered, nonmedicinal ingredient. Possible liver problems were also mentioned in several other secondary sources of information (Foster and Tyler, 1999; NMCD, 2002).

While the use of chaparral may not be widespread, the seriousness of the adverse events and the several authoritative sources citing potential problems, especially liver problems, were considered to be a strong signal requiring the evaluation of the nature of the evidence regarding potential liver and other problems. This is consistent with Chapter 4 guidelines that reports of liver necrosis or acute liver failure be considered in an expedited manner due to their potential for mortality and morbidity.

Initial Review: Considering the Nature of the Evidence

The nature of the case studies and reports to FDA were considered first, as described in Chapter 4. Serious adverse events occurred in individuals

---

[1]Special Nutritional Adverse Event Monitoring System, as available on FDA's website.

[2]This chapter is presented as a review of the prototype monographs as case studies. The actual references for statements made are in the full prototype monographs available at www.iom.edu/fnb.

who reported taking chaparral but no other supplements or drugs, suggesting that the adverse events were not due to concomitantly consumed substances. Reported liver problems were clinically documented. In the case report of jaundice and toxic liver disease, the individual elected to rechallenge and the symptoms recurred. Recurrence of symptoms after rechallenge is considered a convincing factor in assessing strength of association. Thus, the adverse event reports are most consistent with the description of higher concern in the right column in Table 4-1: "Describes a well-documented serious adverse event, with plasma levels at a relevant range (if available) and demonstrates dechallenge and rechallenge (if possible), temporality, and strong attribution."

In addition to the human safety data, there were also indications that persons with pre-existing liver disease might consume chaparral.[3] The fact that the very persons most susceptible to liver problems might be using chaparral should raise the concern level even higher, consistent with the discussion of particularly susceptible subpopulations in Chapter 9.

Given the high level of concern about the human data on liver problems and the additional concern about particularly susceptible subpopulations, the Framework directs FDA to proceed with an integrative evaluation of all available data about chaparral (i.e., other human data, animal data, *in vitro* data, and data about the safety of related substances). In this case, FDA could instead elect to do a focused monograph on the risk of liver adverse effects from chaparral consumption because the evidence available at this point indicates the greatest concern is for liver damage (see discussion of a focused monograph, later in this chapter).

Integrative Evaluation

Although FDA could have chosen to focus its efforts on liver problems, the prototype chaparral integrative evaluation was conducted with a more broad-based strategy. Studies focused on the safety of chaparral were limited in number and value, so the literature search included a search for information about safety problems associated with nordihydroguaiaretic acid (NDGA), a component of chaparral.

The human data considered included information about hepatic adverse events reported to FDA and published as case reports (as discussed in the previous section). Anecdotal information about the traditional use of chaparral as a tea was also considered. This information was only considered relevant to chaparral use as a tea, because as described in the mono-

---

[3]For specifics, see discussion of conditions of use (Section B) in prototype monograph, available at www.iom.edu/fnb.

graph and in Chapters 4 and 6, the similarity of a product form greatly impacts the chemical constituents consumed, and apparent safety associated with one form should not be extrapolated to another form. Specifically, in the case of chaparral, NDGA concentrations are likely to be higher in chaparral products that are not water-extracted teas. Only one of the human adverse events appeared to be associated with chaparral tea use. Thus the integrative evaluation distinguished between safety problems associated with chaparral consumption as a tea and safety problems associated with other chaparral products likely to contain more NDGA.

Animal data included studies about NDGA. They suggested that chaparral and NDGA administration result in anti-implantation activity or inhibition of ovulation and increase resorption of fetuses, respectively. As indicated in Chapter 5, the animal reproductive toxicity effects were deemed particularly important to consider because it is unlikely they would be detected by human use, even with long-term traditional use (see Chapter 4 discussion of "Considering the Relevance of Historical Use"). Also important to the consideration of liver toxicity was the information uncovered about kidney damage, which in addition to indicating a potential risk for renal toxicity might also suggest harm at other sites of NDGA metabolism, such as the liver.

In vitro data relevant to the safety of chaparral were also considered. *In vitro* studies on NDGA provided mechanistic information, such as lipoxygenase and cyclooxygenase inhibition and inhibition of prostaglandin synthesis.

Information about the safety of related substances and the chemical structure of chaparral constituents raised two possible concerns. First, NDGA is *functionally related* (see Chapter 8) to prostanoid pathway inhibitors, which are contraindicated during the first and third trimesters of pregnancy. Second, the chemical structure of NDGA indicates that it is likely to be a substrate for cytochrome P450-dependent quinone formation. Finally, *in vitro* data suggest NDGA is functionally related to 5-α-reductase inhibitors, which are contraindicated in pregnancy due to effects on male development *in utero*.

Finally, the totality of information summarized above is considered according to the scientific principles for evaluating and integrating data, as described in Chapter 10. As stated in Chapter 10, "In the absence of scientific studies designed specifically to test safety of a dietary supplement, concern for public safety may be raised by the presence of even a few reports of possible safety concerns, when viewed together and constituting the weight of available evidence." No scientific studies designed specifically and adequately to test the safety of chaparral were found. The information suggesting safety is limited to the possible historical use of chaparral without documented adverse effects. The information suggesting risk of NDGA-associated reproductive abnormalities is consistent and is biologically plausible. Liver risk is biologically plausible but less consistent given the negative animal data, but lack of observed effects is not considered as important as observation of effects (see Chapter 10). Overall, the weight of the evidence indicates higher concern with NDGA consumption—a concern that is then applied to chaparral consumption, with the possible exception of chaparral tea.

Chromium Picolinate

Presumed Signals

Chromium picolinate was flagged for review because secondary sources mentioned that its use has been reported in cases of renal toxicity, and because secondary sources discussed its purported effect on insulin regulation and theoretical risk when used with insulin by persons with diabetes (NMCD, 2002). Other signals could have brought this dietary supplement ingredient to the attention of FDA as well. For example, the SN/AEMS documented serious adverse events in individuals ingesting chromium picolinate, including severe seizure, ventricular tachyarrhythmia, and jaundice. These adverse events would have been considered a strong indication that chromium picolinate warranted attention. Chromium picolinate's widespread prevalence of use, including its common inclusion in many combination dietary supplements, also suggests value in devoting attention to the risk of the use of chromium picolinate as a supplement ingredient.

Initial Review: Considering the Nature of the Evidence

The renal toxicity cases that signaled chromium picolinate as needing attention were evaluated following the description outlined in Chapter 4. As described in the chromium picolinate prototype monograph, confounders existed, such as concomitant drug consumption and pre-existing conditions, and there was no information about persons experiencing adverse effects ending and then resuming chromium picolinate intake (challenge/rechallenge). Thus, using the criteria from Chapter 4, the concern level about the signal would be relatively low based on the available information.

More context was provided by reviewing additional adverse event reports from the SN/AEMS, which showed two deaths in individuals taking two or more supplements containing chromium. Again, these reports showed that the users consumed a multitude of supplements and did not include information that led to a strong association (see Chapter 4) with chromium picolinate; therefore, the concern level remained lower even though the event is considered most serious.

In addition to the initial signal about renal toxicity, the initial signal of concern about diabetics ingesting chromium picolinate was also considered by reviewing results of a clinical trial. This concern was not deemed a higher concern given that a 10-day trial with 162 diabetic subjects did not reveal changes in clinical parameters associated with glucose regulation problems following insulin administration.

In the case of chromium picolinate, consideration of the nature of the evidence about renal toxicity and glucose regulation signals did not elevate concern to a higher level. Following the Framework, a lower to moderate concern suggests that FDA note what was learned about the signals detected, the serious adverse events, and the insulin regulation concern and then continue to monitor until new signals of concern suggest more consideration is warranted.

Integrative Evaluation

Although not suggested by the review of the two signals above, if FDA did choose to conduct an integrative evaluation of chromium picolinate because of the seriousness of these serious adverse event reports or other reasons, it would be appropriate to follow a broad-based strategy because the serious adverse events reported suggest potential damage to several organ systems. Because chromium picolinate contains a trace element that is poorly excreted, FDA would want to pay particular attention to the impact of dose on safety.

The chromium picolinate prototype monograph preparation process began with a relatively broad-based strategy for identifying risks that might be associated with chromium picolinate ingestion. Specifically, the strategy was to look for information relevant to the major possible toxicities evident from the human data *and* to look for animal and *in vitro toxicity* studies that revealed any other concerns regarding chromium picolinate. This strategy revealed information about carcinogenesis and oxidative stress—information that might not have been apparent in a reactive monitoring approach.

Glucosamine

Presumed Signal

Glucosamine was flagged because secondary sources raised concerns about its use by persons with diabetes (Medical Economics Co., 2001; NMCD, 2002). Animal and *in vitro* data suggested the potential for glucosamine to cause insulin resistance. Use of this information as a signal illustrates that animal and/or *in vitro* data are appropriate signals to identify concern to humans.

In addition, while not a *data* signal *per se*, the high prevalence of glucosamine use among older individuals who are likely to be at risk for type 2 diabetes suggested that if risks are associated with glucosamine and biological activities that interfere with glucose control, they could have large impact on public health as this subpopulation would be particularly vulnerable to insulin problems. Thus this information about a potentially vulnerable subpopulation should encourage the evaluation of glucosamine risk sooner than some other ingredients.

Initial Review: Considering the Nature of the Evidence

The nature of the evidence in the animal studies producing the original signal was reviewed. These studies did indeed confirm that glucosamine can lead to insulin resistance in animals and the *in vitro* studies supported the biological plausibility of such an effect. However, the animal studies that described this effect were experimental investigations on the basic biology of glucosamine, not traditional toxicology studies, and the high blood concentrations of glucosamine (approaching 1 mM) were deemed highly unlikely to be achieved by the amounts ingested orally by humans. The insulin effects would probably be categorized as a Category B (Table 5-1) effect. It is not clear how millimolar blood glucosamine in animals compares with human glucosamine because of significant metabolism: assuming less than 1 percent of orally ingested glucosamine reaches the bloodstream would suggest lower concern, while a 1 to 10 percent assumption would suggest moderate concern.

Additional information was sought to put the animal data's suggestion of insulin regulation problems into context. At this stage in the process, a full literature review was not conducted, but a focused search for human data relevant to insulin resistance was completed. Data from human clinical studies did not suggest an increased risk of insulin resistance, although most of the studies examined (especially older studies) were of relatively short duration and/or did not specifically report on blood or urine glucose levels.

At this point FDA could have decided that the nature of the evidence did not indicate a need to undertake an integrative evaluation, including the development of a monograph, because the level of concern remained lower to moderate. Therefore, instead of an integrative evaluation, this dietary supplement ingredient could have been designated for monitoring of both new signal-generating information and answers to particularly relevant questions. For example, a periodic search for human data suggesting problems of insulin regulation or reporting blood glucosamine levels following ingestion could be put in place. In addition, FDA, working with the National Institutes of Health's (NIH's) Office of Dietary Supplements, could request that laboratory indicators of insulin resistance and diabetes, as well as blood glucosamine levels, be monitored in subsequent clinical studies of glucosamine.

Integrative Evaluation

If FDA chose to proceed with an integrative evaluation for glucosamine, it could follow either a broad-based or a more focused strategy. Glucosamine appears widely used by older individuals, whose baseline incidence rates for several health problems are relatively high. Thus a relatively small increase in risk of any of these conditions associated with glucosamine use might have substantial public health impact, and it might therefore be appropriate to conduct a broad-based evaluation and proactively evaluate all potential risks of harm.

Alternatively, because the signal identified a risk specifically for insulin resistance, FDA could focus its integrative evaluation on insulin resistance and diabetes. In this case, while the topics of a literature search would be fewer than with a more proactive evaluation of all possible risks, it would not be sufficient to look for mention of glucosamine and insulin resistance or glucosamine and diabetes in abstracts of publications. Instead, the literature search would need to identify a wider variety of studies to be read in detail to determine if relevant data on glucosamine and insulin resistance exist. Relevant data might be noted only as a minor point in clinical studies, or it might be revealed only by detailed reading of publications on nonhuman data. In summary, the literature search strategy would need to be sufficiently broad to identify all potentially relevant studies that would then be examined to decide which studies are of importance for the integrative evaluation.

Melatonin

Presumed Signals

Melatonin was flagged because of serious adverse event reports to SN/AEMS. These events were cardiovascular and psychiatric/central nervous system related in nature. Another signal could have been melatonin's regulation as a drug in other countries, a fact signaling that the ingredient's potential risk should be examined.

Initial Review: Considering the Nature of the Evidence

The medical literature was searched to explore cardiovascular and psychiatric types of reports. Case reports indicated that melatonin might exacerbate psychiatric conditions, and it has been reported to cause seizures. Case reports included evidence that supported a causal relationship between melatonin and the occurrence of seizures, including challenge and rechallenge data. Animal data relevant to the issue were also examined. There was little animal data relevant to the behavioral effects, but data describing significant effects on the reproductive axis of animals added to the level of concern. Thus, at this step, multiple factors came together to suggest a higher level of concern regarding the use of melatonin, indicating the need for an integrative evaluation. In addition, there was concern that adverse events such as seizures and psychiatric problems worsened in persons particularly susceptible to these problems.

Integrative Evaluation

The integrative evaluation of melatonin began as a focused effort looking at the initial signal of seizure occurrence in an at-risk population, but the preliminary review to gather additional information yielded other areas of concern related to melatonin's physiological role as a hormone. Once these data were identified, it did not seem appropriate to ignore them as they might also indicate that melatonin was a risk to public health.

Each of the various categories of data (human, animal, *in vitro*, and related substances data) was important to the development of the recommendations and conclusions of the working group. While there was a large amount of human data, it was collected following short-duration exposure to melatonin. Animal studies of some duration helped to put the human data in context. The *in vitro* data were useful for understanding the potential for melatonin to stimulate or inhibit the activity of other hormones. Evidence from human, animal, and *in vitro* studies in which doses far exceeded the usage of melatonin as a dietary supplement were also considered.

Saw Palmetto

Presumed Signals

Saw palmetto was selected for review because of two serious cardiac events reported to SN/AEMS. Other signals of concern could have been evidence that saw palmetto may have or has similar biological activity to a regulated drug (finasteride) and saw palmetto's use as a drug in several

European countries. The finasteride example illustrates how *functional relatedness* can signal concern, as discussed below.

Initial Review: Considering the Nature of the Evidence

The cardiac events reported to FDA were placed in perspective by reviewing whether a pattern of cardiac events existed in clinical trials or published case reports. There was no consistent pattern of serious adverse events reported, and they were largely nonserious or their relevance to saw palmetto was unconvincing. The concern level from the original signal was thus lower and would be unlikely to prompt an integrative evaluation according to the Framework process.

If saw palmetto's drug status and possible mechanistic similarity to the regulated drug finasteride was the original signal, the initial review may have prompted an integrative evaluation. Investigation of this signal would have revealed *in vitro* evidence and animal evidence suggesting antiandrogenic effects, such as 5-α-reductase inhibition. Male human reproductive developmental anomalies are a feature of the congenital deficiency of 5-α-reductase, and the prescription 5-α-reductase inhibitor, finasteride, has been found to cause similar anomalies in male rats. Consequently, labeling of finasteride notes that it is contraindicated in women and children. In summary, the information about saw palmetto's similarity to finasteride and similar drugs should raise concern, consistent with the following guiding principle (see "Constituents Functionally Related to Known Classes of Toxic Compounds" in Chapter 6): "When data (i.e., *in vitro* or animal data) suggest that a dietary supplement constituent targets a receptor, enzyme, or other biological target in a manner similar to a compound known to be toxic, concern is warranted, especially if the dietary supplement constituent is known to reach the biological target in a relevant concentration."

Finally, the high prevalence of saw palmetto use is a modifying factor, suggesting an evaluation of the safety of this dietary supplement ingredient might be of value even if initial review did not result in higher concern if resources are available for such a proactive integrative evaluation. Benign prostatic hyperplasia is a very common condition among older men, and the prevalence of saw palmetto use among individuals with this disease is relatively high, suggesting that if saw palmetto were unsafe, the public health impact might be substantial. On the other hand, available evidence does not suggest this dietary supplement ingredient is frequently used in women or male children, the individuals to which the concerns apply.

Integrative Evaluation

As with all six ingredients selected as prototypes, data on saw palmetto was reviewed in a manner analogous to a proactive integrative evaluation, despite the lower level of concern about the original signal that prompted its selection. This integrative evaluation was relatively broad based in that all information deemed to possibly have anything to do with toxicity was collected in the initial data search.

The impact of a data collection strategy is illustrated in the saw palmetto example. If the data collection had been limited in scope to concerns raised by human data, and the consideration of animal and *in vitro* data had been limited to data from traditional animal toxicity studies and validated *in vitro* studies, testosterone pathway concerns would probably have been overlooked. This is because the information that raised concerns was from mechanistic types of *in vitro* studies and from animal studies that were not classical toxicity studies. In summary, considering data from studies other than animal toxicology and validated *in vitro* studies was useful because the available animal studies were too limited in scope (lacking reproductive toxicology) to detect safety issues.

Shark Cartilage

Presumed Signals

Shark cartilage was flagged because of a case report of hepatitis following ingestion. Another signal of concern could have been information suggesting that shark cartilage had antiangiogenic activity, a mechanism that raises concerns with drugs.

Initial Review: Considering the Nature of the Evidence

Five clinical case reports of adverse liver effects were considered. One SN/AEMS report was confounded by concomitant ingestion of a supplement containing known hepatotoxins. There was not a consistent pattern in the other reports sufficient to overcome the lack of adequate information regarding confounders. Consideration of the limited animal data—summaries of unpublished animal toxicology available in the published literature—did not suggest reason for specific concerns given that no overt signs of toxicity were reported. In summary, a lower level of concern would have resulted from an initial review of shark cartilage's liver effects.

As described above, shark cartilage's purported antiangiogenic mechanism could also have triggered an initial review. An initial review of data relevant to this signal would have uncovered reports of antiangiogenic activity in animal models (non-oral administration) and *in vitro* models suggesting a mechanism by which shark cartilage might possibly lead to serious adverse events, such as teratogenicity. Establishing an appropriate level of concern from these data would have required additional information to place the antiangiogenic activity in perspective. Specifically, information about functionally related antiangiogenic substances would suggest that these agents could potentially cause serious effects, including teratogenic effects. This information indicates that the effect observed in animal data is a Category A effect (severe developmental effects, Table 5-1). Dose comparisons between animals and humans are difficult because of the wide variability in products referred to as shark cartilage, and the fact that the shark cartilage was not orally administered in the reports of antiangiogenic effects in animals. Because the constituent responsible for this purported activity is unknown, its concentration in blood cannot be compared between animals and humans.

In addition to the information presented above, use by a potentially vulnerable subpopulation raises concern. Shark cartilage appears to be used largely and to a significant degree by people with significant and often life-threatening diseases, such as cancer and rheumatoid arthritis, who, as a result of their disease or medical treatments, may be at increased risk for supplement-drug interactions and certain other adverse events, such as liver-related problems. Thus even without signals of higher concern to suggest an integrative evaluation in reaction to signals, a proactive integrative evaluation might be justified if resources are available to proactively conduct them.

Integrative Evaluation

Of the three items mentioned above (liver effects, antiangiogenic potential, and use by vulnerable subpopulations), the antiangiogenic potential raised sufficient concern to warrant a reactive integrative evaluation. The integrative evaluation could therefore be focused on the very limited amount of data addressing this potential concern. The limited amount of data resulted in significant data gaps in the prototype shark cartilage monograph. Conclusions of higher concern were not reached, but the limited amount of data adequately addressing the issue left questions about shark cartilage's antiangiogenic potential in pregnant women. There is no information to suggest that women of child-bearing age are particularly likely to use the ingredient, which appears to be used largely in an effort to treat cancer and age-related conditions.

The shark cartilage prototype monograph also illustrates the wide difference in preparations of some dietary supplement ingredients. Powders could widely differ from extract preparations. Consistent with the guiding principles, safety concerns raised with shark cartilage powder use had to be assumed to occur in extracts as well, given the paucity of data about which constituents might cause effects and whether these constituents would be present in the extracts.

PRINCIPLES IDENTIFIED FROM THE PROTOTYPES

Developing the draft prototype monographs as illustrations of the Framework's integrative evaluation process served to test the process and the scientific principles included in it. The Framework presented in this report was shaped by what was learned. Some of what was identified is important to understanding how to apply each component of the Framework.

Signal Detection

The Framework takes into consideration that a myriad of signals (See Box 11-1) could suggest a potential for harm due to the consumption of a given dietary supplement ingredient. The importance of considering different types of signals is illustrated by the variety of presumed signals that were detected for the prototype supplement ingredients. Some of these signals are scientific information, such as animal data. Others are possible associations between an ingredient and serious adverse events in humans. Some signals of possible risk are not pieces of scientific information *per se* but information that indicates other knowledgeable organizations have expressed concerns about the safety of the ingredient—governments in other countries may control the use of the ingredient or secondary sources may describe potential risks. In summary, a wide variety of signals needs to be considered to some degree to determine which warrant the initiation of a more substantive review (i.e., an integrative evaluation).

BOX 11-1
Examples of Signals

- Serious adverse events reported to FDA's SN/AEMS (chaparral, saw palmetto)
- Clinical trial adverse event reports
- Published case reports (melatonin)
- Animal data (glucosamine)
- *In vitro* data (chromium picolinate)
- Functional relationship to toxic substances (melatonin, saw palmetto)
- Concern from consumer groups or health professional groups
- Known use by physicians for disease treatment (saw palmetto)
- Foreign regulatory action or use as a drug (saw palmetto, melatonin)

Ingredients for the six prototype monographs were selected based on limited knowledge, that is, a signal that a risk *might* exist. In going through the process, it became apparent that it is important initially to evaluate the signal of concern before investing effort and resources to do an exhaustive integrative evaluation. Thus the initial review step in the process was developed to use the guiding principles and spectrum of concern guidelines in Chapters 4 through 8 to efficiently determine if further investigation is warranted (i.e., to set priorities).

Initial Review

The initial review step in the process describes how a relatively cursory review of information about a particular signal will allow FDA to determine a preliminary level of concern as lower, moderate, or higher. The six ingredients illustrate that considering how the information fits into the spectra of concern described at the end of Chapters 4 through 9 will provide enough context to preliminarily determine how much concern the original signal warrants. The prototype ingredients also illustrate that additional information related to the original signal is also often needed to determine how much concern is warranted. If the signal resulted in a moderate concern level, considering other types of data helped determine whether other signals would also suggest value in conducting an integrative evaluation.

Finally, from a public health as well as a limited resources perspective, it is also appropriate to consider the prevalence of use and use by particularly susceptible populations at this stage in the process. An ingredient such as chaparral would not be as likely to affect as many persons, even if harmful, because of its limited current use. Saw palmetto, on the other hand, is used by a large number of U.S. men, warranting its consideration even if the initial review does not characterize concerns as a higher level.

In summary, no decisions regarding the potential for harm are being made in this step; the evaluation at this point is to decide if sufficient concern has been raised by the signal (and/or consideration of other evidence in the case of an initial moderate concern) to suggest an integrative evaluation is warranted. This step in the process allows FDA to set priorities for determining which dietary supplement ingredients require integrative evaluations and when continued monitoring might be a better use of limited resources.

Role of Monitoring

Among the six prototypes developed for this report, only two remained at a higher level of concern after the initial review (chaparral and melatonin).[4] Thus for the other four dietary supplement ingredients, a decision to flag the ingredient for continued monitoring might have been made based on the original presumed signal. Monitoring consists of either *passively* watching for new signals of other concerns about the ingredient or *routinely searching* the scientific literature for new data to address a specific existing concern. For example, if the concerns about glucosamine and insulin regulation were assigned only a lower or moderate concern level because glucosamine's bioavailability in animals and humans is unclear in the data, the scientific literature should be regularly searched to determine if new evidence addresses glucosamine bioavailability in animals or humans. Monitoring might also include working with the National Toxicology Program at the National Institute of Environmental Health Sciences or the Office of Dietary Supplements at NIH to initiate research addressing unanswered questions relative to some of the signals detected.

Integrative Evaluation

Broad-Based Versus Focused Approaches to Integrative Evaluation

If the concern level is moderate or higher, a decision may be made to undertake an integrative evaluation. The integrative evaluations developed into the prototype monographs for this report were comprehensive and hence labor-intensive. This approach did accomplish the objective of gaining enough information to improve and refine the scientific principles included in the Framework, but it also clearly demonstrated that a *broad-based* and comprehensive collection and consideration of all information relevant to the safety of the ingredient can be a resource-intensive undertaking. This is especially true if the ingredient itself or its constituents have been extensively studied, but not in studies particularly designed to address safety (i.e., if studies are designed specifically to evaluate the safety, consideration of these studies may be conclusive and preclude the necessity of collecting related, but less directly relevant, non-safety-focused information).

For many situations, the concern is very specific and can be addressed with an integrative evaluation *focused* on those concerns (documented in a

[4]This is not to say that only chaparral and melatonin raised significant concerns following the prototype integrative evaluation, but rather that they raised concerns following the initial review of the presumed signal. Other possible signals were also discussed for the prototype ingredients. As discussed, these signals might result in a different decision if they were subjected to the initial review.

focused monograph). When concerns center around one type of adverse effect or potential toxicity, it will often be more efficient to focus data collection and analysis efforts on those particular concerns rather than including in the monograph all data about the ingredient. When the focused monograph is prepared, the focus should be clearly described so that the monograph is not interpreted as a complete summary of all risks associated with the ingredient.

Chaparral and saw palmetto are examples of when it may be more practical to focus the integrative evaluation on key issues of concern. Concerns about the safety of chaparral stemmed from a signal of reported hepatotoxic adverse events in humans. Thus all efforts could have focused on collecting and evaluating human, animal, *in vitro*, and related substances data that might have shed light on the relationship between chaparral and liver effects. Similarly, efforts for saw palmetto could have been focused on antiandrogenic concerns. To demonstrate the differences between focused and broad-based integrative evaluations, the chaparral and saw palmetto prototype monographs are presented both ways. The broader-based versions are available for review at http://www.iom.edu/fnb, along with the other full prototype monographs; the *focused* versions are included in Appendixes J (chaparral) and K (saw palmetto).

Data Gathering for the Integrative Evaluation in the Form of a Monograph

The first step in the integrative evaluation is collecting data about the ingredient, usually collated in the form of a monograph without summary and conclusion statements. The most valuable information is studies specifically designed to evaluate toxicity and detect adverse events. Sufficient data of this type rarely exist for dietary supplement ingredients,[5] so relevant information found in studies not focused on safety also needs to be collected. For example, clinical studies on glucosamine and osteoarthritis had to be reviewed to determine if any information was presented regarding the development of insulin resistance in individuals taking glucosamine.

Strategies for collecting the needed information on the prototype dietary supplement ingredients were refined through the development of the six prototype evaluations. Specifically, for chaparral and shark cartilage, the first two ingredients to which the original proposed framework was applied, almost all information was collected and included. The second two ingredients, saw palmetto and glucosamine, were prepared by collecting almost all information that the scientists involved thought could provide

---

[5]Except for some vitamins or minerals; see Chapter 3.

any information about likely toxicities associated with these ingredients. Finally, melatonin and chromium picolinate were prepared by collecting only information relevant to the major possible toxicities in evidence from the human data and animal and *in vitro* toxicity studies. All human data were included in their prototype monographs, but only the animal, *in vitro*, and related substances data that were likely to reveal any targeted toxicities were included in their prototype monographs.

Given that resources are indeed limited, it is more important to *efficiently* collect data for integrative evaluations than to produce an *exhaustive* data collection document. The best approach from the experience with the six prototypes seems to be one between the second and third approaches used. That is, human data that are reasonably available should be collected. Data from animal and *in vitro* studies that are specifically designed to address safety and toxicity should be collected, as should relevant information about related toxic substances. Data relevant to the concerns raised by this information should then be collected. Finally, abstracts or other summaries of *in vitro* and animal data that are not from toxicity studies, or validated *in vitro* studies, *per se*, should be reviewed and used to judge which full reports need to be considered.

Integrating: Considering Consistency and Plausibility and Evaluating Heterogeneous or Seemingly Inconsistent Data

All data relevant to a particular concern often do not agree or point to the same conclusion. In preparing the prototype monographs, it became clear that articulating how to appropriately weave the different types of information together would be helpful. Thus Chapter 10 provides guidance through the difficult and often imprecise process of "weighing the evidence" to reach a scientifically appropriate conclusion about risk. It describes how biological plausibility and consistency are important, as is discounting "negative" data or studies that would not be expected to detect an effect even if it did occur.

Chaparral provides an illustrative example of how concerns raised by knowledge of the substance NDGA found in chaparral and its chemical structure provides biological plausibility to the human adverse events observed and a possible link to the nephrotoxicity observed in animals. Hypothesizing that lipid-soluble NDGA is the problematic substance is also consistent with the fewer number of adverse effects reported with ingestion of chaparral tea (an aqueous extract) as compared with capsules or tablets. As for reproductive effects of chaparral, there is consistency between the *in vitro* effects of NDGA on prostanoid synthesis and the animal effects observed. The reproductive effects, if attributable to NDGA, are also consistent with any claimed safe historical use of tea since it seems unlikely they

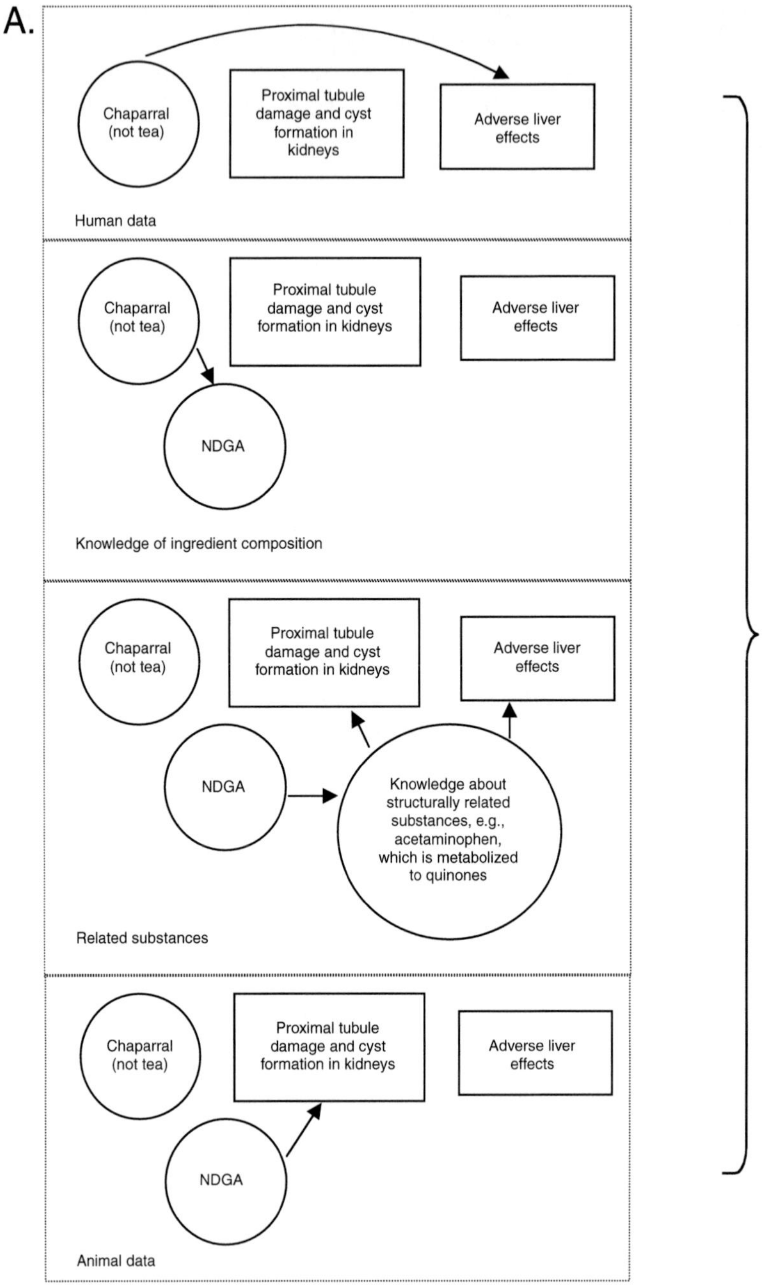

FIGURE 11-1 Causal model diagram illustrating a relationship between chaparral and liver effects in animals and humans.

would be detected with historical use. Similarly, carcinogenic effects are not inconsistent with the historical use information since they would not be expected to be detected if they did occur.

The prototype integrative evaluation process showed that with so many different types of information to process and consider, it is useful to note what is certain and focus on uncertainties. As explained in Chapter 10, causal model diagrams may be useful to visually illustrate what is known and where data gaps exist. In doing so, they can help focus thinking and information searching on remaining questions (as made more obvious by missing or weak linkage arrows). A causal model on the relationship between chaparral and liver effects is presented in Figure 11-1 as an example of the diagram's value. A solid arched arrow illustrates a relationship between chaparral ingestion and adverse liver effects in humans, independent of knowledge about hazards that may be associated with NDGA. Another pathway between chaparral and liver effects is based on the relationship between chaparral and NDGA and knowledge of how chemical structures like NDGA can be metabolized into quinones that subsequently result in adverse liver effects. A related substance with this effect is acetaminophen.

B.

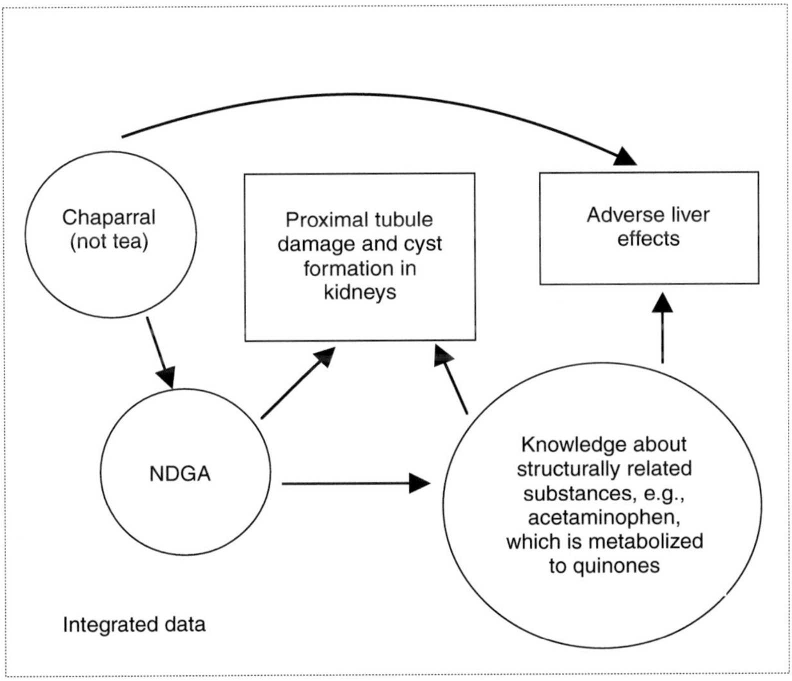

As described in Appendix J, the relationship of chaparral tea to adverse effects is less clear (hence there would be no solid line path between the tea and the adverse livers effect box). It is apparent from Figure 11-1 that if NDGA was found to be a component in chaparral tea, greater concern would be appropriate. Finally, this diagram illustrates how there may be some consistency between the proximal tubule damage observed in rodents following NDGA ingestion and the metabolism of NDGA to an orthoquinone derivative. In summary, it is the pattern of consistency and biological plausibility, illustrated by more than one path from chaparral to adverse liver effects, that raises even more concern about the safety of chaparral, especially when not prepared as a tea and when ingested by subpopulations particularly vulnerable because they have pre-existing liver conditions.

Use of External Advisory Committee

In the prototype development process, external experts were used to simulate the prescribed process of bringing in expertise particular to the ingredient's safety concerns. Consultation with experts on the specific dietary supplement ingredient, the adverse effects of concern, the physiological system of concern, and the categories of data in need of review were all important to the development of relevant conclusions and recommendations, especially when data were sparse, inconsistent, or difficult to interpret. For example, it was helpful to have physicians and scientists very familiar with insulin and glucose regulation to consider glucosamine, experts in melatonin biology and endocrinology for melatonin consideration, experts familiar with metal toxicology and carcinogenicity to help with chromium picolinate, and experts in plant chemistry as chaparral and NDGA were considered. The Framework process outlined in Chapter 11 suggests that FDA may also want to involve external experts when data are not clear-cut, when expertise in particular aspects of human physiology is necessary and when the data to be considered require additional expertise to interpret.

Notably, in the process used to test and improve the Framework, working groups were organized to guide data collection into monographs, but it is not envisioned that FDA will use such working groups to prepare monographs. Instead, FDA will probably choose to collate data into a monograph form in-house or by using outside contractors. Where FDA may choose to involve external experts, if internal expertise needs to be supplemented is in conducting the integrative evaluation (i.e., the actual analysis of how to interpret the data and develop a conclusion).

Review and Updating of Monographs

Once a monograph has been developed, it can serve as a tool for effective monitoring of safety issues in that the monograph can be updated with new information as it becomes available. Thus developing monographs is consistent with developing a proactive, ongoing evaluation system for evaluating risk.

REFERENCES

FDA (Food and Drug Administration). 1992. *Chaparral Warning*. P92-38. December 10. Press Release.

Foster S, Tyler VE. 1999. *Tyler's Honest Herbal. A Sensible Guide to the Use of Herbs and Related Remedies*. 4th ed. New York: Haworth Herbal Press.

McGuffin M, Hobbs C, Upton R, Goldberg A. 1997. *American Herbal Product Association's Botanical Safety Handbook*. Boca Raton, FL: CRC Press.

Medical Economics Co. 2001. *PDR for Nutritional Supplements*. Montvale, NJ: Thomson Medical Economics Company.

NMCD (Natural Medicines Comprehensive Database). 2002. *Natural Medicines Comprehensive Database*. Online. Available at http://www.naturaldatabase.com/. Accessed January 18, 2002.

12

Factors Influencing Use of the Safety Framework

The previous chapters describe a scientifically based framework to evaluate available information and initial indicators of potential safety concerns to determine whether dietary supplement ingredients so evaluated present a significant risk of illness or injury to the consumer. This Framework is the result of (1) extensive revision as the result of comments received from interested stakeholders and the Food and Drug Administration (FDA) after publication of a proposed framework in July 2002; (2) considering the systems used by other organizations to review the safety and effectiveness of dietary supplements ingredients; (3) considering frameworks currently in use for regulating the safety of other ingested substances as described in Chapter 2; and (4) experience gained in using the previously proposed framework to develop six prototype monographs on dietary supplements (described in Chapter 11).

Based on comments on the initial proposed framework (see Appendix B), the approach was modified to have fewer detailed steps in the process and to more explicitly define the indicators of risk across types of information instead of generalized descriptions of how to evaluate these types of data and available evidence. Further, the revised safety Framework now more specifically emphasizes the use of evidence from a variety of sources, in addition to self-reported human data.

FEATURES OF THE FRAMEWORK

This Framework:

a) Incorporates several different types of data that may be available. Utilizing the diverse types of data available (i.e., the different categories) is especially important because the extent of the types of information available are vastly different from one dietary supplement ingredient to another. Using an approach that outlines scientific principles of what constitutes appropriate and useful data informs the decision to determine the extent to which an unreasonable risk may be present—it incorporates data from animal studies, clinical studies, *in vitro* studies, chemistry, and botany, in addition to reported spontaneous adverse events, allowing an integrated assessment of safety and resulting in a qualitative determination of the degree of risk.

b) Integrates the value of different types of evidence, as well as prevalence of use information when reviewing dietary supplement ingredients. The public health perspective that a supplement ingredient used by more individuals warrants greater attention, given similar safety concerns, is included as part of the evaluative process. Consideration of likely users of particular supplement ingredients and the users' characteristics allows a more focused evaluation of risk for groups that might be particularly vulnerable to problems and thus at increased risk.

c) Allows FDA to be both proactive and reactive by responding to information regarding potential adverse consequences of consumption of a dietary supplement ingredient, as well as initiating evaluations for ingredients in use.

d) Identifies a monitoring function that allows FDA to manage new safety concerns and to monitor potential issues as new data become available. When there are suggestions of risk that evolve over time into strong and consistent evidence for safety concerns, the monitoring of concerns that first arise as lower-level indicators should permit identification of a problem at a point at which large-scale public health problems and many adverse events may be prevented.

e) Provides an open and transparent process helpful to the general public and industry in the integrative evaluation step, which includes a mechanism for the public and the relevant industry to provide data and other input voluntarily. Keeping the activity open and transparent also allows the general public to be able to access safety conclusions made by scientists free of conflicts of interest or to know if they are not free of apparent conflicts. For this reason, the safety Framework stresses the value of making safety monographs readily available to the public.

CONSTRAINTS IN USING THE SAFETY FRAMEWORK

Approaches to Safety

The safety Framework presented here does not address the issue of safety within the context of efficacy, an evaluative approach used in other systems and schema that evaluate other types of ingested products, such as over-the-counter drugs used for medicinal purposes.This is because of the boundaries of the Dietary Supplement Health and Education Act (DSHEA)-defined authority given to FDA.

It is also important to recognize that the Framework is a system designed to identify signals from various biological sources that raise the level of scientific concerns about safety of use, not to establish the safety *per se* of a dietary supplement ingredient. Where more immediate concerns are found, the Framework provides a mechanism to develop a comprehensive monograph of information upon which qualified scientists either within or external to FDA can reach a reasoned judgment as to whether or not a significant or unreasonable risk to human health is present when consumed under labeled conditions of use.

Availability of Relevant Data

A core issue that constrains the development and utility of a scientifically based framework for evaluating the safety of dietary supplements is the lack of data readily available for evaluation. Without amendments to DSHEA by Congress, FDA is not empowered to require the submission to the agency of such key information as manufacturers' data on reported adverse events. Further, while FDA has developed a mechanism to receive adverse event reports, such self-reported data that are available on adverse events are known to not reflect the actual incidence of occurrences. The extent to which the public or health care providers have knowledge of the mechanisms for, and an understanding of, the importance of informing FDA of these occurrences is unknown. Thus key information on the occurrence and severity of actual events affecting consumers is very limited and is likely to remain so unless concerted efforts are made to educate the public and health care providers about the importance of reporting these events.

Combinations of Dietary Supplement Ingredients

The heterogeneous and expanding nature of dietary supplements in the United States further constrains the development and utility of a scientifically based framework for evaluating safety. For example, dietary supplement products are increasingly complex rather than comprising single ingredients. Given the current product availability, dietary supplement users are more likely to be ingesting supplements containing multiple ingredients rather than a single dietary ingredient. Further, the epidemiological data on demographic and other characteristics of dietary supplement users indicate that these individuals are also likely to be using over-the-counter and prescribed medications. Information about the effects of combinations and interactions is difficult to obtain and is currently even more limited than information relevant to evaluating the safety of a single ingredient.

Impact of Formulation and Processing

DSHEA does not distinguish the impact of different processing methods or varied formulations on the subsequent characteristics of dietary supplement ingredients; it allows manufacturers to market products containing ingredients that have been produced using manufacturing methods or in formulations altered without prior FDA review. These changes in product manufacture may lead to significant differences in bioavailability and chemical constituents of the resulting product, suggesting a need for reevaluation of any previous safety evaluations. The lack of this reevaluation, amplified by the increasing complexity of ingredients available for use and the lack of premarket examination, hampers the ability of the FDA to have the data needed to evaluate safety within the context of this Framework; this will continue to be the case until DSHEA is amended to require some type of premarket approval or review of any change in manufacturing process or formulation of a marketed product, thus redefining the point at which an ingredient is required to have an agency review for safety.

Availability of Resources

Another key consideration in the utility of this safety Framework, or any data- or information-driven framework, is the evident limitation in resources available to FDA to operate a framework adequately—particularly resources to support the long-term need for monitoring new information as it becomes available. Without increased availability of resources, any framework developed may have limited impact on protecting the health of the public because of a lack of human and material resources to collect, evaluate, and monitor relevant data. The utility and success of the Framework will ultimately depend on FDA being provided adequate resources to fully implement the goals of DSHEA.

Use of Expert Judgment in the Safety Framework

The Framework, by defining and giving examples of data that may elevate or decrease concern, seeks to explicitly evaluate the different components of the data—considering the evidence of possible risk, seriousness of harm, and the potential public health impact as distinct variables. This approach attempts to guide judgments made to assess when an unreasonable risk of illness or injury is likely to result from use of a dietary supplement ingredient. While the determination of safety can be, at least to some extent, a subjective determination dependent upon expert interpretation of the totality of evidence, it is nevertheless important to seek consensus from experts in analyzing evidence available.

The use of expert judgment via an external advisory committee may itself be a difficult issue in that the number of qualified experts not closely associated with industry and thus not having a potential financial incentive for bias may be quite limited. Although avoidance of apparent conflict of interest is necessary, it may be difficult to ensure that all stakeholders in this area have opportunities to contribute to the process while also ensuring that objective judgments of the relevant science result.

Finally, it can be assumed that there may be a need for FDA to act without convening an expert advisory panel or committee and declare a dietary supplement ingredient as inducing significant and unreasonable risk, given the strength and seriousness of the evidence based on review by FDA.

SUMMARY

While the safety Framework outlined in this report is not based entirely on empirical data, it provides a mechanism for FDA to accomplish its goal of using a science-based approach to identify priorities for evaluating the safety of dietary supplement ingredients given available information and needed resources. Some of the factors that make the Framework less than ideal include the heterogeneity of the dietary supplement ingredients as currently defined by law, the shortage of quality studies designed specifically to assess safety, the difficulty in evaluating interactions in combination products using readily available data, and the need for adequate resources to ensure expert judgment is used in making determinations of when available data indicate that consumption of a dietary supplement ingredient presents an unreasonable risk of illness or injury.

13

Findings and Recommendations

The Dietary Supplement Health and Education Act (DSHEA) authorizes the Food and Drug Administration (FDA) to take action only when a dietary supplement ingredient presents a significant and unreasonable risk of illness or injury under conditions of use recommended or suggested in labeling or is adulterated.[1] Outlined in the preceding chapters are guiding principles and recommendations for a process by which FDA can use currently available data to evaluate the safety of dietary supplement ingredients. The guiding principles and process are designed to enhance the ability of FDA to protect consumers from unreasonable risk of harm or injury resulting from use of dietary supplement ingredients. This chapter identifies legal and regulatory barriers and provides recommendations for improvement to enhance the evaluation of the safety of dietary supplement ingredients.

ABILITY TO DETERMINE UNREASONABLE RISK

Judgment of Unsafe Versus Unreasonable Risk

For many dietary supplement ingredients, there is little available information about their safety compared with what is available for new drugs or

[1]DSHEA also gives authority the secretary of the U.S. Department of Health and Human Services to declare that a dietary supplement poses an imminent hazard to public health or safety and thus take action.

food additives. Because of the limited and variable amount and type of data available, definitive statements judging safety may be difficult to completely substantiate scientifically. However, **the standard for demonstrating that a significant or unreasonable risk exists with use of a dietary supplement ingredient does not require the same level of information as is needed to conclusively demonstrate or prove that a substance is unsafe for human consumption.**

The principles used by the scientific community to determine the risk associated with consumption of various substances should also apply to dietary supplement ingredients, bearing in mind that dietary supplements, by virtue of DSHEA, have been *assumed* to be safe, but have not been required to be proven safe. Thus, **the appropriate scientific standard to be used to overturn this basic assumption of safety is to demonstrate significant or unreasonable risk, not *prove* that an ingredient is unsafe.** Many of these scientific principles are outlined in Chapters 4 through 10, but several warrant additional mention here (see Box 13-1).

What Constitutes a Scientific Assessment of Unreasonable Risk?

It is important to consider the relevance and value of information presented by other organizations and regulatory bodies to the regulation of dietary supplement ingredients in the United States. Criteria for evaluating the relevance of other approaches are outlined in Chapter 2. These criteria include the importance of reliance on scientifically based data, consideration of all types of data (including animal data, *in vitro* data, data about chemical and taxonomical relatedness, and as data on human use), and some form of peer review.

To be of use in the safety Framework, conclusions of other regulatory bodies or similar organizations as to the safety of particular dietary supplements should be based on primary informational sources rather than reviews, and standardization and similarity of different preparations containing the active ingredient under study needs to be considered when assessing results. Further, if expert judgments play a significant role in the study conclusions, potential biases and conflicts of interest should be noted, and peer review should be part of the evaluative process.

Approaches taken by diverse organizations and governmental bodies, both within and outside the United States, which evaluate the safety and, at times, efficacy of dietary supplement ingredients, vary in their relevance to the protection of the American public from risks associated with consumption of dietary supplement ingredients.

BOX 13-1
Principles for Evaluating Data to Determine Unreasonable Risk

- **Information that is generally referred to as "safe historical use" should not be used as *prima facie* evidence that the ingredient does not cause harm.**

It is important to carefully consider the actual existence of information about historical use and the relevance of this information, taking into consideration whether the preparations are similarly processed, similar in route of exposure and duration of use, the potential for differences in concurrent use with substances, and whether or not the historical use would have revealed any possible adverse event. Appropriate historical use can then be weighed against the strength of other types of evidence suggesting possible harm (human, animal, and *in vitro* data or information about related substances).

- **Even in the absence of information on adverse events in humans, evidence of harm from animal studies is often indicative of potential harm to humans.**

This indication assumes greatest importance when the route of exposure is oral, the formulation tested is identical or highly similar to that consumed as an ingredient, and more than one species shows the same or similar toxicity.

- **Validated[a] *in vitro* studies can stand alone as independent indicators of risk to human health if a comparative exposure is attained in humans.**

- **It is scientifically appropriate and acceptable to use information about safety concerns of related substances to inform a decision about the risk associated with a dietary supplement ingredient,** by considering whether:

— the ingredient's constituents are compounds with established toxicity, or closely related to compounds with established toxicity, or

— the plant sources of the botanical dietary supplement are taxonomically related to known toxic plants.

[a] In this report, *in vitro* assays are considered validated when their results have been proven to predict a specific effect in animals and/or humans with reasonable certainty.

LEGAL AND REGULATORY BARRIERS TO EVALUATION OF THE SAFETY OF DIETARY SUPPLEMENTS

Through the process of developing the Framework to evaluate the safety of dietary supplement ingredients, a number of legal and regulatory barriers were identified that hamper FDA's ability to protect the public's health. The following findings are designed to enhance the utility of the Framework and enhance the ability of FDA to protect consumers from unreasonable risk of illness or injury.

While some constituents of conventional foods are subject to premarket approval, DSHEA excludes all dietary supplement ingredients from this requirement when labeled as dietary supplements, even though some of these ingredients would be subject to premarket approval as food additives if used in conventional foods. Moreover, while new drugs are subject to premarket approval, DSHEA excludes dietary supplements, despite the fact that they may possess biological activities similar, and in some case identical, to those found in medications and are frequently used by consumers for medicinal purposes according to survey data (Blendon et al., 2001; Chang et al., 2003; Johnson et al., 2000; Martin et al., 2002; Najm et al., 2003; Wood et al., 2003). Further, under the provisions of DSHEA, FDA has no authority to require submission of specific safety data from dietary supplement manufacturers or distributors either before or after their products are made available for sale to the public. (The manufacturer decides what information to provide when notifying FDA 75 days in advance of marketing a dietary supplement containing a new dietary ingredient.)

It is also very challenging to carry out some of the provisions of DSHEA given the limitations on the quantity and quality of the currently available scientific data related to the safety of dietary supplement ingredients. One of the key premises of DSHEA is that history of use is evidence of safety when applied to dietary supplements; as was indicated in the earlier chapters, significant scientific problems with this assumption have been identified. **In line with these findings, some members of the scientific and medical community have strongly advised that the regulatory mechanisms for monitoring the safety of dietary supplements, as currently defined by DSHEA, be revised** (Drazen, 2003; Fontanarosa et al., 2003; Marcus and Grollman, 2002; Palmer et al., 2003). **These constraints imposed on FDA make it difficult for the health of the American public to be adequately protected.**

SPECIFIC FINDINGS AND RECOMMENDATIONS

Prospective Systematic Monitoring and Tracking Mechanism for Dietary Supplement Ingredients

Finding: A prospective, systematic method for recording and monitoring the history of safety issues with specific dietary supplements is necessary to implement a framework for FDA to evaluate the safety of dietary supplement ingredients. During the period of this study, FDA developed a new method of monitoring and tracking adverse event reports—the Special Nutrition/Adverse Event Monitoring System (FDA, 2002). However, a prospective system that enables tracking of information leading to all levels of concern is also needed.

Recommendation: FDA should continue to maintain and refine a prospective system for monitoring and tracking reports of adverse events as well as other information related to safety concerns associated with consumption of dietary supplement ingredients. The system should be open, transparent, and useful for establishing varying levels of concern relating to dietary supplements as outlined in the Framework. Relationships with professional societies, scientific journals, other federal agencies, consumer protection groups, and collaborative scientific groups should be continued and enriched to facilitate the ability of FDA to collect and monitor information regarding the use of dietary supplement ingredients. Resources to support these activities should be provided to FDA.

Adequate Resources to Protect the Consumer Under DSHEA

Finding: While the committee did not conduct an analysis of the cost of implementing this Framework, implementation of any framework for comprehensive safety evaluation generates an additional workload for the responsible staff at FDA. For the framework to be effective, adequate resources must be available to FDA to collect and analyze available information. DSHEA establishes that the determination of the potential for harm from dietary supplement use be done postmarketing, but resources may not be sufficient to fulfill this task.

Recommendation: In order to fully protect the public health, Congress should ensure that FDA is provided with adequate personnel and resources to protect the consumer under DSHEA.

Adverse Event Reporting

Finding: Reports of adverse events are an important source of information by which FDA becomes aware of potential risks to public health from exposure to dietary supplement ingredients. It has been estimated that FDA receives reports of less than 1 percent of all adverse events associated with dietary supplements, according to the Inspector General's Report, *Adverse Event Reporting for Dietary Supplements: An Inadequate Safety Valve*, which also documented the limitations in the reports that are received (OIG, 2001). While spontaneous adverse event reports have recognized limitations, they have considerable strength as potential warning signals of problems requiring attention, making monitoring by FDA worthwhile.

Under DSHEA, there is no requirement for distributors or manufacturers to collect and maintain records of adverse effects associated with the use of dietary supplements. Further, distributors and manufacturers are not required to submit adverse event reports of which they are aware to FDA, thereby significantly compromising the agency's ability to actively monitor dietary supplement safety.

Recommendation: Congress should amend DSHEA to require that manufacturers and distributors report to FDA, in a timely manner, any serious adverse event associated with use of its marketed product of which the manufacturer or distributor is aware. Given that a 15-calendar-day notification of any serious unexpected adverse event to FDA is the standard for medical products,[2] this time frame seems reasonable. Dietary supplements, as for conventional foods, are not expected to be associated with any serious adverse events; therefore, all such events are considered unexpected and should be reported to FDA.

Recommendation: FDA should continue to work with the Poison Control Centers as a source of adverse event reports, and sufficient resources to support this activity should be provided.

Education of Consumers and Health Professionals about Reporting of Adverse Events Related to Dietary Supplement Ingredients

Finding: Consumers and health professionals are not adequately aware of the importance of reporting adverse events to FDA.

Recommendation: FDA should increase efforts to inform health care professionals and consumers that they should use the MedWatch adverse event reporting program to report adverse events associated with the use of dietary supplements. Additional outreach efforts should include:

- Distribution of MedWatch forms with instructions for use for reporting adverse events relating to use of dietary supplements,
- Education of health care professionals to include questions about dietary supplement use when taking diet and drug histories, and
- Education of consumers that dietary supplements are not necessarily safe and adverse events should be reported to their healthcare professional or directly to FDA.

---

[2]It is recognized that with the important exception of drugs that have undergone a switch from prescription status to over-the-counter (OTC) drug status, there is no such reporting requirement for OTC drugs. However, premarket approval following expert review is required for OTC drugs, with such assessments incorporating safety, labeling, purity, and manufacturing, but is not required for dietary supplements. Thus there is a required accumulation of evidence for OTC drug safety that is not required for dietary supplements. This difference in regulatory control results in the need for mandatory reporting of serious adverse events associated with the use of dietary supplement ingredients.

Recommendation: The FDA MedWatch toll-free telephone number should be provided on product labels to facilitate reporting of adverse events by consumers and health care professionals.

Premarket Notification of New Dietary Ingredients

Finding: DSHEA requires that a manufacturer or distributor of a new dietary ingredient notify FDA of its intention to market the ingredient at least 75 days before introducing it into interstate commerce. There appears to be ambiguity regarding the nature and amount of information that must be submitted to FDA for their review in the 75-day period.

Recommendation: To initiate the 75-day premarketing review period, both the distributor and the manufacturer should be required to provide FDA with all available data in their possession, both favorable and unfavorable, regarding safety of the product.

New Formulations and Processes

Finding: Under DSHEA, manufacturers and distributors of dietary supplements are required to provide FDA with information establishing the safety of their product only if it contains new dietary ingredients not marketed before October 1994. Dietary supplement ingredients marketed before 1994 are not subject to this requirement. Yet many dietary supplement ingredients on the market today, though not "new dietary ingredients," are produced in a variety of ways. They have different formulations and are produced through very different processes than related dietary supplement ingredients in traditional products, or even other dietary supplement ingredients bearing the same name. Alterations in formulations and processing of substances that have a history of use as dietary supplements may result in markedly different bioactive substances of potential harm.

Recommendation: When the formulation or processing of a dietary supplement ingredient is changed, it should be considered a new dietary ingredient and subject to regulatory oversight as such.

FDA Proposed Good Manufacturing Practice Guidelines

Finding: While the focus of this report is on developing a framework to evaluate the safety of dietary supplement ingredients *per se*, and not on safety issues related to good manufacturing practice, these are inseparable because variability in content hampers the evaluation of safety. FDA recently proposed current good manufacturing practices (cGMPs), regulations that may be in place by the time this report is released, but the proposed regulations will not establish uniformity across different manufacturers of the same dietary supplement ingredients. The label verification program (USP, 2004) has been a step in the right direction, but this is a voluntary program. While the U.S. Pharmacopeia has developed some standards for content uniformity for dietary supplements (USP, 2004), to date few standards have been published.

Recommendation: The FDA initiative to establish cGMPs for dietary supplement ingredients is supported and additional efforts to develop standards for content uniformity should be undertaken. Sufficient resources to support these efforts should be provided by Congress.

Revision in Requirements for Labeling of Dietary Supplements

Finding: Required label information that would be of use to the consumer in making informed decisions is limited relative to safety of use. Current regulations related to source of a product only require the name and place of business of the manufacturer, packer, or distributor to be provided on the label. In March 2003, the U.S. Department of Health and Human Services Inspector General presented a template for labeling dietary supplements to provide information in a clear and understandable format to help consumers make informed decisions about the safe and appropriate use of dietary supplements (DHHS, 2003b). Several recommendations that relate specifically to the safe use of dietary supplements are provided in a related report, *Dietary Supplement Labels: An Assessment* (DHHS, 2003a).

Recommendation: Adoption of the labeling changes recommended in the report *Dietary Supplement Labels: Key Elements* is urged. In addition, the label should contain the name and place of business of **both** the distributor and manufacturer of the product (e.g., manufactured for Company XX by Company YY) to facilitate tracing the source of the product if adverse events or other problems occur.

Additional Research on the Potential to Cause Harm

Finding: Based on the experience of preparing the prototype monographs for this report, it is evident that as the process for review of ingredients expands, research needs will be identified to address unresolved issues regarding the potential of certain ingredients to cause harm. There is no legal or regulatory requirement that dietary supplement ingredient manufacturers conduct toxicology or safety pharmacology studies on their products or ingredients. Thus the application of any testing of the types described in Chapters 5, 6, and 8 to dietary supplement ingredients will in most cases be initiated by FDA or other federal agencies. A number of collaborative activities between FDA and other governmental bodies have been undertaken and successfully completed.

Recommendation: The continued development of effective working relationships and partnerships between FDA and the National Insti-

tutes of Health is encouraged as one means for fostering more research on the safety of dietary supplement ingredients, especially for high-priority needs identified by FDA when utilizing the framework for safety evaluation.

Recommendation: FDA should ensure that its own National Center for Toxicological Research and the overall Department of Health and Human Services National Toxicology Program are optimally utilized by FDA's Center for Food Safety and Applied Nutrition for investigation into specific concerns of dietary supplement safety. In addition, FDA and the National Institutes of Health should establish clear guidelines for cooperative efforts on high-priority safety issues related to the use of dietary supplements.

Recommendation: All federally supported research on dietary supplements conducted to assess efficacy should be required to include the collection and reporting of all data related to safety of the ingredient under study.

REFERENCES

Blendon RJ, DesRoches CM, Benson JM, Brodie M, Altman DE. 2001. American's views on the use and regulation of dietary supplements. *Arch Intern Med* 161:805–810.

Chang CW, Chu G, Hinz BJ, Grever MD. 2003. Current use of dietary supplementation in patients with age-related macular degeneration. *Can J Ophthalmol* 38:27–32.

DHHS (U.S. Department of Health and Human Services). 2003a. *Dietary Supplement Labels: An Assessment.* Office of Inspector General, OEI-01-01-0012. Online. Available at http://oig.hhs.gov/oei/reports/oei-01-01-00121.pdf. Accessed June 25, 2004.

DHHS. 2003b. *Dietary Supplement Labels: Key Elements.* Office of Inspector General, OEI 01-01-00120. Online. Available at http://oig.hhs.gov/oei/reports/oei-01-01-00120.pdf. Accessed June 25, 2004.

Drazen JM. 2003. Inappropriate advertising of dietary supplements. *N Engl J Med* 348:777–778.

FDA (Food and Drug Administration). 2002. *Letter to Stakeholders. Announcing CAERS—The CFSAN Adverse Event Reporting System.* Online. Available at http://www.cfsan.fda.gov/_dms/caersltr.html. Accessed June 25, 2004.

Fontanarosa PB, Drummond R, De Angelis CD. 2003. The need for regulation of dietary supplements—Lessons from Ephedra. *J Am Med Assoc* 289:1568–1570.

Johnson EM, Wootton JC, Kimzey R, McCullagh L, Wesley R, Byrd DC, Singh KK, Rubino D, Pucino F. 2000. Use of herbal therapies by adults seen in an ambulatory care research setting: An exploratory survey. *J Altern Complement Med* 6:429–435.

Marcus DM, Grollman AP. 2002. Botanical medicines: The need for new regulations. *N Engl J Med* 347:2073–2076.

Martin KJ, Jordan TR, Vassar AD, White DB. 2002. Herbal and nonherbal alternative medicine use in Northwest Ohio. *Ann Pharmacother* 36:1862–1869.

Najm W, Reinsch S, Hoehler F, Tobis J. 2003. Use of complementary and alternative medicine among the ethnic elderly. *Altern Ther Health Med* 9:50–57.

OIG (Office of Inspector General). 2001. *Adverse Event Reporting for Dietary Supplements. An Inadequate Safety Valve.* OEI-01-00-00180. Boston, MA: OIG, Department of Health and Human Services.

Palmer ME, Haller C, McKinney PE, Klein-Schwartz W, Tschirgi A, Smolinske SC, Woolf A, Sprague BM, Ko R, Everson G, Nelson LS, Dodd-Butera T, Bartlett WD, Landszberg BR. 2003. Adverse events associated with dietary supplements: An observational study. *Lancet* 361:101–106.

USP (U.S. Pharmacopeia). 2004. *Overview: USP's Dietary Supplement Verification Program.* Online. Available at http://www.uspverified.org/pinfo/overview.html. Accessed March 10, 2004.

Wood MJ, Stewart RL, Merry H, Johnstone DE, Cox JL. 2003. Use of complementary and alternative medical therapies in patients with cardiovascular disease. *Am Heart J* 145:806–812.

Appendix A

Existing Frameworks or Systems for Evaluating the Safety of Other Substances

The following text provides an overview of existing safety frameworks that have been developed by federal agencies, industries, or other organizations. The descriptions are based on presentations to the committee and information provided by the organizations themselves; the descriptions are not the committee evaluations of the frameworks.

PREMARKET APPROVAL OF FOOD ADDITIVES

"Food additives" include an array of substances that accomplish a variety of technical effects in food. Included are direct food additives (e.g., artificial sweeteners), food-processing aides (e.g., antimicrobials), food contact substances (e.g., food packaging), and, by legal definition, sources of food irradiation. Under the 1958 Food Additives Amendment (FAA, P.L. 85-929) to the Food, Drug, and Cosmetic Act (FDCA), the Food and Drug Administration (FDA) has responsibility for the premarket approval of food additives.[1] The statute, as interpreted by FDA, establishes both the standard of data review (i.e., fair evaluation of the data of record), as well as the standard of safety (i.e., a reasonable certainty of no harm under the intended conditions of use). Notably, the statute exempts from premarket safety evaluation the use of substances in food that are "generally recog-

[1]In 1997 the FDCA was amended to provide for premarket notification, rather than premarket approval, for food contact substances.

nized as safe" (GRAS) by qualified experts in light of scientific procedures or, for substances used prior to 1958, in light of scientific procedures or experience based on common use in food. As discussed in the next section, FDA has in place a process for assessing the worthiness of claims of GRAS status.

FDA conducts safety assessments of new food additives under the principle of establishing a reasonable certainty of no harm by applying a decision framework. This framework uses a risk-assessment approach that includes the compilation of available data and information and the application of toxicological and other types of decision elements.

FDA then reviews the available toxicology studies. It has developed guidelines (*Toxicological Principles for the Safety of Food Ingredients,* commonly known as *The Redbook* [OFAS, 2003]) for interested parties to use when assembling the required data for submission of a food additive petition. *The Redbook* outlines the types of toxicological testing FDA normally expects to be provided in support of the food additive's safety, based initially on the additive's chemical structure and probable human exposure. (*The Redbook* provides guidance; it does not include requirements.) Using the information submitted, FDA assigns additives to initial "concern levels" (or "minimum testing levels") of I, II, or III. In its data review, FDA applies toxicological decision elements to further refine the scope of needed toxicological data.

From the animal studies, FDA determines the highest level of intake associated with no adverse toxicological effect in the most sensitive, longest duration, most relevant animal study. This "highest no-effect level" is then divided by an "uncertainty factor" (or "safety factor"), often a factor of 100, to account for both intra- and interspecies variability. The resulting value is the acceptable daily intake (ADI) for the additive. The ADI is compared to the estimated daily intake to determine whether the proposed use of the additive is consistent with a reasonable certainty of no harm.

For some substances, the traditional risk assessment approach is not applicable. For example, an additive may be so toxicologically inactive that not enough of the additive can be orally ingested by the test animals to elicit a toxic response without perturbing normal nutrition. In such cases it is difficult to determine an ADI. FDA may then employ other types of decision elements. In these cases, increased emphasis may be placed on, for example, chemical identity information and structure-activity relationships; data on absorption, distribution, metabolism, and excretion; and human tolerance studies (to look at physiological and nutritional responses).

Once all the information has been evaluated, FDA concludes whether the proposed use of a food additive is consistent with a reasonable certainty of no harm and can be safely marketed. After a new food additive is on the market, FDA may monitor the substance for safety through examination of available clinical studies and postmarket surveillance (Personal communication, A. Rulis, FDA, January 25, 2002).

SELECT COMMITTEE ON GRAS SUBSTANCES

Based on the 1958 amendment for food additives to the FDCA, FDA developed specific processes to determine whether substances used in foods were safe for their intended use (see previous section). Food additives, as defined in the amendment, are subject to premarket approval by FDA unless they are GRAS or fall within another statutory exception (21 U.S.C. § 321(s)).

Following the passage of the FAA, FDA assumed a lenient approach to dealing with the GRAS exception. In the early 1970s, however, in response to public concern about the apparent carcinogenicity of cyclamate, which FDA had listed as GRAS, FDA adopted a more rigorous approach (Degnan, 2000). In 1972 FDA contracted with the Life Sciences Research Office (LSRO) of the Federation of American Societies for Experimental Biology for assistance with a comprehensive review of GRAS substances. LSRO established a Select Committee on GRAS Substances that examined monographs that provided all known data on physical and chemical properties of a substance, human exposure data, animal and human toxicity data, and reports of special studies on mutagenicity, carcinogenicity, and teratogenicity of each substance. The Select Committee reached one of five conclusions on each GRAS substance reviewed: (1) continue as GRAS, (2) continue as GRAS with limitations, (3) uncertainties exist—issue interim food additive order requiring further testing, but continue as GRAS until tests are evaluated, (4) evidence of adverse effects—establish conditions of safe use or remove GRAS status, or (5) inadequate data precludes evaluation—rescind GRAS status. The review was completed in 1982.

In 1972 FDA also established procedures for petitioning to affirm the GRAS status of a substance, which while still in use have rarely been used due to the significant amount of documentation required. Currently, in order to achieve GRAS status for a substance not used in food prior to 1958, four key criteria must be met: (1) general recognition of safety by qualified experts, (2) the experts must have the scientific training and experience necessary to evaluate the safety of the substance, (3) the experts must base their safety determination on scientific procedures, and (4) GRAS determination must fully consider the intended use of the substance (Hallagan and Hall, 1995).

In 1997 FDA proposed to replace the current GRAS affirmation petition scheme with one of notification, allowing any organization to notify FDA of a self-determination of GRAS. The interim policy allows this method to be used pending issuance of final regulations. The proposed rule would also clarify the types of evidence needed to establish GRAS status (Degnan, 2000).

GRAS DETERMINATION FOR FLAVOR INGREDIENTS: FLAVOR AND EXTRACT MANUFACTURERS ASSOCIATION EXPERT PANEL

Because flavor ingredients are a type of food additive, the flavor industry has to adhere to the requirements laid out in the 1958 FAA. To determine GRAS status for flavoring substances, the Flavor and Extract Manufacturers Association (FEMA), the trade organization of the flavor ingredients industry, created its own independent expert panel. The FEMA Expert Panel, which has been reviewing flavoring substances since soon after the passage of the FAA in 1958, includes qualified experts in toxicology, pharmacology, biostatistics, pharmacokinetics, biochemistry, pathology, nutrition, organic chemistry, medicinal chemistry, and metabolism (Woods and Doull, 1991). The panel evaluates the available data on safety and use of flavoring ingredients and assesses whether the ingredients meet the criteria for GRAS status.

The FEMA Expert Panel has developed a safety assessment evaluation process for determining GRAS status. Once an application for GRAS status is submitted to the panel with a complete literature search, the first step is preliminary assessment of the data for adequacy by FEMA staff. These data are then evaluated by the panel using the following criteria: (1) exposure to the substance in specific foods, (2) natural occurrence in foods, (3) chemical identity and chemical structure, (4) metabolic and pharmacokinetic characteristics, and (5) animal toxicity (Woods and Doull, 1991). The panel examines toxicity and metabolic data on structurally similar compounds and considers the history of use of the substance (Hallagan and Hall, 1995).

Based on the weight of the evidence and expert judgment, the panel reaches one of three conclusions: (1) GRAS, (2) not GRAS, or (3) insufficient data to determine GRAS status. If data are insufficient, the panel will reexamine the substance after more data are available. The designation of GRAS status on a flavor ingredient must be based on a unanimous decision by the panel.

COSMETICS INGREDIENT REVIEW

As is the case for dietary supplements, there is no premarket regulatory system for cosmetic ingredients other than color additives that are regulated directly by FDA. The Cosmetics Ingredient Review (CIR) Program was established in 1976 by the Cosmetic, Toiletry, and Fragrance Association

(CTFA) to review and assess the safety of cosmetic ingredients in the marketplace.

The CIR Program is funded by industry, but its review process is independent and open to public and scientific scrutiny (Bergfeld and Andersen, 2000). Approximately 2,800 cosmetic ingredients were on the market in 1976 when the CIR Program was established. In response, the CIR Program developed a system to prioritize these ingredients before performing the safety review. First it excluded or deferred ingredients being reviewed by other groups, such as fragrances and ingredients being evaluated by FDA, including color additives and over-the-counter (OTC) drug ingredients. The CIR Program then grouped the remaining ingredients into chemically related families and prioritized based on the following factors: frequency of use, ingredient concentration in cosmetic products, area of human exposure, number of products containing the ingredient used by sensitive population subgroups (such as infants and the elderly), biological activity, frequency of consumer complaints, and skin penetration. Using a ranking methodology, ingredients were given a weighted score based on these factors and were then reviewed in priority order. Frequency of use and biological activity were given the most weight in the ranking. This priority listing and ranking methodology is updated periodically.

The safety review starts with a comprehensive literature search by CIR staff. The staff summarizes the available published data and publishes the summaries for public comment. During a 90-day period, interested parties may submit comments or additional data.

Following this comment period, a CIR Expert Panel begins its review of the collected data and determines whether more data are needed. The panel consists of seven scientists and physicians who serve as voting members and three nonvoting liaison members, representing CTFA, FDA, and the Consumer Federation of America. CIR emphasizes that voting members are careful to avoid any perceived or real conflicts of interest. Liaison members serve to keep consumer groups, FDA, and industry informed of the panel's deliberations.

If additional data are required, an informal request is directed toward the cosmetic industry. If data are not forthcoming or are still inadequate for the safety assessment, a formal request is made. Once all the necessary data are received, the panel reviews them and produces a tentative report that is released for public comment. At the end of the comment period, comments are considered and the final report is written.

In determining safety for the final report, the panel looks at all the available data, considers structurally similar substances, and relies on panel members' experience and expertise. The data needed for the safety assessment are dependent on the particular ingredient under review. However, the panel usually considers chemical and physical properties, impurities, extent and type of use, concentration of use, subchronic or chronic toxicity, skin penetration, skin irritation, and skin sensitization.

In each final report, the CIR Expert Panel reaches one of four conclusions on the safety of a cosmetic ingredient: (1) safe as currently used, (2) safe with qualifications, (3) unsafe, or (4) insufficient data. If data are considered insufficient, the panel notes what data are lacking. In practice, this conclusion of insufficient data encourages manufacturers to undertake additional studies.

NEW DRUGS

Unlike dietary supplements, premarket approval of new drugs places the burden of proof regarding safety on the manufacturer rather than on FDA. The evaluation of new drugs, new uses for approved drugs, and classification of OTC drugs is an intensive interactive process that evaluates both safety and efficacy. Manufacturers that want to develop and market a new drug must follow the FDA approval process that is modeled on a risk-benefit approach. Approval of a new drug requires extensive studies of the chemistry, manufacturing, and controls of the drug, toxicology and pharmacology of the compound in animals, and clinical trials of effectiveness and safety in humans. The timeframe and resources for this process are extensive (21 C.F.R. § 300 [2001]).

A key initial step in the drug approval process is submission by the manufacturer of an Investigational New Drug (IND) application to FDA. The IND is a large collection of information that enables FDA to review the safety of the substance before clinical testing in humans is allowed to begin. The IND describes the ingredients, synthesis, manufacturing, purity, and microbiology of the drug product, as well as the stability, packaging, and labeling. Also included in the IND are data from rodent and nonrodent animal studies, such as pharmacokinetic and pharmacodynamic data from animal studies, genotoxicity studies, carcinogenicity studies, reproductive and teratogenic studies, and other toxicological data. When available, the application also includes published or unpublished human data. Because these data help FDA determine whether the human testing process will be allowed to proceed, the manufacturer also provides protocols outlining the Phase I, II, and III clinical studies it plans to conduct. After the IND is submitted, FDA has 30 days to review its content. If FDA does not contact the sponsor within that time, the proposed Phase I study may begin (21 C.F.R. § 312 [2001]).

During Phase I studies, which focus on safety but not efficacy, human volunteers (who are usually healthy) are carefully monitored for tolerability, and pharmacokinetic data are often collected. The aim of Phase II is to evaluate the dose-response relationship and effectiveness of the drug in a few hundred subjects who have the disorder the drug is intended to treat. These studies are usually double-blind and placebo-controlled to minimize investigator and subject bias. Phase III of the investigation consists of well-controlled trials to gather evidence on both effectiveness and safety of the drug and information needed for labeling. These are large trials of several hundred to several thousand subjects.

The data collected in all of the clinical studies enable FDA to approve or disapprove a drug based on a risk-benefit analysis. Once a drug is approved and marketed, additional safety information continues to be collected through mandatory submission of adverse event information from the manufacturer to FDA via MedWatch and other reporting mechanisms. FDA may also require the manufacturer to conduct postmarketing studies.

OVER-THE-COUNTER DRUGS

The process above describes the steps required for a new drug approval (NDA). In the years after proof of effectiveness was added to the NDA requirements, FDA wrestled with how to deal with the thousands of OTC drugs that were on the market though not covered by approved NDAs. Rather than make case-by-case challenges to such products, FDA decided to review them by therapeutic class with the assistance of expert advisory committees. The process that FDA established to accomplish this mission is known as the OTC Drug Review.

In 1972 FDA, with the help of 17 advisory panels, began its review of the more than 700 active ingredients with almost 1,500 uses in marketed OTC drug products. The aim of the review was to prepare monographs establishing the conditions under which OTC drugs would be considered generally recognized as safe and effective, and not misbranded, and thus exempt from the NDA process.

The OTC Drug Review consists of several phases. In the first phase, now complete, the advisory panels made recommendations regarding the categorization of products. Category I was for those drugs that the panel deemed to be generally recognized as safe and effective, and not misbranded if they satisfied specified conditions, including, among others, active ingredients and labeling indications. Category II was for products with active ingredients, labeling claims, or other conditions that resulted in them not being generally recognized as safe or effective or resulted in them being misbranded. Category III was for products with active ingredients, labeling claims, or other conditions for which the data were insufficient and for which further testing was thus required.

In the second phase of the review, FDA published the panels' recommendations as Advanced Notices of Proposed Rulemaking (ANPRs). These ANPRs included proposed monographs establishing the conditions under which OTC drugs in specific therapeutic classes would be generally recognized as safe and effective, and not misbranded (Category I). In the third phase, after considering the public comments received in response to ANPRs, the agency issued proposed rules designated Tentative Final Monographs. In the final step of the process, the agency, after receiving further comments, publishes final monographs. As of March 1, 2001, most, but not all, of these final monographs had been published (CDER, 2001). Final monographs set forth the mandatory conditions for an OTC drug to be considered generally recognized as safe and effective, and not misbranded, including active ingredients, dosages, permitted combinations of ingredients, warnings, and labeling requirements.

NEW CHEMICALS PROGRAM

Under the New Chemicals Program, the Environmental Protection Agency (EPA) is given the authority to regulate the entry and use of new chemicals into the U.S. marketplace. This program, mandated by Section 5 of the Toxic Substances Control Act (TSCA) in 1976, seeks to manage the potential risk from new chemicals both to humans and to the environment. Manufacturers or importers of new chemicals are required under TSCA to notify EPA through a premanufacturer notice (PMN) that must be submitted at least 90 days prior to manufacture or import of the new chemical. New chemicals are defined as those that are not listed on EPA's TSCA Chemical Substance Inventory of existing chemicals. The burden of proof for identifying risk rests with EPA.

EPA receives petitions for approximately 2,000 new chemicals from manufacturers each year (Personal communication, L. Scarano, EPA, October 11, 2001). At submission, the manufacturer provides the PMN, which includes information on chemical and physical identity and properties, product uses, proposed production or importation volume, by-products, human exposure, disposal practices, environmental releases, pollution prevention efforts, and available information on health or environmental effects. A multidisciplinary team of experts is responsible for reviewing the safety information provided in the PMN. The first step is to determine whether the substance is already on the TSCA inventory. If it is not, the team then evaluates chemical structure, how the chemical is synthesized, the intended use of the chemical, and the physical and chemical properties of the chemical. They also check for analogs in an EPA analog database. About 30 percent of the applications are not reviewed after this stage; these substances consist of polymers, which because of their molecular weight and other properties are considered unlikely to present significant hazard potential.

The next step of the process is to estimate the potential environmental and health hazards using analog analysis, quantitative structure activity relationship models, and expert judgment. The structure activity team has identified 54 structural alert categories that may indicate a potential concern for chemicals that fall into these categories (Personal communication, L. Scarano, EPA, October 11, 2001).

The third step is to prioritize the results of the safety evaluations and to decide if further review is warranted. If it is required, the next step is a more detailed standard review. In this step, a risk assessment is conducted, human health hazard information is evaluated, and the chemical is assigned a qualitative determination of the hazard concern level. Evidence of adverse effects in human populations and conclusive evidence of severe effects in animal studies constitute a high hazard concern level. A moderate level of concern results from suggestive animal studies and analog data and knowledge that the chemical class has produced toxicity. The low concern level is for those chemicals for which no concern was identified. At this point, depending on the hazard concern level and considering the estimated exposures and releases, EPA will inform the manufacturer that the chemical presents potential risk issues and that more testing is needed. If EPA does not act to regulate the chemical, the manufacturer may commence production or importation.

REFERENCES

Bergfeld WF, Andersen FA. 2000. The cosmetic ingredient review. In: Estrin NF, Akerson JM, eds. *Cosmetic Regulation in a Competitive Environment.* New York: Marcel Dekker. Pp. 195–216.

CDER (Center for Drug Evaluation and Research). 2001. *Milestone Status of OTC Drug Review Documents as of March 1, 2001.* Online. Food and Drug Administration. Available at http://www.fda.gov/cder/otc/milestone/pdf. Accessed March 28, 2002.

Degnan FH. 2000. *FDA's Creative Application of the Law.* Washington, DC: Food, Drug, and Law Institute. Pp. 19–26.

Hallagan JB, Hall RL. 1995. FEMA GRAS—A GRAS assessment program for flavor ingredients. Flavor and Extract Manufacturers Association. *Regul Toxicol Pharmacol* 21:422–430.

OFAS (Office of Food Additive Safety). 2003. *Redbook 2000. Toxicological Principles for the Safety of Food Ingredients*. Online. Available at http://www.cfsan.fda.gov/~redbook/red-toca.html. Accessed March 28, 2002.

Woods LA, Doull J. 1991. GRAS evaluation of flavoring substances by the Expert Panel of FEMA. *Regul Toxicol Pharmacol* 14:48–58.

Appendix B

Scope of Work and Comments to Initial July 2002 Framework

SCOPE OF WORK

The Food and Drug Administration (FDA) requested that the Institute of Medicine, the National Academies, conduct a study to develop a framework for evaluating the safety of dietary supplement ingredients. The jointly agreed upon scope of work follows:

- The contractor shall work closely with FDA/Center for Food Safety and Applied Nutrition (CFSAN) throughout the period of this contract.
- The focus shall be on the use of ingredients in dietary supplements regulated under food provisions of the law, not as drugs or therapeutic agents.
- The contractor shall develop a framework that includes criteria for how review of dietary supplements and ingredients should be prioritized with regard to safety issues.
- The contractor shall describe a process for developing a monograph system with specifications for evaluating the safety of dietary supplement ingredients and shall develop at least six prototype monographs as examples.
- The contractor shall solicit public input on the proposed framework and relative to their plans for monograph development.
- The contractor shall consider the relevance/lack of relevance of the way in which other expert bodies have categorized and reviewed supplement safety issues.

- The description of the framework and criteria for categorizing the safety of dietary supplement ingredients shall contain sufficient information to describe the rationale used.
- The prototype monographs shall contain information to document the science base and rationale for the conclusions and recommendations contained in these documents.
- The framework shall outline approaches to be used to conduct the review of available research regarding the safety of each dietary supplement ingredient.

The project shall be conducted in several phases:

Phase I. The contractor shall identify a framework for categorizing and/or classifying ingredients based on safety concerns. Across and within the categories, the contractor shall give criteria for how ingredient reviews should be prioritized. The contractor shall publish its proposed framework and rationale for this framework and shall also solicit public comment on these.

Phase II. The contractor shall develop prototype monographs for at least six of the most critical risk categories. The prototype monographs shall consist of, but are not limited to, (a) a description of the ingredient under review, (b) a critical evaluation of the state-of-the-art science relative to the adverse effects of the ingredient, (c) a review of the research on the ingredient's chemical and pharmacological properties and use conditions that could adversely affect health, (d) identification of research needed to further characterize its adverse effects, and (e) conclusions as to what is known and unresolved issues about the safe use conditions for this ingredient when included as part of a dietary supplement.

The contractor shall publish a final report for the proposed framework and rationale.

COMMENTS RECEIVED ON THE PHASE I FRAMEWORK

As part of the requirements noted in the scope of work for this project, a proposed framework was released for comment. The committee received more than 20 oral or written comments from various stakeholders related to the proposed framework. Below is a summary of the comments that were the most useful to the committee as they revised the framework.

Comments are summarized into four broad areas: scientific concepts that need to be addressed or addressed in more detail, process related, regulatory situation of dietary supplements, and testing the framework.

Scientific Concepts

The comments received suggested that some scientific concepts in the framework report should be addressed or addressed in more detail, as described below.

Dose-Response Relationship

Several comments mentioned that more consideration should be given to the relationship between the dose consumed of a dietary supplement ingredient and adverse effects.

Historical Use Information

Comments suggested that guiding principles on human data outlined in the framework should give more consideration to historical use. However, industry stakeholders and a consumer interest group agreed that historical data are not *prima facie* evidence that a supplement is harmless.

Adverse Event Reports

A consumer interest group commented that priority should be given to credible adverse event reports but that an absence of these reports should not be an assurance of safety. In addition, a consumer interest group suggested that there should be further investigation and evaluation of adverse events that are reported. Some industry stakeholders expressed that adverse event reports should not be used to reach conclusions about causality. Other comments were received suggesting that the benefits of dietary supplement ingredients should also be taken into account when evaluating the incidence and severity of adverse events. In addition, comments were made recommending that if clinical data indicate conditions of safe use, then the dose-response relationship needs to be considered when evaluating adverse event reports.

Vulnerable Subpopulations

Some of the comments indicated that more attention needs to be focused on the use of dietary supplement ingredients among subgroups of the population that may be more susceptible to serious adverse effects.

Prevalence of Use in the Population

Several of the comments received mentioned that more attention needs to be focused on dietary supplements that are widely used among the general population. While some of the comments received from industry stakeholders agreed that these supplements should be a higher priority for a safety evaluation, some also noted that wide use alone should not warrant a safety evaluation.

Weighing the Evidence

Comments emphasized that more discussion is needed on how the key factors outlined in the framework are to be used to weight the evidence for evaluating the safety of dietary supplement ingredients. More specifically, several comments expressed concern that too much emphasis was placed on human data.

Some stakeholders interpreted the report as indicating that human data are to be relied on, which caused a concern because of the opinion that adequate human data may not be available. Comments were also received expressing that the weight placed on animal data, *in vitro* data, and the biological activity of structurally related or taxonomically related substances needs to be reconsidered in the screening process. In addition, comments were received stating that consideration should also be given to genotoxic data. One comment mentioned that genotoxic data should be weighed differently from data about structure-activity relationships and should be considered sooner in the process. It was also mentioned that more emphasis should also be placed on biological activity in the key factors.

Finally, several comments suggested that more guiding principles describing the appropriate weighing of evidence needed to be outlined in the report.

Process-Related Comments

The comments received relating to the evaluation process outlined in the draft framework are summarized below.

General Comments

A few of the comments received recommended that the framework process should be initiated by having experts develop a priority list.

Comments also criticized the "other concerns" screening category. Some stakeholders were concerned that this category would allow unsubstantiated expressions of concern or letters of concern to trigger a critical safety evaluation.

It was also recommended that the first step in evaluating safety should be to determine if there is an imminent danger that requires immediate action or a limitation on use.

Industry stakeholders suggested that industry input should be sought earlier in the evaluative process and that this process should be transparent.

Some comments expressed concerns that the proposed framework would not be cost-effective for FDA to implement.

In addition, comments were made suggesting that more discussion is needed on how the other approaches used to evaluate the safety of dietary supplements are or are not applicable in the proposed framework.

One comment stated that, while a good description of other approaches on the safety of botanicals was given, little attention was given to approaches used for vitamins, minerals, and other nutritional ingredients.

Prioritization Scoring System

Comments about the sorting matrix used in the priority-setting process to categorize ingredients are described below.

Concerns were raised over the complexity of the scoring system and whether FDA has enough resources to implement the proposed system.

A few stakeholders expressed concerns that the quantitative nature of the scoring system may give the false impression of numerical precision.

Furthermore, several industry stakeholders were concerned that the numerical scoring system for prioritization may be misused in legal cases against manufacturers.

It was also mentioned that the scoring criteria needed to be more clearly defined in the report to reduce subjectivity and variability.

Monographs

Comments were made suggesting that more guiding principles on how to develop the monographs are needed.

It was also suggested that the monographs should be considered to be in "draft" form until public input can be made.

One industry stakeholder suggested that FDA and not the advisory committee described in the report should develop conclusions for the monographs. It was suggested that FDA should base its conclusions on the advisory committee's recommendations about the data.

Comments were also expressed over the extensive nature of the draft prototype monographs developed as part of this document. Some questioned whether FDA has the resources to develop monographs that are as extensive as the examples developed.

Expertise Needed

Several comments were received indicating that particular expertises needed to be added to the suggestions for who should be included in an expert committee. It was suggested that a representative for consumers and an expert on evidence-based analysis be included in the advisory group. It was also suggested that pharmacognosists and others with experience with botanical products also be included.

Regulatory Situation of Dietary Supplements

Several comments received applied more to the appropriateness of the current regulatory situation that to the report itself, an issue that the committee did not specifically address in the first report.

Comments were received stating that the risks and benefits of dietary supplements should be considered in evaluating the safety of dietary supplements.

A few comments were also received questioning whether FDA had the legal authority under the Dietary Supplement Health Education Act to develop monographs on dietary supplements and whether the study commissioned is scientifically valid.

One comment was also received suggesting that the description for the 75-day advanced notice for new dietary supplements should be compared with the self-declaration of "generally recognized as safe" used for conventional food ingredients.

Testing the Framework

A few comments called for a description on how the six supplements chosen for monograph development as part of this report came through each of the steps of the proposed framework.

Appendix C

Plant Family Information

This appendix provides additional information about the genera listed in Table 6-1. Discussions are organized by families rather than genera because characteristics may be common to a particular family, but inclusion of a family in this list does not necessarily indicate toxicity. Instead, whether belonging to a particular family is sufficient to raise concern should be informed by the text describing which families are generally considered unsafe, which may include only a few unsafe members, and which contain both commonly ingested foods and toxic members.

GENERAL REFERENCES CONSULTED

The information in the following section was generated by committee members knowledgeable in botanicals by consulting the following resources:[1]

Cheeke PR. 1998. *Natural Toxicants in Feeds, Forages, and Poisonous Plants,* 2nd ed. Danville, IL: Interstate Publishers, Inc.

Colegate SM, Dorling PR, eds. 1994. *Plant-Associated Toxins: Agricultural, Phytochemical and Ecological Aspects.* Wallingford, UK: CAB International.

[1]Kingsbury's (1964) *Poisonous Plants of the United States and Canada* is an especially useful resource and, while not consulted for all the families below, Dewick (2002) is also especially helpful.

Everist SL. 1981. *Poisonous Plants of Australia.* London: Angus & Robertson Publishers.

Garland T, Barr AC, eds. 1998. *Toxic Plants and Other Natural Toxicants.* Wallingford, UK: CAB International.

James LF, Keeler RF, Cheeke PR, Bailey EM, Hegarty MP, eds. 1992. *Poisonous Plants.* Ames, IA: Iowa State University Press.

Keeler RF, Tu AT, eds. 1983. *Handbook of Natural Toxins. Volume 1. Plant and Fungal Toxins.* New York: Marcel Dekker.

Keeler RF, Tu AT. 1991. *Handbook of Natural Toxins. Volume 6. Toxicology of Plant and Fungal Compounds.* New York: Marcel Dekker.

Keeler RF, Van Kampen KR, James LF, eds. 1978. *Effects of Poisonous Plants on Livestock.* New York: Academic Press.

Kellerman TS, Coetzer JAW, Naudé TW. 1988. *Plant Poisonings and Mycotoxicoses of Livestock in Southern Africa.* Cape Town, South Africa: Oxford University Press.

Kingsbury JM. 1964. *Poisonous Plants of the United States and Canada.* Englewood Cliffs, NJ: Prentice-Hall.

Seawright AE, Hegarty MP, Keeler RF, James LF, eds. 1985. *Plant Toxicology.* Brisbane, Australia: Queensland Poisonous Plants Committee.

INFORMATION ON TOXICITY IN SELECTED PLANT FAMILIES

The **Agavaceae** is of primary concern for the species *Agave lecheguilla* (lechuguilla), which causes secondary (hepatogenic) photosensitization; sheep and goats are frequently poisoned. The toxin is a saponin that is hepato- and nephrotoxic (Camp et al., 1988). Damage to the liver results in incomplete metabolism of chlorophyll, leading to peripheral circulation of phylloerythrin with excessive absorption of solar radiation (Keeler and Tu, 1983). Also, *Nolina texana* (sacahuista, bear grass) has been responsible for poisoning in livestock, especially the buds, blooms, and fruits, which are readily consumed (Cheeke, 1998; Keeler and Tu, 1983). In sheep, a toxic dose is 1.1 percent of the animal's body weight (Kingsbury, 1964). Primary damage is to the liver, with progressive deterioration and death, but the toxin is unknown.

The **Amaryllidaceae**, especially the genera *Amaryllis, Crinum, Galanthus, Haemanthus, Narcissus*, and *Nerine*, have caused poisonings in humans and animals when consumed during times of food shortages (Kingsbury, 1964). The bulbs of these species contain galanthamine, a competitive cholinesterase inhibitor, as well as other related alkaloids (Lopez et al., 2002).

The **Anacardiaceae** contains a number of species that produce alkenylcatechol derivatives capable of producing severe allergic dermatitis (Everist, 1981; Keeler and Tu, 1983). *Toxicodendron* species (poison ivy, poison oak, and poison sumac) contain these alkenylcatechol allergens, the major constituent of which is urushiol, in all parts of the plant (Cheeke, 1998; Keeler and Tu, 1983). Most adverse reactions reported from this plant family are through dermal contact (Cheeke, 1998), but there is reason to be concerned about ingestion of plants containing urushiol and its analogs. Some cases of severe damage to gastric mucosa and death have been reported in humans ingesting these species (Kingsbury, 1964). Presumably, the severe reactions have occurred in response to internal immune/allergic response. Given that individual susceptibility to dermal reactions in humans varies widely, but most animals are not affected (Cheeke, 1998), it would probably not be prudent to regard lack of adverse effects following animal ingestion of dietary supplement ingredients containing these compounds as an indication of safety in humans.

The **Apiaceae** contains plants commonly consumed as vegetables or condiments, such as carrots, parsnips, celery, and dill (*Anethum, Apium, Daucus, Pastinaca* species). The phytochemicals of concern in this family include piperidine alkaloids, polyacetylenes, and coumarins (Cheeke, 1998; Everist, 1981). Conium (piperidine) alkaloids are of concern because they can cause nervousness, nausea, vomiting, ataxia, coma, and death due to respiratory failure in many different animals, including humans (Cheeke, 1998; Colegate and Dorling, 1994). Alkaloid levels vary considerably with plant growth stage and are particularly high in flowers and seeds. Poisoning in humans has resulted from mistaking *Conium maculatum* (poison hemlock) for parsley or anise seeds (Kingsbury, 1964). The most toxic alkaloid, γ-coniceine, has an LD_{50} in a mouse bioassay of 2.5 mg/kg (Burrows and Tyrl, 2001).

Some polyacetylenes are acutely toxic, resulting in rapid death due to complete paralysis and respiratory failure. The compounds act on the central nervous system, causing extremely violent convulsions, abdominal pain, and delirium in humans (Cheeke, 1998). Levels of the toxin (cicutoxin) are very high in roots of *Cicuta* species and a single root is capable of killing a cow (Kingsbury, 1964). There are structurally related compounds in carrot roots, although evidence of toxicity in humans from these compounds is minimal, probably because of extremely low levels (Cheeke, 1998). Simple coumarins can block the vitamin K pathway, thus inhibiting blood coagulation, and also can cause photosensitivity on exposure to sunlight. Photosensitivity, resulting in severe sunburn, has been observed following ingestion of celery soup, and sensitivity also occurs via dermal contact with the vegetable (Boffa et al., 1996; Seligman et al., 1987). Celery oil and celery root are also known causes of acute food-induced anaphylaxis (Pauli et al., 1988).

The **Apocynaceae** contains three genera (*Apocynum*, *Nerium*, and *Thevetia*) that are of concern because some species are acutely toxic to livestock and humans (Cheeke, 1998; Colegate and Dorling, 1994; Kellerman et al., 1988). Accidental poisoning of children has been frequent and it has been estimated that a single leaf of oleander (*Nerium oleander*) can be fatal (Cheeke, 1998; Everist, 1981; Keeler et al., 1978). The toxins are cardiac glycosides with symptoms similar to digitalis toxicity and may occur at up to 4 percent of the weight of the plant (Kingsbury, 1964).

Plant species in the **Araceae** that are toxic contain crystals of calcium oxalate (Cheeke, 1998; Everist, 1981; Keeler et al., 1978). In humans, this compound produces numbness of the mouth and throat (Cheeke, 1998; Keeler et al., 1978), resulting in the common name, dumbcane, for *Dieffenbachia seguine*. Death due to nephritis occurs on occasion in humans, but is more common in cats and laboratory animals (Burrows and Tyrl, 2001). *Colocasia esculenta* (taro, dasheen) leaves are generally recognized as being toxic (Burrows and Tyrl, 2001).

The **Araliaceae** is of concern primarily because of the species *Hedera helix* (English ivy), ingestion of the berries having been reported to poison children (Kingsbury, 1964). There have been occasional reports of poisoning in cattle when large amounts of the vine have been consumed, and the toxicity has been attributed to the saponin hederagenin (Kingsbury, 1964). In addition, *H. helix* contains the polyacetylene falcarinol, which also occurs in a number of species in the Apiaceae and is responsible for contact dermatitis in some individuals (Keeler and Tu, 1991). Falcarinol has structural affinities to the extremely toxic cicutoxin of water hemlock (*Cicuta virosa*). No toxicity appears to have been associated with the many other *Hedera* species. The only other potentially toxic species in the Araliaceae is the Devil's walking stick (*Aralia spinosa*), which has been suspected of poisoning livestock (Kingsbury, 1964).

The **Arecaceae** encompasses a number of palm species growing in Asia and the Indian subcontinent. Betel nuts, the seeds of *Areca catechu*, are of concern, but the plant family is not considered to be of concern. Betel nuts are chewed when mixed with lime and wrapped in leaves of the betel pepper (*Piper betle*). This has a stimulant effect and produces slight intoxication. The seed contains approximately 0.45 percent of several tetrahydropyridine alkaloids, the primary active alkaloid being arecoline, an agonist of muscarinic acetylcholine receptors; it is used as an anthelmintic in humans (Hirschhorn, 1983). Betel quid chewing is an etiologic factor for oral cancer, and arecoline is suspected to contribute to the pathogenesis of cancer by producing mucosal inflammation and growth of oral epithelial cells (Keeler and Tu, 1983).

The **Aristolochiaceae** has a number of *Aristolochia* species that contain the nephrotoxic nitrophenanthrenes aristolochic acids, such as *A. serpentina* (snakeroot). These plants have been used in traditional medicines, especially in Chinese and Indian herbal remedies, which are consumed only for short periods. In European use, where the plant was consumed over several weeks, there is good evidence based on misidentification that they are responsible for acute kidney failure and possibly urothelial carcinoma (Cosyns et al., 1998; Violon, 1997).

The **Asclepidaceae** is known to contain a considerable number of *Asclepias* species (milkweeds) that are acutely toxic to livestock and domestic fowl (Cheeke, 1998; James et al., 1992). As little as 0.05 percent of an animal's weight of green *A. labriformis* can result in death; most species are toxic at 0.25 to 1 percent (Kingsbury, 1964). Poisoning is characterized by symptoms of weakness, staggering, seizures, and coma, appearing within a few hours, followed by death within 1 or 2 days (Everist, 1981; James et al., 1992). The toxins are usually cardiac glycosides (cardenolides) structurally related to digitoxigenin (Cheeke, 1998).

The **Asteraceae** encompass a significant number of genera that contain hepatotoxic unsaturated pyrrolizidine alkaloids. Among these are *Eupatorium* species (gravelroot) and *Tussilago farfara* (coltsfoot) (Keeler and Tu, 1983). Others such as *Packera candidissima* (hierba de milagro) (Bah et al., 1994) and *Senecio longilobus* (gordolobo yerba) are also hepatotoxic, with the latter having been documented as causing severe hepatic fibrosis and death in infants and children (Cheeke, 1998; Stillman et al., 1977) *Senecio* species have a particular propensity to accumulate high levels of the alkaloids (up to 18 percent dry-weight basis in *S. riddellii*), and are a frequent cause of poisoning in livestock (Kingsbury, 1964; Molyneux and Johnson, 1984). Seeds of *Senecio* and *Heliotropium spp* have caused large-scale poisonings of humans in southern Africa, central Asia, and India (Cheeke, 1998; Colegate and Dorling, 1994; Kellerman et al., 1988). The alkaloids can also be sequestered in milk, eggs, and honey (Colegate and Dorling, 1994; Keeler et al., 1978). Pyrrolizidine alkaloid toxicity is characterized primarily by progressive hepatic cirrhosis (veno-occlusive disease) (Everist, 1981; Garland and Barr, 1998). The alkaloids have been demonstrated to be genotoxic and mutagenic, and cause cancer in rats, but evidence is insufficient to establish carcinogenicity in humans (Garland and Barr, 1998;

Keeler and Tu, 1983). The progressive nature of the poisoning is such that symptoms are not readily apparent and are slow to appear, and it has been categorized as an "iceberg disease" (Everist, 1981). Acute toxicity is rarely observed, but trichodesmine, senecionine, and seneciphylline have LD_{50} values in rats of 25, 50, and 77 mg/kg respectively (Mattocks, 1986). It is important to note that not all pyrrolizidine alkaloids are toxic *per se*; they become so only after dehydrogenation by P450 enzymes in the liver. In the plant they exist as a mixture of the free base forms and N-oxides. Although the N-oxides cannot be directly transformed into the toxic forms by P450 enzymes, they can be reduced to the free base in the gut and thence metabolized to the dehydro-alkaloids. It has been estimated that 3 percent of flowering plants worldwide contain some level of pyrrolizidine alkaloids (Colegate and Dorling, 1994).

Within the Asteraceae family, certain *Baccharis* species are acutely toxic to cattle, horses, and sheep (Colegate and Dorling, 1994; Garland and Barr, 1998). Poisoning is characterized by tachycardia, restlessness, recumbancy, and death; lesions are found primarily in the digestive tract (Garland and Barr, 1998). Doses as low as 0.25 to 5.0 g/kg of the green plant can be fatal (Garland and Barr, 1998). The toxicity is probably due to macrocyclic trichothecenes of the roridin and verrucarin type (Colegate and Dorling, 1994). The LD_{50} intravenous administration of verrucarin A in rabbits is 0.54 mg/kg (O'Neil et al., 2001). These sesquiterpenes are known to be produced by fungi and there is evidence that the DNA of the fungus is transferred to the plant. Their occurrence in *Baccharis* may be due to the presence of a fungal endophyte, possibly *Myrothecium verrucaria* (Colegate and Dorling, 1994; James et al., 1992).

Centaurea solstitialis (yellow star thistle) produces nigropallidal encephalomalacia ("chewing disease") in horses, resulting in failure in prehension; as a result, animals usually die of starvation or thirst (Colegate and Dorling, 1994).

Eupatorium and *Haplopappus spp.* on occasion have caused epidemic poisoning of humans in certain parts of the United States. The disease, known as "milksickness," is characterized by weakness, nausea, muscular tremors, prostration, and death, and is caused by consumption of milk from animals that have consumed the plant (Colegate and Dorling, 1994; James et al., 1992). The toxicity is attributed to tremetone, an acetyl dihydrobenzofuran, but concrete evidence for its toxicity is lacking (Cheeke, 1998; Garland and Barr, 1998).

Gutierrezia (broomweed) is toxic to cattle and sheep but is of primary concern for its abortifacient activity in cattle (Cheeke, 1998; Colegate and Dorling, 1994). The amount of plant causing this effect is highly variable, but as little as 20 lb of the fresh plant can produce abortion in cattle (Kingsbury, 1964). Signs of poisoning are very similar to those of "pine needle abortion," caused by *Pinus* species (vide infra), and broomweed contains diterpene acids structurally similar to isocupressic acid, established as the abortifacient constituent of pine needles (Cheeke, 1998; Colegate and Dorling, 1994). Both *Solidago* species (goldenrods) and *Tanacetum vulgare* (tansy) have been used as abortifacients by humans and have been reported to produce abortions in cattle (Kingsbury, 1964). The latter two species have also been associated with death of cattle, sheep, and horses, but the active constituents are unknown (Kingsbury, 1964).

Helenium (sneezeweed) and *Hymenoxys* species (rubberweeds, pingue) have been responsible for serious losses of livestock, especially sheep (Keeler and Tu, 1983). Poisoning is characterized by severe vomiting, depression, emaciation, and death (James et al., 1992; Kingsbury, 1964). *Helenium tenuifolium* has been implicated in human poisoning (Kingsbury, 1964). The toxins have been shown to be structurally related sesquiterpene lactones, especially helenalin and hymenovin (Keeler and Tu, 1983; Keeler et al., 1978). *Psilostrophe* species also have been found to poison sheep, producing a similar vomiting syndrome, but the toxin is unknown (Kingsbury, 1964).

Rudbeckia species (coneflowers) are toxic to pigs, sheep, and horses, and occasionally cattle (Kingsbury, 1964). Poisoning is characterized by aimless wandering and incoordination. Deaths in laboratory animals are characterized by fatty degeneration of the liver (Kingsbury, 1964). The nature of the toxin is unknown (Kingsbury, 1964). In spite of the coincidence in the common names, these species should not be confused with the purple coneflower (*Echinacea purpurea*), which is sold as an herbal remedy.

Tetradymia species cause secondary photosensitization in sheep, known as "bighead," and is toxic at 0.5 percent of the animal's weight (Kingsbury, 1964). Light-skinned animals are the most sensitive and areas of the body not covered by hair, particularly around the muzzle, become severely inflamed and enlarged. The photosensitization is due to circulation of phylloerythrin, produced from chlorophyll due to liver damage (Keeler and Tu, 1983). The toxins are tetradymol (Cheeke, 1998) and related furanoeremophilane terpenes (Keeler and Tu, 1983).

Xanthium species (cockleburs) are toxic to a number of livestock, but especially pigs (Cheeke, 1998). The primary effects are acute nephritis and hepatitis (Everist, 1981). The main toxic compound is concentrated particularly in the seeds, as well as in plants at the cotyledonary growth stage, and has been identified as carboxyatractyloside, a kaurene (diterpene) glycoside (James et al., 1992; Keeler and Tu, 1983).

In the **Berberidaceae** family, the mayapple or mandrake (*Podophyllum peltatum*) has caused occasional poisoning in cattle, sheep, and pigs, although animals generally will not eat it (Kingsbury, 1964). The plant, especially the root, has been used by American Indians and early settlers for medicinal purposes. Poisoning in humans has resulted from overuse of such preparations, and occasionally from use as an herb, resulting in gastroenteritis and vomiting (Kingsbury, 1964). Contact with the milled root can cause ulceration of the skin and conjunctivitis (Kingsbury, 1964). The bioactive constituents are lignans (podophyllotoxin, 4'-demethylpodopyllotoxin, and α- and β-peltatins) (Canel et al., 2000).

The **Boraginaceae** family encompasses a number of plant genera that produce hepatotoxic pyrrolizidine alkaloids (Keller and Tu, 1983). The toxic effects are essentially the same as those discussed for the pyrrolizidine alkaloids occurring in genera of the Asteraceae (vide supra). Of particular concern for poisonings in humans are *Heliotropium* and *Symphytum* species. The seeds of *H. lasiocarpum* and *H. popovii* have caused extremely large-scale poisonings (as many as 7,800 cases of veno-occlusive disease) when they have contaminated wheat and have been consumed as bread (Mattocks, 1986). Similarly, problems have resulted from *H. europaeum* contaminating feed grains at 0.6 percent by weight (Mattocks, 1986).

Symphytum species (comfrey) of the Boraginaceae family have been used for medicinal purposes since antiquity, primarily for external use to promote healing of wounds. Modern usage has involved internal consumption, either as a salad vegetable or as a tea, both of which have resulted in deaths of humans (Stickel and Sietz, 2000). Teas have been prepared not only from the leaves, but also from roots, which contain higher levels of the alkaloids. It has been determined that a single cup of comfrey root tea contains as much as 8.5 mg of total alkaloids (Roitman, 1981).

The **Brassicaceae** contains a number of plant species, especially *Brassica*, which are used as vegetables or condiments. Other species are used for forage or are weed species to which livestock may be exposed. All of these contain either cyanogenic or goitrogenic substances (Kellerman et al., 1988).

Armoracia rusticana (horseradish) contains glucosinolates, especially glucobrassicin, which generate isothiocyanates, the pungent principles of horseradish on hydrolysis by myrosinase (Shapiro et al., 1998). Glucosinolates are also present in most *Brassica* species, including *B. nigra* (black mustard), *B. napus* (rape), *B. rapa* (turnip), and varieties of *B. oleracea* (cabbage, broccoli, Brussels sprouts, and kale) (Keeler and Tu, 1991; Stoewsand, 1995). Under certain conditions, hydrolysis of glucosinolates can also generate thiocyanates or nitriles (Kellerman et al., 1988). Other hydrolysis products from glucosinolates, namely oxazolidine-2-thiones, are potent inducers of goiter (enlargement of the thyroid gland) (Stoewsand, 1995). This effect cannot be treated by administration of iodine. The toxicity of isothiocyanates, thiocyanates, and nitriles, as well as the goitrogenic activity of glucosinolates, suggests that excessive consumption of *Brassica* and related species should be avoided. Poisoning of livestock by many of these plants when used as forage or feedstuff has been reported, especially when the seeds, which contain the highest levels of glucosinolates, are included (Kellerman et al., 1988). In addition, *B. napus* (rape) causes respiratory, digestive, nervous, and urinary syndromes and hemolytic anemia in livestock, which may be caused by factors other than glucosinolates; some of these syndromes have also been observed with wild radish (*Raphanus raphanistrum*) (Kingsbury, 1964). Severe haemolytic anaemia in cattle caused by feeding kale has been shown to be due to the hydrolysis product of S-methyl cysteine sulfoxide, a common constituent of *Brassica* species (Everist, 1981).

Buxus sempervirens (common box), a cultivated ornamental shrub in the **Buxaceae** family, has been associated with mortality in many types of livestock worldwide (Kingsbury, 1964). Poisoning is usually associated with animals being exposed to clippings of the plant, with as little as 1.5 lbs being lethal to a horse (Kingsbury, 1964). Poisoning is characterized by gastroenteritis, convulsions, and respiratory failure. The toxic constituents are steroidal and triterpene alkaloids that occur in all parts of the plant, including the roots (Atta-ur-Rahman et al., 1997). Korean box (*B. microphylla*) contains analogous alkaloids and is also planted widely in the United States as an ornamental (Kingsbury, 1964).

The **Campanulaceae** is of concern because of *Lobelia* species, which are wild and cultivated plants that contain piperidine alkaloids, the most common of which is lobeline (Everist, 1981). *Lobelia inflata* in excessive doses has proved to be toxic (Kingsbury, 1964). Lobeline has a similar activity to nicotine, but is less potent in stimulating nicotinic receptor sites. Indian tobacco is toxic to sheep at 0.5 percent of the animal's weight, with symptoms of salivation and nasal discharge, ulceration of the mouth, and coma (Kingsbury, 1964). These symptoms are consistent with those produced by the pure alkaloid, lobeline.

The elderberries (*Sambucus* species) are reputed to be poisonous species in the **Caprifoliaceae** family. The most common in North America are *S. canadensis* and *S. pubesn;* the European elderberry is *S. nigra*. There have been reports of toxicity to cattle and pigs, and children have been poisoned by using the stems as pea shooters (Kingsbury, 1964). The most poisonous parts of the plant appear to be young growth and the roots (Kingsbury, 1964). The berries can be consumed after cooking, but fresh berries cause nausea and vomiting (Kingsbury, 1964). The toxic constituents include a number of cyanogenic glycosides, especially sambunigrin and prunasin (Buhrmester et al., 2000). The content and presence of these glycosides appears to be highly variable from one population to another.

The **Caryophyllaceae** family has many genera that contain triterpenoid saponins, namely *Agrostemma githago* (corn cockle), *Drymaria* species (inkweed, alfombrilla), and *Saponaria* species (soapwort, cow cockle) (Cheeke, 1998; Everist, 1981). The saponins are present in all parts of the plant but are highest in the seeds, comprising 5 to 7 percent of *A. githago* seeds (Everist, 1981). Less than 0.25 percent of the animal's weight of ground corn cockle seed was fatal in cattle and hogs, and 0.5 percent of inkweed or alfombrilla green plant was also lethal (Kingsbury, 1964). Symptoms are severe gastroenteritis, vomiting, diarrhea, coma, and death (Kingsbury 1964).

A large number of *Euonymus* species occur in the **Celastraceae**, some of which have been incriminated as poisonous plants. These plants occur as both wild and ornamental plants in the form of shrubs, vines, and ground covers. The spindle tree (*E. europaeus*) and burning bush (*E. atropurpureus*) are reported as toxic to children and livestock, causing violent purgation, vomiting, and unconsciousness (Kingsbury, 1964). Poisoning in humans has most commonly been attributed to consumption of the fruit, but the bark and leaves are also toxic (Kingsbury, 1964). Various *Euonymus* species have been shown to contain cytotoxic cardioglycosides, as well as sesquiterpene pyridine alkaloids and a phytohemaglutinin (Jinbo et al., 2002; Kuo et al., 2003). Poisoning has also been attributed to another member of the Celastraceae, the viny bittersweet (*Celastrus scandens*), and other *Celastrus* species have been shown to contain sesquiterpene pyridine alkaloids and biologically active agarofuran sesquiterpenes (Jin et al., 2002). The Chinese herb *Tripterygium wilfordii* (lei gong teng), also a member of the Celastraceae, has been shown to be immunosuppressant and to decrease spermatogenesis. It contains triptolide and related highly epoxidized diterpenoids, which are most likely to be the bioactive constituents (Qui and Kao, 2003).

The **Convolvulaceae** encompasses species of the genera *Calystegia* and *Convolvulus* (bindweeds) and *Ipomoea* (sweet potato) that contain polyhydroxy alkaloid glycosidase inhibitors. The most common of these are the calystegines, nortropane alkaloids with varying degrees of hydroxylation, that are potent inhibitors of glycosidases, especially β-glucosidase and β-galactosidase (Cheeke, 1998; Garland and Barr, 1998). Ingestion of these alkaloids results in inhibition of glycoprotein processing with consequent accumulation of oligosaccharides, particularly in cells of the cerebellum, classified as a lysosomal storage disease (Elbein and Molyneux, 1998). Consumption of *Ipomoea* species by sheep in Australia and goats in Mozambique has resulted in a neurological syndrome characterized by muscle-twitching, trembling, staggering, and incoordination (de Balogh et al., 1999). In addition to the calystegines, these *Ipomoea* species also contain the polyhydroxy indolizidine alkaloid swainsonine, the causative agent of locoweed poisoning produced by certain *Astragalus*, *Oxytropis*, and *Swainsona* species of the Fabaceae (vide infra) (Colegate and Dorling, 1994; Garland and Barr, 1998). The polyhydroxy alkaloids have also been shown to occur in the edible tubers of sweet potato (*I. batatas*), but no episodes of poisoning in humans from this source appear to have been recorded (Asano et al., 1997). The seeds of some species of *Ipomoea* and *Rivea* contain D-lysergic acid diethylamide-related alkaloids (Everist, 1981). The alkaloid levels in all of the genera of concern in the Convolvulaceae are very low, but the extraordinary potency of their glycosidase inhibitory properties and cumulative effects results in chronic toxicity. It is reasonable to assume that glycosidase inhibition could also interfere with digestive processes, leading to malabsorption and emaciation. Although the calystegines are structurally related to tropane alkaloids (e.g., scopolamine), they do not have any similarity in their mode of action to the latter class.

The **Coriariaceae** is a very small plant family consisting of the single genus *Coriaria*. Accidental poisoning by the Mediterranean shrub *C. myrtifolia* has been reported following ingestion of the fruits, which may be mistaken for blackberries. Toxicity is characterized by vomiting and abdominal pain, convulsions, and respiratory disorders; death has resulted on occasion (Skalli et al., 2002). The picrotoxin-like sesquiterpene lactones coriamyrtin and corianin, together with structurally related compounds, have been identified in a number of *Coriaria* species (Aguirree-Galviz and Templeton, 1990; Kariyone and Okuda, 1955; Reyes et al., 1980; Wei et al., 1998).

The **Cupressaceae** encompasses cypress and juniper trees. The Monterey cypress (*Cupressus macrocarpa*) is a native of North America that has been introduced into New Zealand, where it has caused third-trimester abortion and other pregnancy disorders in sheep and cattle that consumed small amounts of the leaves (Everist, 1981). The toxin has been shown to be the labdane diterpene isocupressic acid, identical to that in *Pinus* species (Pinaceae) that produce the same syndrome (Cheeke, 1998). Relatively high levels of isocupressic acid have also been measured in common juniper (*Juniperus communis*) and Rocky Mountain juniper (*J. scopulorum*), which have also been incriminated in abortions (Gardner et al., 1998).

The **Cycadaceae** includes *Cycas* species, palm-like in appearance, that are native to tropical Asia, Australia, and Polynesia; some of the plants have been introduced as ornamentals in subtropical regions or are cultivated in glasshouses. The sago palm (*C. revoluta*) and *C. circinalis* are the most commonly seen. In Australia, consumption of leaves, or seeds of a number of other *Cycas* species, commonly known as Zamia palms, has produced poisoning in livestock and humans (Keeler and Tu, 1983). Animals are generally poisoned by eating the leaves, and the typical syndrome is irreversible ataxia in the hindquarters known as "Zamia staggers" or "wobbles," although consumption of as little as 0.6 kg of the seeds led to progressive weakness and death in a steer (Hall, 1987). Poisoning in man is more likely to occur from eating the raw seeds and is characterized by neurological problems, carcinogenicity, and hepato- and nephrotoxicity (Keeler and Tu, 1983). Indigenous peoples have a history of preparing a starch from the seeds by extensive cooking, soaking, or fermenting procedures. Cycads have been shown to contain a number of azoglycosides, including cycasin and neocycasins, each of which has the same aglycone methylazoxymethanol (Keeler and Tu, 1983). The latter is highly toxic in experimental animals and acts as a potent methylating agent. Identification of the specific toxic agent is complicated by the co-occurrence of low levels of α-amino-β-methylaminopropionic acid, which is also neurotoxic in rats (Keeler and Tu, 1983).

The **Ephedraceae** has a number of *Ephedra* species that contain the phenylalanine-derived alkaloid (–)-ephedrine, its diastereomer (+)-pseudoephedrine, and their demethyl analogs. The botanical preparation Ephedra, or Ma Huang, is prepared from one or more of the species *E. sinica, E. equisetina, E. intermedia, E. major*, and *E. gerardiana*. Typical alkaloid levels are 0.5 to 2.0 percent, with (–)-ephedrine predominating, except in *E. intermedia*, in which (+)-pseudoephedrine is the major alkaloid (Dewick, 2002). The alkaloids are peripheral vasoconstrictors; they do not act directly on α-adrenergic receptors like noradrenaline, but displace the latter from storage vesicles, thereby elevating blood pressure. There is evidence that these effects of *Ephedra* species have resulted in death in humans (Samenuk et al., 2002).

Three genera of the **Ericaceae** are of particular concern, *Azalea, Kalmia,* and *Rhododendron* species, with periodic severe loss of life in livestock. The poisonous constituents are grayanotoxins, highly hydroxylated polycyclic diterpenes; the specific grayanotoxins vary with the plant species (Cheeke, 1998; Puschner et al., 2001). The grayanotoxins bind to the group II receptor site of sodium channels in cell membranes, localized on a region of the sodium channel that is involved in the voltage-dependent activation and inactivation. The compounds prevent inactivation so that nerve and muscle cells are maintained in a depolarized state, permitting entry of calcium into the cells (Temma et al., 1986). All species of *Kalmia* appear to be similarly toxic in animals, and *K. angustifolia* (lambkill) or *K. latifolia* (mountain laurel) are reported to have been used by American Indians to commit suicide (Kingsbury, 1964). An amount of 0.2 percent by weight of green leaves is sufficient to induce toxicity in animals, with gastroenteritis, vomiting, diarrhea, abdominal pain, and tremors (Kingsbury, 1964). Cardiac irregularities and convulsions may occur, followed by coma and death. A tea made from 2 oz of mountain laurel produced symptoms of toxicity, but not death, in humans. The intoxication generally lasts for less than 24 hours and is rarely fatal. Symptoms are dizziness, weakness, excessive perspiration, nausea, and vomiting. Cardiac irregularities that can occur are low blood pressure or shock, bradyarrhythima, sinus bradycardia, anomalous atrioventricular excitation, and complete atrioventricular block (Onat et al., 1991).

The **Euphorbiaceae** has numerous *Euphorbia* species (spurges) that produce a milky sap with vesicant properties, blistering the skin, mouth, and digestive tract, consequently having a purgative action. The toxic effects are due to esters of phorbol, diterpene esters, which activate protein kinase C, a phosphorylating enzyme (Cheeke, 1998). Permanent activation of this enzyme results in cell proliferation and tumor promotion (cocarcinogen activity) (Cheeke, 1998). *Croton spp.* contain structurally similar compounds and have similar effects (Cheeke, 1998).

The *Aleurites* species, *A. fordii* (tung nut) and *A. moluccana* (candle nut), have been shown to be toxic to cattle, producing hemorrhagic lesions in the gastrointestinal tract (Everist, 1981). In humans, a single tung nut can cause severe vomiting, diarrhea, cyanosis, respiratory depression, weakness, and possibly death (Everist, 1981). Necrosis of the digestive tract is similar to that in animals. The candle nut is also toxic when eaten raw, but can be consumed after roasting.

The manchineel tree (*Hippomane mancinella*) possesses a very irritant and toxic sap, which may cause temporary blindness (Kingsbury, 1964). Caribbean Indians used the sap as an arrow poison. The fruit has poisoned humans who ate it, producing vomiting, hemorrhagic diarrhea, and occasional death (Kingsbury, 1964). The toxin is unknown, but may be related to the phorbol esters present in *Euphorbia* species.

Jatropha species, which include *J. curcas* (Barbados nut) and *J. multifida* (physic nut), contain a purgative oil similar to that of croton or castor oils (Everist, 1981). Poisoning of humans by ingestion of *J. curcas* seeds has been reported, with the number of seeds producing toxicity being highly variable, but as few as three producing symptoms (Everist, 1981; Kellerman et al., 1988). Severe gastroenteritis is the primary toxic effect, with associated diarrhea (Kingsbury, 1964).

Manihot esculenta (cassava, tapioca) contains cyanogenic glycosides that can produce lethal amounts of hydrocyanic acid on ingestion (Cheeke, 1998; Kellerman et al., 1988). However, it is general knowledge that peeling, grating, and soaking the root removes the toxin, and the cooked product can be eaten safely (Kingsbury, 1964). Although the discarded peelings may be toxic to livestock, human poisonings are likely to be accidental.

Ricinus communis (castor bean) is probably the most toxic plant known. The toxin is the polypeptide ricin, present only in the seeds, consisting of A and B chains linked by a disulfide bond (Keeler and Tu, 1991). The B chain is a lectin that binds to specific sugars in cellular glycolipids or glycoproteins and enables entry of the ribosomal-inactivating A chain into the cytosol, where it stops protein synthesis. Ricin comprises about 5 percent of the protein content of a seed, and the amount in a single seed, approximately 250 μg, is sufficient to kill an adult human; the toxic dose by injection is as low as 1 μg/kg (Bradberry et al., 2003; O'Neil et al., 2001). Poisoning is accompanied by hemorrhage of the digestive tract, convulsions, and circulatory collapse. Animals vary in susceptibility, with consumption of 0.01 to 0.2 percent of the weight of the animal being fatal (Everist, 1981).

The extremely large legume family, **Fabaceae**, encompasses many valuable food plants (peas and beans), in addition to numerous genera that are toxic. Thus it is necessary to examine individual species. The jequirity bean (*Abrus precatorius*) is extremely poisonous, containing a polypeptide toxin, abrin, similar in its mode of action to ricin (vide supra) (Kellerman et al., 1988). A single seed is sufficient to kill an adult human (Kellerman et al., 1988), and children have been killed from chewing on necklaces made from the attractive red and black beans (Gunn, 1969). A dose of 2 oz of the powdered seed is sufficient to kill a horse (Kingsbury, 1964). *Robinia pseudoacacia* (black locust) contains a similar toxin and there are reports of human poisoning, especially in children, either from eating the seeds or chewing on the bark (Kingsbury, 1964). The extreme toxicity of these toxins indicates extremely serious concerns for use of any part of these plants in the human diet.

Certain *Astragalus* and *Oxytropis* species (locoweeds), and *Swainsona* species (poison peas), contain the trihydroxy indolizidine alkaloid swainsonine, a potent inhibitor of α-mannosidase (Cheeke, 1998). The alkaloid is also found in *Ipomoea* species (Convolvulaceae) (vide supra), accompanied by the glycosidase-inhibitory calystegines (Garland and Barr, 1998). Swainsonine is chronically toxic, producing a multitude of symptoms depending on the physiological state of the animal (Keeler et al., 1978). The primary syndrome is a neurological deficit (locoism) characterized by depression, solitariness, startling, and visual misperceptions. Reproductive deficits are common in both males and females, and pregnant animals may abort or give birth to offspring with limb deformities (Keeler and Tu, 1983). As with the calystegines, the mode of action is inhibition of glycoprotein processing and accumulation of oligosaccharides in various cells (Cheeke, 1998). It has been estimated that swainsonine levels of 0.001 percent in the plant are sufficient to cause poisoning if consumed over a sufficient period of time (Garland and Barr, 1998). *Castanospermum australe*, the Moreton Bay chestnut or black bean (actually not a chestnut, but a bean), contains structurally similar tetrahydroxy indolizidine and pyrrolizidine alkaloids, known as castanospermines and australines, respectively (Garland and Barr, 1998). These alkaloids are potent inhibitors of α- and β-glucosidase. The large seeds of *C. australe* poison livestock in Australia (Cheeke, 1998), and there have been fatal poisonings of humans who have mistaken the seeds for a type of chestnut (Everist, 1981). The most common symptom of poisoning is severe gastrointestinal upset (Cheeke, 1998).

Baptisia, Cytisus, Laburnum, Lupinus, and *Sophora* species contain a variety of quinolizidine alkaloids that have produced major poisoning episodes in livestock (Kingsbury, 1964). Symptoms are generally labored breathing, tremors, convulsions, coma, and death (Kingsbury, 1964). Poisoning by lupines has been responsible for losses of over 1,000 sheep in a single episode (Kingsbury, 1964). Teratogenicity, with scoliosis and bowed front limbs ("crooked calf disease") has been observed in calves born from cows eating certain lupines in the seeding stage (Keeler and Tu, 1983). There is some evidence that babies have been born with similar defects, caused by their mother drinking milk from goats that were grazing on lupine (Colegate and Dorling, 1994). Some species and varieties of lupines ("sweet" lupines) contain no or insignificant amounts of the alkaloids and are cultivated as feed grains. *Laburnum anagyroides* (golden-chain tree) contains the tricyclic quinolizidine alkaloid, cytisine, and it has been implicated in numerous human poisonings (Cheeke, 1998).

Canavalia ensiformis (jack bean) is toxic to cattle due to the presence of the nonprotein amino acid canavanine (Cheeke, 1998). Symptoms are severe diarrhea, with nephritis and pulmonary emphysema (Kingsbury, 1964). *In vivo* experiments have shown that canavanine hydrochloride, fed to rats at 0.004 percent body weight over a 6-week period, produces signs of hepatotoxicity (Everist, 1981). Mature jack beans contain free hydrogen cyanide, probably derived from cyanogenic glycosides (Laurena et al., 1994). *Indigofera endecaphylla* (creeping indigo) is toxic to numerous animal species and fowl, causing a variety of syndromes, including abortion, corneal opacity, depression, emaciation, and death (Kingsbury, 1964). Indigo also contains the nonprotein amino acid indospicine, which is present at up to 0.5 percent in the leaves and 2.0 percent in the seeds, and has been detected in seeds of 32 *Indigofera* species (Everist, 1981). Indospicine is an analog of arginine and acts as an inhibitor of arginase and arginine decarboxylase in the liver, blocking incorporation of arginine and reducing incorporation of other amino acids into liver proteins (Everist, 1981). Canavanine is also found in many species of *Indigofera* (Everist, 1981).

The genus *Crotalaria* contains pyrrolizidine alkaloids, the most common of which is monocrotaline, similar in structure to those present in the Asteraceae (vide supra), but of slightly different ring size (Colegate and Dorling, 1994). The slight change in ring size of the macrocyclic diester moiety results in cardiopulmonary toxicity rather than the more generally observed hepatotoxicity; however, metabolic activation by the liver is still required. Human poisoning in the West Indies from the use of "bush teas," prepared primarily from *C. fulva*, was at one time common (McDermott and Ridker, 1990).

Lathyrus and *Vicia* species contain amino-butyric and amino-propionic acids and their corresponding nitriles. The most common of these in *L. sativus* (grass pea or Indian pea), α-amino-β-oxalylaminopropionic acid, occurs at up to 2.5 percent dry weight in the seeds (Everist, 1981). This and other *Lathyrus* species have been associated with a neurological disease in livestock characterized by irreversible paralysis of the legs and occasionally death, neurolathyrism, as well as osteolathyrism, involving severe skeletal deformities (Cheeke, 1998; Everist, 1981). *Vicia sativa* (common vetch) and other *Vicia* species contain β-cyano-L-alanine and its γ-glutamyl derivative, which is not only cyanogenic, but also neurotoxic (Cheeke, 1998; Everist, 1981). In certain individuals, consumption of broad beans (*V. faba*) can cause acute toxic hepatitis (Everist, 1981; Kellerman et al., 1988; Kingsbury, 1964).

Beans of mesquite (*Prosopsis juliflora*) are poisonous to cattle when consumed over extended periods and as the primary sources of feed. Poisoning is characterized by indigestion, rumen stasis, and eventual degenerative changes in the liver and kidney, and death (Kingsbury, 1964).

Leucaena leucocephala contains the toxic amino acid mimosine in high levels in young leaves (8–10 percent dry weight) and seeds (3–5 percent dry weight) (Everist, 1981). Mimosine is reduced to 3-hydroxy-4(1H)-pyridone, a goitrogen that inhibits the binding of iodine in ruminants (Colegate and Dorling, 1994). Fetal resorption and birth defects resulted from feeding lecaena to swine (Kingsbury, 1969). It is not known whether a similar reproductive process can occur in humans. The pyridone may interfere with enzyme systems responsible for inactivating adrenalin and noradrenalin, causing hyperactivity (Keeler et al., 1978). In livestock, mimosine causes reduction in weight gain and loss of hair, and possibly reproductive defects and cataracts (Cheeke, 1998; Keeler et al., 1978).

Melilotus alba (sweet clover) contains coumarin (Kellerman et al., 1988). Although this compound is not toxic *per se*, when the plant is moldy the dimer dicoumarol, which is a potent anticoagulant, is formed (Kellerman et al., 1988). Animals consuming moldy hay made from sweet clover frequently die from internal or external bleeding (Cheeke, 1998).

Phaseolus lunatus (lima bean) is commonly eaten by humans. The commercial varieties generally contain low levels of the cyanogenic glycoside phaseolunatin, with a hydrogen cyanide potential of < 0.01 percent; cooking greatly reduces the cyanogenic glycoside potential (Keeler and Tu, 1983). However, tropical or wild varieties have much higher potential for generating hydrogen cyanide and have poisoned humans even after cooking.

Sesbania species (coffeebean, mescalbean, frijolito) contain toxic quinolizidine alkaloids. The seeds have fatally poisoned livestock at levels as low as 0.05 percent of the animal's weight, with hemorrhage of the intestinal tract, rapid and shallow respiration and pulse, and coma (Kingsbury, 1964). Mescalbeans (*S. secundiflora*) are known to be toxic to humans with a single seed being regarded as a lethal dose (Kingsbury, 1964).

Trifolium species are valuable crops, cultivated as forage for livestock. Some contain coumestrol, its 4-methoxy derivative, and a number of isoflavones (Keeler et al., 1978). Symptoms of poisoning in animals have been severe photosensitization and estrogenic effects (clover disease). The coumestrols are probably responsible for liver damage, causing secondary photosensitization (Kingsbury, 1964). The estrogenic effects are primarily due to metabolism of the isoflavone formononetin to equol, resulting in reduced and often permanent infertility in sheep (Kellerman et al., 1988). Levels of formononetin in excess of 0.8 percent dry weight have been shown to produce these effects, but levels below 0.3 percent are considered to be safe (Reinli and Block, 1996).

The seeds and pods of *Wisteria* species have been responsible for poisoning in humans, especially children (Kingsbury, 1964). It is estimated that one or two seeds are sufficient to induce severe gastroenteritis, vomiting, and diarrhea (Kingsbury, 1964). The toxic principle is unknown, but canavanine is a common constituent of the seeds of all species of *Wisteria*, as in *Canavalia* species.

The **Illiciaceae** is a small family consisting of the single genus *Illicium,* of which *I. anisatum* (Japanese star anise) and *I. floridanum* are grown in the southeastern United States. There have been a number of reports of neurological syndromes, described as epileptic-type seizures, after consumption of herbal teas prepared with Japanese star anise (Johanns et al., 2002). The toxicity appears to be attributable to anisatin, a noncompetitive γ-aminobutyric acid antagonist that can cause hyperactivity of the central nervous system and tonic-clonic seizures (Schmidt et al., 1998). Prezizaane-type sesquiterpenes structurally related to anisatin have been identified in a number of other *Illicium* species (Kuriyama et al., 2002).

In the **Juncaginaceae**, the arrowgrasses (*Triglochin* species) are of concern because of high levels of cyanogenic glycosides (Kingsbury, 1964). These species have been listed as edible plants for backcountry hikers. While cooking may reduce the cyanogenic potential, the raw plants, which are relatively palatable, have frequently poisoned sheep and cattle (Kingsbury, 1964). The same considerations apply as in other plant species that are capable of generating high levels of hydrogen cyanide (e.g., *Sorghum* species in the family Poaceae).

The family **Lamiaceae** is also often referred to as the **Labiatae** and contains a number of aromatic herbs useful for culinary purposes, including *Rosmarinus officinalis* (rosemary), *Salvia officinalis* (sage), *Origanum vulgare* (marjoram), *Thymus vulgaris* (thyme), and various mints (*Mentha* species). Nevertheless, some native species of *Salvia* have been incriminated in livestock poisonings (Kingsbury, 1964). In addition, *Stachys arvensis* (stagger weed or mintweed) causes a staggering gait and shivering in cattle, sheep, and horses (Kingsbury, 1964). Iridoids are characteristic constituents of *Stachys* species, but the causative agent for the neurological syndrome has not been established (Munoz et al., 2001). The major species of concern in this plant family is *Teucrium chamaedrys* (germander), which has been incriminated in a number of cases of acute hepatotoxicity when used as an herbal remedy (Larrey et al., 1992). Liver transplantation for acute liver failure was reported as being required after ingestion of *Teucrium polium* (Mattei et al., 1995). The toxic constituents may be clerodane diterpenoids, a number of which have been isolated from *T. chamaedrys* and are also present in other *Teucrium* species (Bedir et al., 2003).

The **Lauraceae** includes *Sassafras albidum* (sassafras), which has been used as a flavoring agent in beverages. However, the major component of sassafras oil, safrole, has been shown to be a carcinogen in laboratory animals due to its propensity to undergo hydroxylation or epoxidation in the allyl side chain (Dewick, 2002). These metabolic products form covalent bonds with cellular DNA.

Leaves of the avocado (*Persea americana*), another member of the Lauraceae, are cardiotoxic to numerous livestock species, domestic animals, laboratory animals, and even fish (Garland and Barr, 1998;

Kingsbury, 1964). In cattle and goats, a severe noninfectious mastitis with reduction in lactation can also occur. The active constituent is persin, a monoacetylated dihydroxy-heneicosadienone (Garland and Barr, 1998).

The **Liliaceae** includes a large number of species that contain toxic compounds of various structural types. The only edible plants of significance are the *Allium* species (onions, chives, leeks, garlic). In cattle and horses, moderate amounts of raw or cooked onions (*A. cepa*), both cultivated and wild (*A. canadense*), have produced severe anemia and death (Kellerman et al., 1988; Kingsbury, 1964). An amount of 0.5 percent of the body weight in the diet was sufficient to produce the same symptoms in dogs (Kingsbury, 1964). Chives (*A. schoenoprasum*) produced similar symptoms in horses (Kingsbury, 1964). The toxic principle is N-propyl disulfide, which primarily produces hemolysis of erythrocytes (Kellerman et al., 1988). There are no reports of anemia being produced in humans at normal consumption levels.

Colchicum autumnale (autumn crocus) has been known since historical times as a toxic plant to humans and animals. All parts of the plant are poisonous, but the highest levels of the toxic alkaloid colchicine occur in the seed and corm, comprising approximately 0.7 percent by weight (Dewick, 2002). The alkaloid is found in other *Colchicum* species and also in *Gloriosa* species. *Ornithogalum umbellatum* contains colchicine or structurally similar compounds, and children have been poisoned by eating the onion-like bulbs (Kingsbury, 1964).

Convallaria majalis (lily-of-the-valley) has long been considered to be a poisonous plant. It contains cardioactive glycosides, the major constituent being the rhamnoside of strophanthidin, known as convallatoxin (Kingsbury, 1964).

Urginea maritima (squill) contains approximately 4 percent bufadienolides, a class of cardiac glycosides; the closely related *Scilla* species contain similar compounds (Dewick, 2002). The cardiac effect in humans has short duration of action and large doses are distasteful and induce vomiting, so it is rarely fatal (Kingsbury, 1964).

Veratrum species have been considered to be poisonous plants since ancient times. A large number of steroidal alkaloids have been identified from *Veratrum* species (Colegate and Dorling, 1994). *V. californicum* (false hellebore, corn lily) and *V. viride* are noteworthy for their teratogenicity in sheep (Keeler et al., 1978). Ewes consuming the plant on the fourteenth day of gestation produce lambs with cyclopia, a single eye in the center of the forehead (Seawright et al., 1985); when the plant is consumed at later periods, limb defects and tracheal stenosis are observed (Colegate and Dorling, 1994). Cyclopia was originally thought to be a genetic defect confined to certain herds, but the involvement of the plant was established in the 1950s and the toxin responsible established as the C-nor-D-homosteroid alkaloid, cyclopamine (11-deoxojervine) (Keeler and Tu, 1991). The alkaloid has been shown to experimentally induce cyclopia in sheep (Keeler et al., 1978), rabbits, and chick embryos (Seawright et al., 1985). Cyclopia is observed in human births and is one extreme of the general class of birth-defect syndromes known as holoprosencephaly (Roessler et al., 1996). However, the causes of these defects are not known and could be either genetic or dietary. Given the experience with cyclopia in sheep, and in particular the very restricted and early period of insult, a dietary component can reasonably be expected. Any consumption of *Veratrum* species should be a cause for extreme concern.

Zygadenus species (death camas) have caused catastrophic losses in livestock, especially sheep herds, and frequently poisoned American settlers and even indigenous tribes aware of their toxic nature (Garland and Barr, 1998; Kingsbury, 1964). The bulbs are easily confused with those of wild onions or the edible camas (*Camassia* species; Liliaceae). Flour made from the bulbs of death camas caused serious illness to members of the Lewis and Clark expedition (California Academy of Sciences, 2003). The minimum toxic dose of above-ground parts of the plant in sheep is 0.4 to 2 percent of the animal's body weight, with symptoms appearing in as little as 1.5 hours; the bulbs may be significantly more toxic (Burrows and Tyrl, 2001). The toxic principles are steroidal glycoalkaloids, particularly zygacine (Cheeke, 1998) and zygadenine (O'Neil et al., 2001). The difficulty of identifying bulbs of *Zygadenus* species indicates that extreme caution is warranted in consuming even edible species such as camas. The problem of identification would be compounded if ground material is used and alcoholic extracts would be expected to concentrate the alkaloids.

Strychnos nux-vomica is the pre-eminent toxic species in the **Loganiaceae**. The seeds contain up to 5 percent alkaloids by weight, consisting primarily of strychine and brucine (Dewick, 2002). Strychnine is extremely toxic, affecting the central nervous system and causing convulsions. Approximately 100 mg of strychnine is fatal to an adult human resulting in death by asphyxia (Dewick, 2002). Other *Strychnos* species also contain strychnine, brucine, and structurally related alkaloids. The fruit pulp surrounding the seed contains high levels of the iridoid glycoside loganin, a biosynthetic precursor of strychnine.

There are a number of reports of animal poisoning associated with ingestion of *Gelsemium sempervirens* (Carolina jessamine or yellow jessamine), characterized by neurological symptoms, progressive weakness, convulsions, and death through respiratory failure. Poisoning has been reported in children who have sucked nectar from the flowers and there is evidence that honey made from the nectar may also be toxic (Kingsbury,

1964). The plant contains many alkaloids of the terpenoid indole and oxindole types, structural classes that are also found in other *Gelsemium* species (Burrows and Tyrl, 2001).

The **Loranthaceae** contains a number of *Phoradendron* species (mistletoes—the plants are parasitic on oak trees), as well as the European mistletoe (*Viscum album*). These plants have proved to be toxic to cattle, and eating the berries has caused fatalities in humans (Kingsbury, 1964). A tea brewed from the berries caused acute gastroenteritis and cardiovascular collapse, with death occurring after about 10 hours (Kingsbury, 1964). The toxic compounds are probably the pressor amines tyramine and β-phenylethylamine (Kingsbury, 1964). Individuals taking monoamine oxidase inhibiting drugs would be especially sensitive to such compounds because their detoxification is suppressed by these drugs (Dewick, 2002).

The **Menispermaceae** is chiefly of concern because of *Anamirta cocculus*, an East Indian flowering vine, the seeds of which are known as "cocculus indicus" or "fish berries" because they can be used to poison fish. The toxin is the intensely bitter principle picrotoxin, which is composed of two molecular entities, the nontoxic picrotin and the toxic picrotoxinin, causing vomiting and muscular twitchings progressing to epileptiform convulsions, followed by unconsciousness and death (O'Neil et al., 2001).

The **Musaceae** is chiefly of concern because it includes the genus *Strelitzia*; there have been suggestions that the latter should be classified into a separate family, Strelititziaceae. The bird of paradise plant, *S. reginae*, contains phenalenones that can induce gastroenteritis and vertigo (Holscher and Schneider, 2000). Related compounds have been isolated from the rhizomes of the edible banana species *Musa acuminata* and *Ensete ventricosum* (Luis et al., 1996).

The nutmeg *Myristica fragrans* is a member of the **Myristicaceae** and contains the allyl phenols myristicin (methoxysafrole) and safrole. Ground nutmeg is mildly hallucinogenic, possibly because the myristicin is metabolized via amination to methoxymethylenedioxyamphetamine. Intoxications have been reported after an ingestion of approximately 5 g of nutmeg, corresponding to 1 to 2 mg myristicin/kg body weight (Dewick, 2002). Safrole, which also occurs in *Sassafras albidum* (sassafras; Lauraceae family), is a reported carcinogen (Cheeke, 1998).

The **Myrtaceae** includes the finger-cherry (*Rhodomyrtus macrocarpa*), which has been known to induce blindness in livestock. In the early 1900s, there were a number of reports in northern Queensland of permanent blindness in school children and the government issued warnings against the practice of eating the fruit (Everist, 1981). The toxicity appears to be related to the presence of one or more of a series of highly substituted dibenzofurans, known as rhodomyrtoxins (Everist, 1981).

The privets (*Ligustrum* species), used as ornamental shrubs, hedges, and windbreaks, are classified in the **Oleaceae**; the common privet, *L. vulgare*, is particularly widespread. Consumption of the foliage and berries has caused severe gastroenteritis, vomiting, and death in many classes of livestock (Kingsbury, 1964). Children who consumed the berries had similar symptoms, together with drowsiness and difficulty in movement (Burrows and Tyrl, 2001). The plants contain monoterpene, glycosides, but the toxin is not established (Burrows and Tyrl, 2001).

The **Papaveraceae** encompasses *Argemone* (prickly poppy, Mexican poppy), *Chelidonium* (celandine), *Sanguinaria* (bloodroot), and *Papaver* (poppies, wild and cultivated) species, in addition to others. *Argemone* species contain isoquinoline alkaloids of the berberine and sanguinarine (Cheeke, 1998). Sanguinarine has been shown to be a quantitative DNA intercalator *in vitro* that might cause tumors (Allen et al., 2001). However, *Argemone* seeds have been shown to be toxic to fowl, and experimental oral administration of sanguinarine hydrochloride to rats at a dose of 1 mg per day for 7 days was shown to be fatal (Burrows and Tyrl, 2002). In humans, consumption of grains containing *Argemone* seeds has induced dropsy and glaucoma (Cheeke, 1998). *Sanguinaria canadensis* and *Chelidonium majus* contain many of the same isoquinoline alkaloids, and poisoning of livestock and humans has been reported on occasions (Kingsbury, 1964).

In addition to the isoquinoline alkaloids, *Papaver* species are renowned for the morphinan alkaloids, such as morphine, codeine, and thebaine (Dewick, 2002). The highest levels occur in the opium poppy (*P. somniferum*), the mature fruits of which contain approximately 0.5 percent total alkaloids (Dewick, 2002). The concentrated form, opium, contains up to 25 percent of the alkaloids (Dewick, 2002). When used habitually or to excess, it produces euphoria, nausea, vomiting, and addiction (Dewick, 2002). Withdrawal symptoms are severe and can lead to physical dependence. Although poppies are generally unpalatable to livestock, death has resulted in livestock from feeding poppy seed residue after extraction of the oil and when the plant has been mixed with more palatable feed (Kingsbury, 1964). Poisoning is characterized by excitement, ataxia, gastroenteritis, and coma (Kingsbury, 1964). Species in the Papaveraceae family should be looked at carefully for toxicity potential in almost every case.

The **Phytolaccaceae** includes *Phytolacca americana* (syn. *P. decandra*), the pokeweed, the leaves of which are eaten as a vegetable after boiling. The fruits have been reported to be toxic to children (Burrows and Tyrl, 2001). Livestock, especially pigs, are known to be poisoned by eating the roots, and extreme irritation can be caused in humans by inhalation of root powder. The berries and roots have been shown to contain saponins (Kang and Woo, 1980).

Ponderosa pine (*Pinus ponderosa*) is a member of the **Pinaceae** that has frequently produced third-trimester abortion in pregnant cattle grazing the needles (Cheeke, 1998). Anecdotal evidence indicates that under rangeland conditions, as little as 1 lb of the green needles can induce the effect in as little as 24 hours with virtually the whole herd being affected. The syndrome is generally known as "pine needle abortion," but is more properly described as premature parturition since the calves are born live but generally do not survive without exceptional supportive treatment (Cheeke, 1998). Isocupressic acid (a diterpene), together with its acetyl and succinyl esters, has been shown to be the agent responsible for the observed effects by feeding trials with the purified compound; the esters are rapidly hydrolyzed to the acid in the rumen (Cheeke, 1998). Lodgepole pine (*P. contorta*) and Jeffrey pine (*P. jeffreyi*) also contain significant amounts of isocupressic acid, the needles of which have been reported to cause abortion (Garland and Barr, 1998). A number of other *Pinus* (Pinaceae) and *Juniperus* (Cupressaceae) species contain lower levels of the isocupressic and related diterpene acids and may be capable of inducing pregnancy disorders (Garland and Barr, 1998).

The **Poaceae** encompasses many cultivated species used as a staple food source as grains or flour. Both cultivated and wild grasses are used as forage for livestock, and poisoning episodes are not uncommonly observed in certain situations, especially when a single species is grazed almost exclusively. Toxic levels of nitrates, strongly influenced by factors such as soil type and environmental conditions, can occur in *Avena sativa* (oats), cultivated and wild *Sorghum* species, *Secale cereale* (rye), and *Zea mays* (corn) (Kellerman et al., 1988). Nitrate levels exceeding 1.5 percent potassium nitrate equivalents are considered to be fatal to livestock (Kingsbury, 1964). In the gut, nitrate is reduced to nitrite, which is approximately 10 times more toxic than nitrate, and ultimately to ammonia (Kellerman et al., 1988).

Cultivated *Sorghum* species are produced either as grain sorghums (milo) or forage sorghums. All of these, and also wild species, contain cyanogenic glycosides, in particular the glucoside dhurrin (Cheeke, 1998).

At levels of 0.34 percent cyanide potential, 0.5 lb of forage could prove fatal in grazing animals (Kingsbury, 1964).

Additional concerns arise with certain species in the Poaceae due to the ability of endophytic fungi to produce toxic compounds. *Cynodon dactylon* (Bermuda grass) and related species produce high levels of cyanogenic glycosides, but the syndrome known as "Bermuda grass tremors" is caused by the presence of the parasitic fungus *Balansia epichloe* (Bacon, 1995). The fungus produces nonpeptide ergot alkaloids such as agroclavine, which produce symptoms in livestock (especially horses) ranging from muscle twitching to paralysis of the hind limbs (Bacon, 1995). Peptide-derived ergot alkaloids, based on (+)-lysergic acid, are produced by the fungus *Claviceps purpurea* growing on rye (*Secale cereale*) (Dewick, 2002). *Claviceps* species infect many other cereals and grasses and the risk of ergotism is therefore always present. Ergot alkaloids of the ergopeptine class, produced by infection of *Festuca* species by the endophyte *Acremonium coenophialum*, are responsible for "fescue foot," a lameness and gangrene in the hind feet of cattle (Kellerman et al., 1988).

A disease known as "perennial ryegrass staggers" in livestock is produced by infection of Lolium perenne by *Claviceps paspali* (Cheeke, 1995) and *Acremonium lolii* (Cheeke, 1998; Garland and Barr, 1998). The toxins are complex tremorgenic mycotoxins (penitrems and lolitrems) (Cheeke, 1998) that are potent inhibitors of calcium-activated potassium channels (Cavanagh et al., 1998). The disease is characterized by tremors, severe incoordination, and collapse.

The estrogenic macrolide zearalenone is produced by the fungus *Gibberella zeae* (*Fusarium graminearum*) growing on corn (*Zea mays*) and has produced vulvovaginitis, especially in pigs (Cheeke, 1998).

The **Polygonaceae** includes the genera *Fagopyrum*, *Rheum*, *Rumex*, *Halogeton*, and *Sarcobatus*. Most of these contain high levels of soluble oxalates, which have caused death in livestock and humans, and also significant amounts of nitrate (Kingsbury, 1964).

Fagopyrum sagittatum (buckwheat) is cultivated as a minor grain crop, generally for milling into flour or as a forage for animals. It has produced photosensitization in humans and animals known as fagopyrism, which appears to be of the primary type rather than secondary since there is no evidence of liver damage (Kellerman et al., 1988). The photoactive pigment is probably fagopyrine, a naphthodianthrone structurally related to hypericin in St. John's wort (*Hypericum perforatum*) (Kellerman et al., 1988). Many cases of buckwheat poisoning in humans are the result of an allergic reaction to the plant, and ingestion or inhalation can induce an allergenic reaction (Kingsbury, 1964).

The **Polypodiaceae** includes the bracken fern *Pteridium aquilinum*, which is worldwide in distribution and is established as acutely and chronically toxic to livestock and laboratory animals. The plant contains the enzyme thiaminase, which results in anorexia and ataxia in horses, bright blindness in sheep due to retinal neuroepithelium degeneration, and depression of bone marrow in cattle (Cheeke, 1998). The plant also produces carcinoma of the upper alimentary tract and urinary bladder, caused by ptaquiloside (Cheek, 1998). A number of other structurally related illudane-type sesquiterpene glucosides have been isolated and identified (Nagao et al., 1989). There is evidence that carcinoma can result in calves from ingestion of the toxin through the milk of cows grazing bracken fern (Smith and Seawright, 1995). Epidemiological studies in Japan and Brazil have suggested a close association between bracken frond (fiddleheads) consumption and cancers of the upper alimentary tract (Alonso-Amelot and Avendano, 2001; Brown et al., 1999), but there is evidence that fiddleheads processed by salting can be eaten safely; other routes of exposure may therefore be a factor (Hirono et al., 1972).

The **Ranunculaceae** includes *Aconitum* (aconite, wolfsbane, monkshood) and *Delphinium* (larkspur) species that are acutely toxic to livestock (Kingsbury, 1964). Dried roots of aconite were historically used as an external application for treatment of pain, such as from rheumatism. The plant has been used to poison baits for pest animals, for execution of criminals, and for homicidal purposes. Accidental deaths have been caused by mistaking the root for that of horseradish (Kingsbury, 1964). The dried root can contain up to 1.5 percent by weight of alkaloids with the primary toxic constituent being the diester diterpenoid alkaloid aconitine, comprising approximately 30 percent of the total (Dewick, 2002). Aconitine is acutely toxic, with an oral LD_{50} in mice of 1 mg/kg, and has been used to produce heart arrhythmia in experimental animals (O'Neil et al., 2001). The root of *A. ferox* (Indian aconite) is extremely toxic and very small quantities can produce fatal cardiac depression (Klasek et al., 1972). The major alkaloid constituent is pseudoaconitine (Klasek et al., 1972). The extreme toxicity of *Aconitum* species indicates that use of any parts of the plant or preparations thereof should be a matter of extreme concern.

Delphinium (larkspur) species also contain norditerpene alkaloids and have produced large-scale losses of cattle, especially when grazed in the early growth and flower/seed stage (Cheeke, 1998). Death is often rapid, preceded by staggering gait, recumbancy, muscle twitching, and rapid and irregular pulse (Cheeke, 1998). *Delphinium* species contain over 40 different diterpenoid alkaloids with highly variable compositions and concentrations (Cheeke, 1998). A major constituent is deltaline, generally in excess of 50 percent of the total alkaloid content, with an intravenous LD_{50}

in mice of about 200 mg/kg (Garland and Barr, 1998). The most toxic alkaloids are those possessing an N-(methylsuccinyl)-anthranoyl ester substituent on the basic norditerpenoid skeleton, of which methyllycaconitine is the most common, comprising 0.2 percent of the dry weight of *D. barbeyi* (Manners et al., 1995). These alkaloids reversibly bind and block nicotinic acetylcholine receptors (Garland and Barr, 1998). Whereas methyllycaconitine has a binding constant (KI_{50}) of 1.7 nM, that of its parent, lycoctonine, is only 2,800 nM. Their LD_{50} values, when administered intravenously to mice, are 4.0 and 444 mg/kg, respectively (Manners et al., 1993). The range in toxicities of these various alkaloids and their tendency to change rapidly from one plant species to another, and within a species in response to growth stage and environmental conditions, makes an assessment of risk problematic.

Anemone and *Ranunculus* species are known to be irritant to livestock and toxic on occasion (Kingsbury, 1964). The plants contain ranunculin, the glucoside of 5-methylene-2(5H)-furanone or protoanemonin (Kingsbury, 1964). Enzymatic hydrolysis of ranunculin releases protoanemonin as a volatile, irritant oil that is unstable and rapidly polymerizes to give a resin of which the dimer, anemonin, is a major constituent (Cheeke, 1998). Anemonin is relatively nontoxic with an LD_{50} value when administered intraperitoneally to mice of 150 mg/kg (O'Neil et al., 2001). Protoanemonin can be transferred into the milk of lactating animals, on which it confers a bitter taste (Burrows and Tyrl, 2001).

The coyotillo or tullidora, *Karwinskia humboldtiana*, a member of the **Rhamnaceae** growing in the border areas of the United States and Mexico, has been established as toxic to children and livestock for two centuries (Garland and Barr, 1998). Over 50 confirmed cases of poisoning in humans were reported in Mexico in a 3-year period from 1991 to 1993 (Garland and Barr, 1998). The toxicity is characterized by progressive and symmetrical noninflammatory paralytic neuronopathy, initially in the lower limbs and progressing to respiratory and bulbar paralysis (Burrows and Tyrl, 2001). The fruits contain a series of cytotoxic hydroxyanthracenones known as peroxisomicines and karwinols (Galindo and Waksman, 2001). Administration of a mixture of karwinols to a laboratory animal caused quadriplegia (Garland and Barr, 1998).

The **Rosaceae** contains a number of *Prunus* species (bitter almond, cherries, peaches, plums), the kernels of which contain cyanogenic glycosides, the most representative being amygdalin, a diglucoside (Kingsbury, 1964). Crushing of the tissue releases glucosidases that hydrolyse amygdalin to the monoglucoside prunasin and subsequently to mandelonitrile, which undergoes aqueous hydrolysis to benzaldehyde and hydrogen cyanide (Kingsbury, 1964). Consumption of the foliage of wild cherries and other *Prunus* species is a frequent cause of poisoning in livestock (Kingsbury, 1964). Symptoms are typical of hydrogen cyanide poisoning, with heart and respiratory failure, as previously discussed. It has been reported that 7 to 10 bitter almond kernels were fatal to a 3-year-old child and 40 to 60 kernels were fatal for a man (Burrows and Tyrl, 2001).

The dried leaflets, known as pilocarpus or jaborandi, of various *Pilocarpus* species belonging to the **Rutaceae** family, contain up to 1 percent of imidazole alkaloids, the chief of which is pilocarpine (Dewick, 2002). The salts of this alkaloid are useful in ophthalmic practice for the treatment of glaucoma. Pilocarpine has a structural analogy to muscarine and acetylcholine. Toxicity due to ingestion of the plant can occur due to its activity as a cholinergic agent and as a muscarinic agonist (Dewick, 2002). The main source of pilocarpus is *P. microphyllus*.

The **Sapindaceae** includes the species *Blighia sapida* (akee), the fruit and oil of which are edible if properly prepared by parboiling and frying. However, it has been the cause of a disease in undernourished humans, especially children, known as "vomiting sickness" (Cheeke, 1998). The causative agent is hypoglycin-A, a cyclopropane amino acid that causes severe hypoglycemia (Cheeke, 1998). Toxicity is characterized by violent vomiting, convulsions, coma, and death in most cases (Cheeke, 1998). In rats, hypoglycin-A has been shown to be teratogenic (Persaud, 1968). These effects may be due to a reduction in the rate of fatty acid oxidation due to inhibition of a flavin-dependent acyl dehydrogenase (Tanaka et al., 1971). The severe toxicity suggests a high concern for use of this plant itself or its aqueous and alcoholic extracts.

The family **Scrophulariaceae** contains *Castilleja* (paintbrush) and *Pedicularis* (lousewort) species that have been found to contain relatively low levels of pyrrolizidine alkaloids. The hepatotoxicity of these alkaloids has been discussed in detail under the Asteraceae. There is evidence that these alkaloids are not biosynthesized *de novo* within the plants, but acquired from other plant species by root parasitism (James et al., 1992). Alkaloid levels are therefore likely to be low, but the unpredictable nature of such parasitism and the cumulative nature of pyrrolizidine alkaloid toxicity raises the level of concern regarding use of these plants.

Digitalis purpurea (foxglove) has a long history as a medicinal plant for treatment of heart disease, especially to increase the force of contraction and prolong the duration of diastole (Cheeke, 1998). The plant contains over a dozen cardenolide-type cardiac glycosides, the most important of which are digitoxin and digoxin, yielding digitoxigenin and digoxigenin, respectively, on hydrolysis (Kingsbury, 1964). Although the active compounds are the glycosides, the sugar residues serve an important function in conferring sufficient solubility for oral administration (Kingsbury, 1964). Toxicity is characterized by nausea, vomiting, drowsiness, delirium, hallucinations, and death (Kingsbury, 1964). In humans, poisoning occurs from overdose or too frequent use of the drug, which accumulates in tissues (Kingsbury, 1964).

The **Solanaceae** includes some of the most valuable food plants used by humans, while at the same time encompassing a large number of toxic plant species. The edible plants are confined to the genera *Solanum* and *Lycopersicon* and include potato (*S. tuberosum*), eggplant (*S. melongena*), tomato (*L. esculentum*), and other minor vegetables. Even among these foods, certain plant parts are poisonous and should not be consumed. In particular, green sprouting potatoes are known to be toxic and have on occasion caused fairly large-scale poisoning in humans (Burrows and Tyrl, 2001; Cheeke, 1998). The toxicity has been attributed to steroidal glycoalkaloids, typified by solasonine, solanine, and tomatine, which give rise to the aglycones solasodine, solanidine, and tomatidine, respectively, on hydrolysis (Cheeke, 1998; Keeler and Tu, 1991). Glycoalkaloid contents above 140 ppm confer a bitter taste on potatoes and a burning sensation in the throat (Burrows and Tyrl, 2001). The solanine content in fresh potato sprouts is approximately 0.04 percent (400 ppm); potatoes are considered to be toxic to humans at glycoalkaloid levels above 200 ppm, producing vomiting, abdominal pain, diarrhea, and sometimes death (Burrows and Tyrl, 2001). The alkaloids cause membrane disruption in the digestive system and have anticholinesterase activity on the central nervous system; they have also been shown to be potentially teratogenic (Cheeke, 1998). However, recent studies have shown that many food plants in the Solanaceae also contain significant levels of calystegines, which are polyhydroxytropane alkaloids that are potent inhibitors of glucosidases (Asano et al., 1997). These alkaloids may therefore also be involved in digestive disturbances through inhibition of gut enzymes.

Atropa, *Brugmansia*, *Datura*, *Duboisia*, and *Hyoscyamus* are all genera that have been recorded as poisoning livestock. Humans appear to be particularly susceptible to poisoning by these plants as well. All species contain tropane alkaloids, mainly scopolamine and hyoscamine (Cheeke, 1998; Kingsbury, 1964; Seawright et al., 1985). Typical content of total alkaloids ranges from 1 to 3.5 percent in the leaves (Dewick, 2002). The tropane alkaloids act as anticholinergics, binding to the muscarinic site of the parasympathetic nervous system and thus competing with acetylcholine (Dewick, 2002). As a consequence, they have a depressant effect on the central nervous system, they suppress salivary secretions, they have an antispasmodic effect on the gastrointestinal tract, and they dilate the pupil of the eye. Poisoning from ingestion of plant parts or preparations thereof is relatively common and small quantities of the plant will produce observable adverse effects and even death (Cheeke, 1998). It has been calculated that 4 to 5 grams of leaf or seed of *Datura* is equivalent to a fatal dose for a child (Burrows and Tyrl, 2001). Most of these species have recently been shown to contain glycosidase inhibitory calystegines, as in the *Solanum* species.

The **Taxaceae** includes a number of *Taxus* species, all parts of which are acutely toxic to humans and livestock (Garland and Barr, 1998). The most extensive studies on toxicity have been conducted with the English yew *T. baccata*, native to Europe although it is widely grown as an ornamental plant in North America. Discarded clippings from a garden plant were recently reported to have resulted in the death of 43 cattle in a single night (Panter et al., 1993). Immediate fatalities are due to heart and circulatory failure, although less severely poisoned animals may show trembling, dyspnea, and collapse prior to succumbing (Garland and Barr, 1998; Kingsbury, 1964). The discovery of the Pacific yew *T. brevifolia* as a source of the anticancer drug, taxol, has stimulated extensive phytochemical examination of various *Taxus* species and over 100 diterpenoid taxanes have been characterized (Kingston et al., 2002).

Daphne species, members of the **Thymelaeaceae**, have been long recognized as poisonous plants. The most commonly seen is *D. mezereum*, cultivated as an ornamental, but also naturalized in some areas of the United States. The plants have attractive berries that have poisoned children, and it has been reported that only three berries each resulted in the death of six piglets (Kingsbury, 1964). Chewing on the bark has also caused fatalities in humans, and livestock have been killed by prunings from ornamental plantings (Burrows and Tyrl, 2001; Kingsbury, 1964). The toxic principles are daphnetoxins and mezerein, diterpenes of the phorbol ester type, which may also be cocarcinogenic and allergenic (Burrows and Tyrl, 2001).

The **Verbenaceae** contains *Lantana* species, which are toxic to sheep and cattle in Australia, South Africa, and the United States (Kellerman et al., 1988). Children are suspected of having been poisoned by consumption of the berries (Kingsbury, 1964). Principle among the poisonous species are *L. camara* and *L. montevidensis* (Burrows and Tyrl, 2001; Garland and Barr, 1998). Toxicity is highly variable, and in Australia there have been attempts made to classify the hazard on the basis of their flower color. Primary signs of acute poisoning in livestock is gastroenteritis, but in chronic poisoning secondary photosensitization due to liver damage may be apparent (Cheeke, 1998; Seawright et al., 1985). The toxic principles are lantadenes and hepatoxic triterpene acids (Cheeke, 1998).

The **Zamiaceae** is closely related to the Cycadaceae and consumption of the leaves or seeds produces similar neurological defects in man and animals. *Macrozamia* (burrawang, Zamia palm, or wild pineapple) are the most common species in this family and contain azoglycosides, especially macrozamin, consisting of the aglycone methylazoxymethanol, glycosylated with various sugars (Everist, 1981). *Zamia integrifolia* (Florida arrowroot) is a woody, fern-like plant common in peninsular Florida and has been reported to poison cattle in South America; the seeds are suspected of being poisonous to humans (Kingsbury, 1964).

Larrea tridentata, a member of the **Zygophyllaceae** found in the American Southwest and northern Mexico and known as creosote bush or tarbush, has an ethnobotanic reputation as a beneficial plant. A number of reports have shown that products containing *L. tridentata* induce hepatotoxicity and nephrotoxicity in humans (Garland and Barr, 1998; Lambert et al., 2002). Nordihydroguaiaretic acid, a lignan occurring at up to 10 percent dry weight in the leaves and twigs of the plant, has been demonstrated to be the toxic constituent (Burrows and Tyrl, 2001).

Other species of the Zygophyllaceae known to be toxic to livestock are *Peganum harmala* (African rue), a plant introduced into the United States from deserts of Africa, and *Tribulus terrestris* (puncture vine or caltrop). *P. harmala*, although generally unpalatable, causes death in cattle and the ground seed was lethal to guinea pigs at 0.15 percent of the animals' weight (Kingsbury, 1964); the plant contains β-carboline alkaloids, which are responsible for its toxicity (Burrows and Tyrl, 2001). *T. terrestris* causes hepatogenic photosensitization in livestock and is a major cause of this disease in sheep, known as bighead or geeldikkop, in Australia and South Africa, respectively (Cheeke, 1998; Kellerman et al., 1988). The plant contains steroidal saponins which have been postulated as the hepatotoxins responsible (Cheeke, 1998).

REFERENCES

Aguirre-Galviz LE, Templeton W. 1990. Toxic sesquiterpenoid lactones from the leaves of *Coriaria microphylla*. *Planta Med* 56:244.

Allen CL, Loudon J, Mascarenhas AK. 2001. Sanguinaria-related leukoplakia: Epidemiologic and clinicopathologic features of a recently described entity. *Gen Dent* 49:608–614.

Alonso-Amelot, ME, Avendano M. 2001. Carcinogenic activity of *Pteridium aquilinum* var latiusculum in humans. Possible association between gastric cancer and bracken fern in Venezuela: An epidemiological study. *Int J Cancer* 91:252–259.

Asano N, Kato A, Matsui K, Watson AA, Nash RJ, Molyneux RJ, Hackett L, Topping J, Winchester B. 1997. The effects of calystegines isolated from edible fruits and vegetables on mammalian liver glycosidases. *Glycobiology* 7:1085–1088.

Atta-ur-Rahman, Noor-e-ain F, Choudhary MI, Parveen Z. 1997. New steroidal alkaloids from *Buxus longifolia. J Nat Prod* 60:976–981.

Bacon CW. 1995. Toxic endophyte-infected tall fescue and range grasses: Historic perspectives. *J Anim Sci* 73:861–870.

Bah M, Bye R, Pereda-Miranda R. 1994. Hepatotoxic pyrrolizidine alkaloids in the Mexican medicinal plant *Packera candidissima* (Asteraceae: Senecioneae). *J Ethnopharmacol* 43:19–30.

Bedir E, Manyam R, Khan IA. 2003. Neo-clerodane diterpenoids and phenylethanoid glycosides from *Teucrium chamaedrys* L. *Phytochemistry* 63:977–983.

Boffa MJ, Gilmour E, Ead RD. 1996. Celery soup causing severe phototoxicity during PUVA therapy. *Br J Dermatol* 135:334.

Bradberry SM, Dickers KJ, Rice P, Griffiths GD, Vale JA. 2003. Ricin poisoning. *Toxicol Rev* 22:65–70.

Brown L, Zahm SH, Hoover RN, Fraumeni J. 1999. Bracken fern consumption and human bladder cancer. *J Epidemiol Comm Health* 53:653.

Buhrmester RA, Ebinger JE, Seigler DS. 2000. Sambunigrin and cyanogenic variability in populations of Sambucus cyanogenic variability in populations of *Sambucus canadensis* L. (Caprifoliaceae). *Biochem Syst Ecol* 28:689–695.

Burrows GE, Tyrl RJ. 2001. *Toxic Plants of North America.* Ames, IA: Iowa State University Press.

California Academy of Sciences. 2003. *California Wildflowers: Death Camas.* Online. Available at http://www.calacademy.org/research/botany/wildflow/comfrm.htm. Accessed December 11, 2003.

Camp BJ, Bridges CH, Hill DW, Patamalai B, Wilson S. 1988. Isolation of a steroidal sapogenin from the bile of a sheep fed *Agave lecheguilla. Vet Hum Toxicol* 30:533–535.

Canel C, Moraes RM, Dayan FE, Ferreira D. 2000. Podophyllotoxin. *Phytochemistry* 54:115–120.

Cavanagh JB, Holton JL, Nolan CC, Ray DE, Naik JT, Mantle PG. 1998. The effects of the tremorgenic mycotoxin peniterem A on the rat cerebellum. *Vet Pathol* 35:53–63.

Cheeke PR. 1995. Endogenous toxins and mycotoxins in forage grasses and their effects on livestock. *J Anim Sci* 73:909–918.

Cheeke PR. 1998. *Natural Toxicants in Feeds, Forages, and Poisonous Plants.* 2nd ed. Danville, IL: Interstate Publishers.

Colegate SM, Dorling PR, eds. 1994. *Plant-Associated Toxins: Agricultural, Phytochemical and Ecological Aspects.* Wallingford, UK: CAB International.

Cosyns JP, Goebbels RM, Liberton V, Schmeiser HH, Bieler CA, Bernard AM. 1998. Chinese herbs nephropathy-associated slimming regimen induces tumours in the forestomach but no interstitial nephropathy in rats. *Arch Toxicol* 72:738–743.

de Balogh KKIM, Dimande AP, van der Lugt JJ, Molyneux RJ, Naude TW, Welmans WG. 1999. A lysosomal storage disease induced by *Ipomoea carnea* in goats in Mozambique. *J Vet Diagn Invest* 11:266–273.

Dewick PM. 2002. *Medicinal Natural Products. A Biosynthetic Approach, 2nd ed.* New York: John Wiley and Sons.

Elbein AD, Molyneux RJ. 1998. Inhibitors of glycoprotein processing. In: Stutz AE, ed. *Iminosugars as Glycosidase Inhibitors-Nojirimycin and Beyond.* New York: Wiley-VCH.

Everist SL. 1981. *Poisonous Plants of Australia.* London: Angus & Robertson Publishers.

Galindo VR, Waksman N. 2001. Cytotoxic hydroxyanthracenones from fruits of *Karwinskia parvifolia. Nat Prod Lett* 15:243–251.

Gardner DR, Panter KE, James LF, Stegelmeier BL. 1998. Abortifacient effects of lodgepole pine (*Pinus contorta*) and common juniper (*Juniperus communis*) on cattle. *Vet Hum Toxicol* 40:260–263.

Garland T, Barr AC, eds. 1998. *Toxic Plants and Other Natural Toxicants*. Wallingford, UK: CAB International.

Gunn CR. 1969. *Abrus precatorius*: Pretty but poisonous. *Science* 164:245–246.

Hall WT. 1987. Cycad (Zamia) poisoning in Australia. *Aust Vet J* 64:149–151.

Hirono I, Shibuya C, Shimizu M, Fushima K. 1972. Carcinogenic activity of processed bracken used as human food. *J Natl Cancer Inst* 48:1245–1249.

Hirschhorn HH. 1983. Botanical remedies of the former Dutch East Indies (Indonesia). Part II: Dicotyledones up to and including leguminosae. *J Ethnopharmacol* 8:65–96.

Holscher D, Schneider B. 2000. Phenalenones from *Strelitzia reginae*. *J Nat Prod* 63:1027–1028.

James LF, Keeler RF, Cheeke PR, Bailey EM Jr, Hegarty MP, eds. 1992. *Poisonous Plants*. Ames, IA: Iowa State University Press.

Jin HZ, Hwang BY, Kim HS, Lee JH, Kim YH, Lee JJ. 2002. Antiinflammatory constituents of *Celastrus orbiculatus* inhibit the NF-kappaB activation and NO production. *J Nat Prod* 65:89–91.

Jinbo Z, Mingan W, Wenjun W, Zhiqing J, Zhaonong H. 2002. Insecticidal sesquiterpene pyridine alkaloids from *Euonymus* species. *Phytochemistry* 61:699–704.

Johanns ES, van der Kolk LE, van Gemert HM, Sijben AE, Peters PW, de Vries I. 2002. An epidemic of epileptic seizures after consumption of herbal tea. *Ned Tijdschr Geneeskd* 146:813–816.

Kang SS, Woo WS. 1980. Triterpenes from the berries of *Phytolacca americana*. *J Nat Prod* 43:510–513.

Kariyone T, Okuda T. 1955. Studies on the toxic components of *Coriaria japonica* A. Gray. *Acta Sch Med Univ Kioto* 33:45–55.

Keeler RF, Tu AT, eds. 1983. *Handbook of Natural Toxins. Volume 1. Plant and Fungal Toxins*. New York: Marcel Dekker.

Keeler RF, Tu AT. 1991. *Handbook of Natural Toxins. Volume 6. Toxicology of Plant and Fungal Compounds*. New York: Marcel Dekker.

Keeler RF, Van Kampen KR, James LF, eds. 1978. *Effects of Poisonous Plants on Livestock*. New York: Academic Press.

Kellerman TS, Coetzer JAW, Naudé TW. 1988. *Plant Poisonings and Mycotoxicoses of Livestock in Southern Africa*. Cape Town, South Africa: Oxford University Press.

Kingsbury JM. 1964. *Poisonous Plants of the United States and Canada*. Englewood Cliffs, NJ: Prentice-Hall.

Kingston DG, Jagtap PG, Yuan H, Samala L. 2002. The chemistry of taxol and related taxoids. *Fortschr Chem Org Naturst* 84:53–225.

Klasek A, Simanek V, Santavy F. 1972. Alkaloids from Aconitum plants. I. Isolation of bikhaconitine, chasmaconitine, indaconitine and pseudaconitine from *Aconitum ferox*. *Lloydia* 35:55–60.

Kuo YH, Huang HC, Chiou WF, Shi LS, Wu TS, Wu YC. 2003. A novel No-production-inhibiting triterpene and cytotoxicity of known alkaloids from *Euonymus laxiflorus*. *J Nat Prod* 66:554–557.

Kuriyama T, Schmidt TJ, Okuyama E, Ozoe Y. 2002. Structure-activity relationships of seco-prezizaane terpenoids in gamma-aminobutyric acid receptors of houseflies and rats. *Bioorg Med Chem* 10:1873–1881.

Lambert JD, Zhao D, Meyers RO, Kuester RK, Timmermann BN, Dorr RT. 2002. Nordihydroguaiaretic acid: Hepatotoxicity and detoxification in the mouse. *Toxicon* 40:1701–1708.

Larrey D, Vial T, Pauwels A, Castot A, Biour M, David M, Michel H. 1992. Hepatitis after germander (*Teucrium chamaedrys*) administration: Another instance of herbal medicine hepatotoxicity. *Ann Intern Med* 117:129–132.

Laurena AC, Revilleza MJR, Mendoza EMT. 1994. Polyphenols, phytate, cyanogenic glycosides and trypsin inhibitor activity of several Philippine indigenous food legumes. *J Food Compost Anal* 7:194–202.

Lopez S, Bastida J, Viladomat F, Codina C. 2002. Acetylcholinesterase inhibitory activity of some Amaryllidaceae alkaloids and Narcissus extracts. *Life Sci* 71:2521–2529.

Luis JG, Quinones W, Echeverri F, Grillo TA, Kishi MP, Garcia-Garcia F, Torres F, Cardona G. 1996. Musanolones: Four 9-phenylphenalenones from rhizomes of *Musa acuminata*. *Phytochemistry* 41:753–757.

Manners GD, Panter KE, Ralphs MH, Pfister JA, Olsen JD, James LF. 1993. Toxicity and chemical phenology of norditerpenoid alkaloids in the tall larkspurs (*Delphinium* species). *J Agric Food Chem* 41:96–100.

Manners GD, Panter KE, Pelletier SW. 1995. Structure-activity relationships of norditerpenoid alkaloids occurring in toxic larkspur (*Delphinium*) species. *J Nat Prod* 58:863–869.

Mattei A, Rucay P, Samuel D, Feray C, Reynes M, Bismuth H. 1995. Liver transplantation for severe acute liver failure after herbal medicine (*Teucrium polium*) administration. *J Hepatol* 22:597.

Mattocks AR. 1986. *Chemistry and Toxicology of Pyrrolizidine Alkaloids*. Orlando, FL: Academic Press.

McDermott WV, Ridker PM. 1990. The Budd-Chiari syndrome and hepatic veno-occlusive disease. Recognition and treatment. *Arch Surg* 125:525–527.

Molyneux RJ, Johnson AE. 1984. Extraordinary levels of production of pyrrolizidine alkaloids in *Senecio riddellii*. *J Nat Prod* 47:1030–1032.

Munoz O, Pena RC, Montenegro G. 2001. Iridoids from *Stachys grandidentata* (Labiatae). *Z Naturforsch* 56:902–903.

Nagao T, Saito K, Hirayama E, Uchikoshi K, Koyama K, Natori S, Morisaki N, Iwasaki S, Matsushima T. 1989. Mutagenicity of ptaquiloside, the carcinogen in bracken, and its related illudane-type sesquiterpenes. I. Mutagenicity in *Salmonella typhimurium*. *Mutat Res* 215:173–178.

Onat FY, Yegan BC, Lawrence R, Oktay A, Oktay S. 1991. Mad honey poisoning in man and rat. *Rev Environ Health* 9:3–9.

O'Neil MJ, Smith A, Heckelman PE, eds. 2001. *The Merck Index: An Encyclopedia of Chemicals, Drugs, and Biologics*. 13th ed. Whitehouse Station, NJ: Merck and Co.

Panter KE, Molyneux RJ, Smart RS, Mitchell L, Hansen S. 1993. English yew poisoning in 43 cattle. *J Am Vet Med Assoc* 202:1476–1477.

Pauli G, Bessot JC, Braun PA, Dietemann-Molard A, Kopferschmitt-Kubler MC, Thierry R. 1988. Celery allergy: Clinical and biological study of 20 cases. *Ann Allergy* 60:243–246.

Persaud TV. 1968. Teratogenic effects of hypoglycin-A. *Nature* 217:471.

Puschner B, Holstege DM, Lamberski N, Le T. 2001. Grayanotoxin poisoning in three goats. *J Am Vet Med Assoc* 218:573–575, 527–528.

Qui D, Kao PN. 2003. Immunosuppressive and anti-inflammatory mechanisms of triptolide, the principal active diterpenoid from the Chinese medicinal herb *Tripterygium wilfordii* Hook. f. *Drugs RD* 4:1–18.

Reinli K, Block G. 1996. Phytoestrogen content of foods—A compendium of literature values. *Nutr Cancer* 26:123–148.

Reyes AG, Martinez RJ, Bartulin J. 1980. Coriamyrtin and other metabolites of *Coriaria ruscifolia*. *J Nat Prod* 43:532–533.

Roessler E, Belloni E, Gaudenz K, Jay P, Berta P, Scherer SW, Tsui LC, Muenke M. 1996. Mutations in the human Sonic hedgehog gene cause holoprosencephaly. *Nat Genet* 14:357–360.

Roitman JN. 1981. Comfrey and liver damage. *Lancet* 1:944.
Samenuk D, Link MS, Homoud MK, Contreras R, Theohardes TC, Wang PJ, Estes NAM III. 2002. Adverse cardiovascular events temporally associated with ma huang, an herbal source of ephedrine. *Mayo Clin Proc* 77:12–16.
Schmidt TJ, Schmidt HM, Muller E, Peters W, Fronczek FR, Truesdale A, Fischer NH. 1998. New sesquiterpene lactones from *Illicium floridantum*. *J Nat Prod* 61:230–236.
Seawright AE, Hegarty MP, Keeler RF, James LF, eds. 1985. *Plant Toxicology*. Brisbane, Australia: Queensland Poisonous Plants Committee.
Seligman PJ, Mathias CG, O'Malley MA, Beier RC, Fehrs LJ, Serrill WS, Halperin WE. 1987. Phytophotodermatitis from celery among grocery store workers. *Arch Dermatol* 123:1478–1482.
Shapiro TA, Fahey JW, Wade KL, Stephenson KK, Talalay P. 1998. Human metabolism and excretion of cancer chemoprotective glucosinolates and isothiocyanates of cruciferous vegetables. *Cancer Epidemiol Biomarkers Prev* 7:1091–1100.
Skalli S, David JM, Benkirane R, Zaid A, Soulaymani R. 2002. Acute intoxication by Redoul (*Coriaria myrtifolia* L.). Three observations. *Presse Med* 31:1554–1556.
Smith BL, Seawright AA. 1995. Bracken fern (*Pteridium* spp.) carcinogenicity and human health—A brief review. *Nat Toxins* 3:1–5.
Stickel F, Seitz HK. 2000. The efficacy and safety of comfrey. *Public Health Nutr* 3:501–508.
Stillman AS, Huxtable R, Consroe P, Kohnen P, Smith S. 1977. Hepatic veno-occlusive disease due to pyrrolizidine (Senecio) poisoning in Arizona. *Gastroenterology* 73:349–352.
Stoewsand GS. 1995. Bioactive organosulfur phytochemicals in *Brassica oleracea* vegetables—A review. *Food Chem Toxicol* 33:537–543.
Tanaka K, Miller EM, Isselbacher KJ. 1971. Hypoglycin A: A specific inhibitor of isovaleryl CoA dehydrogenase. *Proc Natl Acad Sci USA* 68:20–24.
Temma K, Akera T, Ng YC. 1986. Effects of inotropic agents on isolated guinea pig heart under conditions that modify calcium pools involved in contractile activation. *Can J Physiol Pharmacol* 64:947–953.
Violon C. 1997. Belgian (Chinese herb) nephropathy: Why? *J Pharm Belg* 74:11–36.
Wei H, Zeng FJ, Lu, MY, Tang RJ. 1998. Studies on chemical constituents from the root of Coriaria nepalensis wall (*Coriaria sinica*). *Yao Xue Xue Bao* 33:688–692.

OTHER RESOURCES THAT MAY BE USEFUL

ARS (Agricultural Research Service). 2003. *Poisonous Plant Research Laboratory*. Online. U.S. Department of Agriculture. Available at http://www.pprl.usu.edu. Accessed July 8, 2003.
Chang HM, But PPH, eds. 1986. *Pharmacology and Applications of Chinese Materia Medica*. Vol. 1. Philadelphia, PA: World Scientific.
Chang HM, But PPH, eds. 1987. *Pharmacology and Applications of Chinese Materia Medica*. Vol. 2. Singapore: World Scientific.
Cornell University. 2002. *Poisonous Plants Informational Database*. Online. Available at http://www.ansci.cornell.edu/plants/index.html. Accessed July 8, 2003.
Lampe K, McCann MA. 1985. *American Medical Association's Handbook of Poisonous and Injurious Plants*. Chicago: American Medical Association.
Leikin JB, Paloucek FP. 1998. *Poisoning and Toxicology Compendium with Symptoms Index*. Washington, DC: Lexi-Comp Inc., Ohio and American Pharmaceutical Association.
Lemmens RHMJ, Bunyapraphatsara N, eds. 2003. *Plant Resources of South-East Asia. Medicinal and Poisonous Plants. 3*. Leiden, The Netherlands: Backhuys Publishers.
Watt JM, Breyer-Brandwijk MG. 1962. *The Medicinal and Poisonous Plants of Southern and Eastern Africa*. 2nd ed. Edinburgh, Scotland: E&S Livingstone.

Appendix D

Chaparral: Prototype Monograph Summary[1]

V. SUMMARY AND CONCLUSIONS

A. Summary

Reports of chaparral toxicity are inconsistent. Native populations in the southwest United States appear to have used chaparral tea for decades without reported evidence of toxicity. In addition, a clinical study looking at the use of chaparral tea and nordihydroguaiaretic acid (NDGA) in advanced incurable cancer patients showed no evidence of hepatotoxicity. Limitations of this study included a lack of detail on those who did not

[1]This is a summary of a prototype monograph, prepared for the purpose of illustrating how a safety review of a dietary supplement ingredient might be prepared following the format described in this report. While it was prepared as a prototype using the processes described in the report, it was not conducted under the auspices of the Food and Drug Administration utilizing all the resources available to the agency. Thus some pertinent information not available to the Committee could be of importance in evaluating safety to determine if use of this dietary supplement ingredient would present an unreasonable risk of illness or injury. Also, the development and review of this prototype was conducted by individuals whose backgrounds are in general aspects of evaluating science and whose expertise is not necessarily focused specifically on this dietary ingredient, although significant additional assistance was provided by consultants with relevant expertise. Therefore, this prototype monograph, while extensive, does not represent an authoritative statement regarding the safety of this dietary supplement ingredient. The full prototype monograph and its data tables on chaparral may be accessed at http://www.iom.edu/fnb.

complete the trial (25 percent of the subjects). This evidence is somewhat inconsistent with other information on chaparral use.

There are nine reported cases of definite hepatotoxicity temporally related to chaparral use as a single known agent; there are an additional six cases of possible hepatotoxicity. Five of the exhibited documented recovery after cessation of chaparral use and one exhibited abnormal liver function upon rechallenge. One patient required an orthotopic liver transplant, but had major confounding variables, such as hepatitis C and prior drug and ethanol abuse. In all the other cases, liver function tests became significantly abnormal with clinically evident jaundice that reversed upon discontinuation of chaparral use. In at least three cases of chaparral-associated hepatotoxicity, the patient had prior history of alcohol abuse or underlying liver disease and may represent a vulnerable population.

In determining causation, one looks for a dose-response relationship. The amount of chaparral ingested ranged from 0.3 to 6 g/day over periods ranging from 20 days to "many years." There appeared to be no dose-response relationship, although evidence of toxicity was clearly reflected in abnormal liver function tests. The absence of pharmacokinetic data or even characterization of the formulations ingested made it difficult to determine actual dose in the various case reports.

Another important factor in determining causation is characterization of the product responsible for the adverse effect. In most of the reported cases, the product ingested by the subject was simply described as chaparral capsules or tablets. This description does not reveal whether the contents of the capsule or tablet were dried, ground plant material or dried extract. Ideally, if the contents were an extract, then the solvent should have been described as well as the ratio of solvent to plant material. This is all assuming that the plant material was properly identified and that the plant parts used were fine leaves/stems. In addition, no chemical profiles were available for the products, making it difficult to compare the different doses ingested by the subjects. Further, without examination of the quality of the product, contamination or adulteration cannot be ruled out.

In only one of the 15 case reports of chaparral-associated hepatotoxicity was it reported that a chaparral tea had been ingested. This is important because the chemical profile of the product will depend upon the preparation used. Chaparral tea contains very little NDGA or other lipophilic compounds as compared with other preparations such as a dried extract prepared with an organic solvent. If NDGA is the causal agent, the content of NDGA in various preparations becomes an important variable in determining causality.

Animal studies evaluating chaparral did not show hepatotoxicity. Animal studies evaluating NDGA did not exhibit hepatotoxicity, but instead exhibited renal proximal tubular damage and cyst formation. In other studies, rodents exhibited both renal and hepatic toxicity in response to the toxic quinone imine from acetaminophen; this involves proximal tubular damage, but not cyst formation. A plausible mechanism in both hepatotoxicity and nephrotoxicity is the cytochrome P450-dependent metabolism of NDGA to a toxic quinone with failure to remove this reactive metabolite by conjugation if glutathione is limiting. The link between the nephrotoxicity of NDGA in animals and the hepatotoxicity of chaparral in humans is not definite, but similar links have been shown with structurally related chemicals, such as the quinone imine of acetaminophen.

While the human data strongly suggest an association between chaparral consumption and hepatotoxicity, a number of confounding factors also require consideration. The temporal clustering of the majority of the hepatotoxicity cases (1992–1993) provides some suggestion of a localized contamination problem. Inadequate characterization of the preparations used by individual patients does not allow determination of possible product contamination during harvesting/processing or natural alterations in composition of chaparral plants due to environmental factors. If typical chaparral preparations contained hepatotoxic principles, it is possible that many more reports of human hepatotoxicity during the period of significant chaparral use (1970–1992) would have emerged. Pre-existing liver disease, including excessive alcohol use, hepatitis, or chronic acetaminophen use, may have predisposed some of the individuals to hepatotoxicity. Such possibilities are hypothetical, but the quality of the data provided in the case reports is inadequate to rule out such possibilities.

B. Conclusions and Recommendations About the Safety of the Ingredient Based on the Strength of the Scientific Evidence

Conclusions (concerns and caveats): The available literature raises concern for hepatic, renal, and reproductive toxicity. The reasons for concern about hepatotoxicity/nephrotoxicity can be summarized as case reports showing a pattern of hepatotoxicity, nephrotoxicity in rats given NDGA, and *in vitro* studies showing that NDGA exhibited cytotoxic activity.

While the human data strongly suggest an association between chaparral consumption and hepatotoxicity, a number of confounding factors also require consideration. There was a clinical study (published in 1970) in which serum glutamicoxaloacetic transaminase (SGOT), a marker of liver damage, was evaluated; this was an uncontrolled, poorly designed study, yet no elevation in SGOT was reported. However, the subjects were critically ill cancer patients and 15 of the subjects (25 percent of the total number of subjects in the study) were removed from the study. At the time of this study there was no awareness of a possible relationship between chaparral ingestion and hepatotoxicity; these individuals could have been removed from the study because elevations in SGOT were used to indicate a measure of general health and appropriateness, a possible criteria to remain in the study.

Hepatotoxicity: The temporal clustering of the majority of the hepatotoxicity cases (1992–1993) provides some suggestion of localized contamination or a variation in constituent concentration, probably due to inadequate characterization or lack of standardization. It is unfortunate that animal studies were not conducted at the time this cluster of hepatotoxic events was reported. During a period of 20 years (1973–1993), 200 tons of chaparral was sold on the U.S. market, equivalent to 500 million doses at 500 mg/dose. If typical chaparral preparations contained hepatotoxic principles, it is possible that many more reports of human hepatotoxicity during the period of significant chaparral use (1970–1992) would have emerged. Traditional uses of chaparral tea by native populations have not revealed reports of hepatotoxicity. It is possible that some of the individuals who experienced the adverse events had pre-existing liver disease, including excessive alcohol use, hepatitis, or chronic acetaminophen use, which predisposed them to hepatotoxicity. Since the quality of the data provided in the case reports is inadequate to rule them out, such possibilities remain hypothetical.

The evidence for toxicity of chaparral in humans is supported by a similar toxicity observed in animal studies using NDGA. Classic toxicity studies with NDGA were conducted in several species; toxicity over a range of doses was a common finding (Ashby, 2002). Of the animal studies reported, only two identified hepatic effects following administration of NDGA to rats or mice; the one mouse study used intraperitoneal administration of NDGA and is confounded by coadministration of endotoxin, a known hepatotoxin. Thus minimal hepatotoxicity was exhibited in animals treated with NDGA. However, if toxicity of a compound is related to the site of its metabolism, hepatotoxicity would be expected because the liver is the major site of xenobiotic metabolism. Instead, nephrotoxicity was the major toxicity found in rats treated with NDGA; this nephrotoxicity is discussed in detail below (Kacew, 2001).

The *in vitro* data on chaparral are incomplete and do not provide the necessary details either to generate hypotheses of mechanisms or to determine doses that might cause toxicity in intact animals. In a large number of *in vitro* studies, NDGA was used at pharmacological doses as a scientific tool to inhibit lipoxygenase in basic research. This lyoxygenase inhibition, at pharmacological doses, while indicating a possible pathway of NDGA action, was not viewed as particularly helpful in assessing the safety of chaparral because the degree to which enzyme inhibition would occur with chaparral consumption was not readily apparent. However, this inhibition of a prostanoid pathway does provide a mechanistic explanation for the reproductive effects observed in animals (see below).

Of the 15 reported cases of chaparral-associated hepatotoxicity, only one case was associated with ingestion of chaparral tea, whereas 11 cases were associated with ingestion of capsules or tablets containing chaparral. If NDGA contributes to the toxicity, it is important to note that it and other nonpolar compounds, including lignans, appear to be minimal in a water extract/tea in contrast to an alcoholic extract (Obermeyer et al., 1995). This differential extraction of lignans by water extraction versus alcohol extraction (Obermeyer et al., 1995) is explained by the lipophilic character of lignans. Therefore, alcoholic extracts of leaf or other aerial plant parts would contain larger amounts of NDGA and other lipophilic compounds than a water extract/tea.

Nephrotoxicity: There are no reports of renal damage following chaparral ingestion in humans or in relevant animal feeding studies. Toxicology studies of NDGA administration in rodents have repeatedly shown nephrotoxicity, including proximal tubular damage and cyst formation.

NDGA can be expected to be a substrate for cytochrome P450-dependent quinone formation based on its chemical structure, as well as on evidence discussed by Obermeyer and colleagues (1995). A plausible mechanism of cytotoxicity of NDGA is cytochrome P450-dependent metabolism of NDGA to a toxic quinone with failure to remove this reactive metabolite by conjugation if glutathione is limiting. It is possible that there is a link between the nephrotoxicity of NDGA in animals and hepatotoxicity of chaparral in humans based on the fact that both the renal proximal tubules and the liver are major sites of xenobiotic metabolism. A parallel finding has been demonstrated in rodents; both renal and hepatic toxicity develop in response to the toxic quinone imine from acetaminophen.

Reproductive toxicity: Since reproductive effects are less likely to be detected in humans, animal data deserve careful consideration. Reproductive toxicity has been demonstrated by one group studying chaparral administered to female rats and three groups studying NDGA administered to female rats or mice. The chaparral study identified anti-implantation activity while the NDGA studies identified inhibition of ovulation and increased resorption of fetuses. These data are supported by the findings that NDGA inhibits prostaglandin synthesis, cyclooxygenase, and lipoxygenases. Because of the important role of eicosanoids in reproduction and fetal development, inhibitors of prostanoid pathways are contraindicated during the first and third trimesters of pregnancy (Mikuni et al., 1998).

Summary of the conclusions: Although substantial limitations exist in the available information, concerns about the safety of chaparral remain based on the weight of the evidence discussed above. The most significant concern is hepatotoxicity, but some concerns also exist for reproductive and renal toxicities. This is especially applicable for certain groups, including those with pre-existing hepatic or renal problems, those taking drugs that affect liver function, those with current or prior alcohol abuse, and women of child-bearing age. There is more concern with ingestion of chaparral preparations containing leaves/stems or alcoholic extracts than with the ingestion of aqueous extracts (i.e., teas) because of the higher content of NDGA and other lipophilic compounds in the former preparations.

C. Data Gaps and Future Research Recommended

Concern for possible adverse effects in American Indian and Hispanic populations that use local botanical remedies prompts the panel to propose research needs that will help in the evaluation of the human clinical data. This concern would be increased if a resurgence in public interest in chaparral occurs.

Detailed toxicity studies in animals are needed to explore the possible dose-response relationship in the development of hepatotoxicity and nephrotoxicity as the result of chaparral ingestion. In animal studies, pair feeding should be included in the experimental protocol due to possible aversion to the chow if NDGA has been added (Goodman et al., 1970). Ideally, studies should compare the different preparations of chaparral (powdered leaf, alcoholic extract, and water extract). The differences in the chemical composition of the various preparations of chaparral need to be explored. The literature shows that a preponderance of toxicities were associated with preparations other than tea; hepatotoxicity was not reported in a clinical trial of cancer patients drinking chaparral tea. This suggests that there are differences in the bioavailability of the components of chaparral that result from differences in the chemical composition of the various preparations. These differences need to be explored in detail.

In all further research, it is important to carry out careful product characterization. A qualified taxonomist should identify the plant material and a botanical sample should be retained in an herbarium for future reference. It is important to carefully describe the plant part utilized. As an example, newer leaves should be distinguished from older leaves because newer leaves contain a higher proportion of the NDGA-containing resin. Chaparral roots contain a quinone not reported to be present in the aerial parts of the plants and, thus, roots should be carefully excluded. The plant material should be chemically profiled, including quantitative determination of NDGA and other lignans. As a quality measure, there should be an analysis of metals since chaparral plants concentrate metals from the soil (Gardea-Torresdey et al., 2001). Furthermore, when reporting human experience with ingesting chaparral, the formulation is important to note. The formulation can best be critically evaluated if the manufacturer, date, and lot number are reported.

REFERENCES

Ashby J. 2002. Scientific issues associated with the validation of *in vitro* and *in vivo* methods for assessing endocrine disrupting chemicals. *Toxicology* 181–182:389–397.

Gardea-Torresdey JL, Arteaga S, Tiemann KJ, Chianelli R, Pingitore N, Mackay W. 2001. Absorption of copper(II) by creosote bush (*Larrea tridentata*): Use of atomic and x-ray absorption spectroscopy. *Environ Toxicol Chem* 20:2572–2579.

Goodman T, Grice HC, Becking GC, Salem FA. 1970. A cystic nephropathy induced by nordihydroguaiaretic acid in the rat. Light and electron microscopic investigations. *Lab Invest* 23:93–107.

Kacew S. 2001. Confounding factors in toxicity testing. *Toxicology* 160:87–96.

Mikuni M, Yoshida M, Hellberg P, Peterson CA, Edwin SS, Brännström M, Peterson CM. 1998. The lipoxygenase inhibitor, nordihydroguaiaretic acid, inhibits ovulation and reduces leukotriene and prostaglandin levels in the rat ovary. *Biol Reprod* 58:1211–1216.

Obermeyer WR, Musser SM, Betz JM, Casey RE, Pohland AE, Page SW. 1995. Chemical studies of phytoestrogens and related compounds in dietary supplements: Flax and chaparral. *Proc Soc Exp Biol Med* 208:6–12.

Appendix E

Glucosamine: Prototype Monograph Summary[1]

V. SUMMARY AND CONCLUSIONS

A. Summary

Glucosamine is an amino monosaccharide that is derived from cellular glucose metabolism and is also found in the body as a simple component of cartilage macromolecules. Glucosamine is widely used as a dietary supplement for chronic joint pain, often recommended at amounts of 500 to 2,000 mg/day.

In humans glucosamine has been tested against placebo or nonsteroidal anti-inflammatory drugs (NSAIDs) in 11 randomized, double-blind,

[1]This is a summary of a prototype monograph, prepared for the purpose of illustrating how a safety review of a dietary supplement ingredient might be prepared following the format described in this report. While it was prepared as a prototype using the processes described in the report, it was not conducted under the auspices of the Food and Drug Administration utilizing all the resources available to the agency. Thus some pertinent information not available to the Committee could be of importance in evaluating safety to determine if use of this dietary supplement ingredient would present an unreasonable risk of illness or injury. Also, the development and review of this prototype was conducted by individuals whose backgrounds are in general aspects of evaluating science and whose expertise is not necessarily focused specifically on this dietary ingredient, although significant additional assistance was provided by consultants with relevant expertise. Therefore, this protoype monograph, while extensive, does not represent an authoritative statement regarding the safety of this dietary supplement ingredient. The full prototype monograph and its data tables on glucosamine may be accessed at http://www.iom.edu/fnb.

placebo-control (7 studies) or reference-control (4 studies) clinical trials ranging in duration from 1 to 36 months and including a total of 716 participants (in the glucosamine arms). Many of these trials presented incomplete information about the systematic collection of data on adverse effects, and many did not examine or report clinical laboratory values systematically. Many of the trials relied only on passive reporting. In the placebo-controlled trials, the incidence of adverse effects among the treatment arms was almost identical, while in the NSAID comparison trials, adverse effect rates were higher among those taking NSAIDs (range of 15–35 percent). In general, the adverse effects reported were mild and most often related to gastrointestinal complaints. No data are available on the safety of glucosamine use in pregnant or lactating women or in children.

Classical animal toxicity studies for glucosamine have not been published; however, reviewers citing only unpublished data state that no toxicity was observed with glucosamine administered by oral administration or by gavage. These findings are corroborated by findings of only minimal toxicity with glucosamine administered by other routes of administration. For glucosamine, as for other substances endogenous to the body, LD_{50} values could not be determined due to the lack of toxicity observed except when supraphysiologic amounts were administered.

Animal studies using infusion of glucosamine in rats at high doses (approaching 1 mM in blood) and in *in vitro* studies (using the addition of glucosamine to cell-culture media at high concentrations) found that glucosamine inhibited the ability of pancreatic islet cells to increase insulin secretion in response to an increased concentration of glucose. It should be emphasized that these studies were designed to test hypotheses about the intracellular signaling pathways by which glucose exerts its regulatory effects and were not designed to examine the "toxicity" of glucosamine *per se*.

The pharmacokinetics of glucosamine become important to assessing its risk, as discussed below. Orally ingested glucosamine appears to be rapidly absorbed, but it is largely metabolized before it reaches the bloodstream.

The primary source of glucosamine in the United States is chitin, derived from shellfish (e.g., shrimp, crab). There may be a risk for antigen exposure if the product is incompletely purified. There is no systematic surveillance of contaminants of these products, and only a subset of the manufacturers apparently comply with U.S. Pharmacopeia (USP) standards.

B. Conclusions and Recommendations About the Safety of the Ingredient Based on the Strength of the Scientific Evidence

From the evaluation of the available data, there appears to be no evidence that use of 1.5 g of glucosamine per day poses a substantial risk in nonpregnant adults. However, given the uncertainty of the minimum glucosamine exposure required for adverse effects on insulin regulation in individuals who are predisposed to glucose regulation problems, glucosamine may present a risk in individuals with, or at risk for, insulin resistance and/or glucose intolerance who ingest it as a dietary supplement for long periods of time. Notably, the available data do not include sufficient studies powered to evaluate safety parameters (e.g., studies measuring relevant blood chemistry parameters following oral administration to animals and humans). These conclusions are therefore based on (1) interpretation of animal and human data indicating that very little intact glucosamine is found in the bloodstream following oral ingestion and thus the secretion problems observed following millimolar blood concentrations in rats would not occur in humans following ingestion,[2] and (2) lack of many consistent overt serious effects reported in clinical trials.

However, individuals with shellfish allergy should be cautious about use of glucosamine products, many of which are derived from shellfish.

C. Unresolved Issues and Uncertainties in the Available Data

- As mentioned above, few animal or human studies have been designed for evaluating the safety of glucosamine intake. In some studies, data concerning adverse effects was obtained by passive reporting, which is not optimal.
- The impact of increased glucosamine intake during pregnancy and lactation, especially in the context of insulin resistance, is unknown.
- The impact of increased glucosamine intake in the individual with liver disease, especially in the context of insulin resistance, is unknown.
- The impact of increased glucosamine intake in children is unknown.

D. Data Gaps and Future Research Recommended

- The impact of glucosamine on insulin secretion needs further animal and human study at doses relevant to human oral intake.
- Details of the metabolism of glucosamine are still unclear and, as mentioned above, the conclusions about glucosamine safety are dependent on glucosamine being only minimally bioavailable in the bloodstream.

[2]The highest blood concentration possible from ingestion of 1.5 g of glucosamine per day is 1 mM (assuming 7 liters blood volume), assuming no loss due to lack of absorption or metabolism. However, glucosamine does appear to be extensively metabolized.

- Long-term safety evaluation of glucosamine as a dietary supplement is needed (beyond 3 years of usage).

All future trials should have a systematic collection, evaluation, and reporting of adverse events, and key data relevant to addressing the gaps in knowledge should be collected and reported.

Appendix F

Melatonin: Prototype Monograph Summary[1]

V. SUMMARY AND CONCLUSIONS

A. Summary

Melatonin, a substance normally produced in the human body, is a dietary supplement available in the United States in a synthetic form. Upon stimulation by norepinephrine, pinealocytes synthesize melatonin from serotonin. In humans, under normal circumstances, the synthesis of melatonin has a circadian rhythm. The levels of endogenous melatonin can be decreased due to various disease states or physiological conditions. It is common to find decreased levels of melatonin in people with insomnia.

---

[1]This is a summary of a prototype monograph, prepared for the purpose of illustrating how a safety review of a dietary supplement ingredient might be prepared following the format described in this report. While it was prepared as a prototype using the processes described in the report, it was not conducted under the auspices of the Food and Drug Administration utilizing all the resources available to the agency. Thus some pertinent information not available to the Committee could be of importance in evaluating safety to determine if use of this dietary supplement ingredient would present an unreasonable risk of illness or injury. Also, the development and review of this prototype was conducted by individuals whose backgrounds are in general aspects of evaluating science and whose expertise is not necessarily focused specifically on this dietary ingredient, although significant additional assistance was provided by consultants with relevant expertise. Therefore, this prototype monograph, while extensive, does not represent an authoritative statement regarding the safety of this dietary supplement ingredient. The full prototype monograph and its data tables on melatonin may be accessed at http://www.iom.edu/fnb.

The literature on melatonin includes reports of adverse effects reported with human melatonin use at 10 mg/day or less to include central nervous system effects (e.g., somnolence, headaches, increased frequency of seizures, nightmares), cardiovascular effects (e.g., hypotension or hypertension), gastrointestinal effects (e.g., diarrhea, abdominal pain), and dermatological effects. In addition, melatonin use at higher doses (240–1,000 mg/day) in a small number of subjects was associated with hormonal changes that were inconsistent among the different reports. This summary explores the quality and other factors that may have contributed to serious adverse events.

The available data on melatonin safety in humans are based mostly on reports of studies with small numbers of participants that were not designed to evaluate the safety of melatonin. This monograph is based on 48 studies and reports of melatonin use in humans that included over 1,000 subjects (in the melatonin arms). The range of melatonin doses used in these studies is wide, 0.1 to 1,000 mg. These studies vary from one-time ingestion of melatonin to 6 months of daily ingestion. Many studies omit statements about adverse effects or state that no adverse effects were observed without describing the safety parameters monitored. Moreover, there is insufficient information on interactions of melatonin with drugs or other dietary supplements. Most available studies were conducted with adults, and little information is available for infants and young children regarding adverse effects, specifically concerning possible melatonin-induced alterations of pubertal development. Likewise, there is no information on safety of melatonin use by pregnant or lactating women.

The LD_{50} of melatonin in animal models (1–3 g/kg body weight for oral doses in rats and mice) far exceeded the typical doses used as a dietary supplement in humans (0.5–10 mg/d). At a dose of 20 mg/L in drinking water, melatonin was associated with an increased rate of spontaneous tumors in one strain (CBA) of female mice. However, more recent studies by the same group showed the same amount of melatonin administered to another strain (SHR) of female mice had no effect on tumor rate. Thus the data on the effect of melatonin on tumor incidence in mice is inconclusive and this area of investigation should continue to be monitored. (This monograph focus is on understanding and interpreting these data, as limited resources were instead focused on human data.) In addition, it has been well established that melatonin has significant effects on the reproductive axis in animals (Reiter, 1991; Rivest et al., 1986). These effects might be undesirable if they occured in humans.

B. Conclusions and Recommendations About the Safety of the Ingredient Based on the Strength of the Scientific Evidence

Based on the available data, it appears that short-term use of melatonin in a daily amount of 10 mg or less does not raise concern of harm for healthy adults who are not taking concurrent medications or other dietary supplements. The basis for each of these qualifications is explained below. Long-term use of melatonin increases the level of concern because use for periods longer than a few weeks has not been documented except in a small number of subjects or for therapeutic uses (e.g., entrainment of blind individuals). Use of melatonin in amounts above 10 mg per day increases the level of concern because there are only a few clinical studies using these amounts and, in some, serious adverse effects were observed. Use of melatonin in populations other than healthy adults increases the level of concern based in part on the observation that serious adverse effects reported at 10 mg or less of melatonin per day generally occurred in humans with pre-existing medical or psychological conditions that may have contributed to the ill effects. Specifically, concern of harm exists for individuals with one or more of the following: (1) past or current depression; (2) cardiovascular problems; (3) seizure disorders; (4) immune system disorders; (5) chronic liver disease; (6) chronic kidney disease; (7) predisposition to headaches; especially migraine headaches; and (8) concurrent use of anticonvulsant, sedative, hypnotic, or psychotropic medications. One exception to the lack of concern of harm in healthy adults is that women attempting to become pregnant should be aware that melatonin may affect reproductive function, including possible effects on hormone levels (Forsling et al., 1999; Ninomiya et al., 2001; Okatani and Sagara, 1993; Pawlikowski et al., 2002). Use of melatonin by children cannot be recommended without supervision by a physician due to the lack of data available for individuals below the age of 18 years and possible effects on hormone levels (Forsling et al., 1999; Luboshitzky et al., 2002; Ninomiya et al., 2001; Okatani and Sagara, 1993; Pawlikowski et al., 2002; Valcavi et al., 1987).

Even among healthy adults, caution about use of melatonin should be considered for (1) individuals participating in functions that require alertness (e.g., operating a motor vehicle or machinery), (2) lactating women, and (3) individuals ingesting medications or other dietary supplements.

C. Unresolved Issues and Uncertainties in the Available Data

Uncertainty about potential for harm with the use of melatonin remains because of the following factors:

- Human data are from very short-term and relatively short-term treatment studies that were not designed to examine safety. Few studies included children.
- Many of the available studies in humans included small numbers of participants and varied greatly in duration of treatment, from a single dose to dosing for a few weeks or months.
- Few investigators described systematic collection of adverse effects in clinical trials.
- There is uncertainty in the dose-response relationship for adverse effects.
- The risk of harm from doses greater than 10 mg/day is unknown.

D. Data Gaps and Future Research Recommended

- All future clinical trials should include systematic collection and evaluation of adverse effects.
- Dose-dependent safety studies in adults and children are needed. These studies should include investigations of the potential for harm in individuals taking more than 10 mg of melatonin per day.
- The literature should continue to be monitored for signs of melatonin effects on tumors and testes.
- The long-term safety of melatonin use in adults and children needs further study. These studies should include close monitoring of individuals with cardiovascular disease, specifically hypotension.
- More information is needed concerning possible interactions between melatonin and drugs, particularly various cardiovascular, psychotropic, and anticonvulsant drugs.

REFERENCES

Forsling ML, Wheeler MJ, Williams AJ. 1999. The effect of melatonin administration on pituitary hormone secretion in man. *Clin Endocrinol (Oxf)* 51:637–642.

Luboshitzky R, Shen-Orr Z, Nave R, Lavi S, Lavie P. 2002. Melatonin administration alters semen quality in healthy men. *J Androl* 23:572–578.

Ninomiya T, Iwatani N, Tomoda A, Miike T. 2001. Effects of exogenous melatonin on pituitary hormones in humans. *Clin Physiol* 21:292–299.

Okatani Y, Sagara Y. 1993. Role of melatonin in nocturnal prolactin secretion in women with normoprolactinemia and mild hyperprolactnemia. *Am J Obstet Gynecol* 168:854–861.

Pawlikowski M, Kolomecka M, Wojtczak A, Karasek M. 2002. Effects of six months melatonin treatment on sleep quality and serum concentrations of estradiol, cortisol, dehydroepiandrosterone sulfate, and somatomedin C in elderly women. *Neuroendocrinol Lett* 23:17–19.

Reiter RJ. 1991. Pineal gland: Interface between the photoperiodic environment and the endocrine system. *Trends Endocrinol Metab* 2:13–19.

Rivest RW, Aubert ML, Lang U, Sizonenko PC. 1986. Puberty in the rat: Modulation by melatonin and light. *J Neural Transm Suppl* 21:81–108.

Valcavi R, Dieguez C, Azzarito C, Edwards CA, Dotti C, Page MD, Portioli I, Scanlon MF. 1987. Effect of oral administration of melatonin on GH responses to GRF 1-44 in normal subjects. *Clin Endocrinol (Oxf)* 26:453–458.

Appendix G

Chromium Picolinate: Prototype Monograph Summary[1]

V. SUMMARY AND CONCLUSIONS

Chromium picolinate is chromium(III) trispicolinate, the chromium salt of three picolinic acid molecules. The chemical formula of chromium picolinate is $C_{18}H_{12}CrN_3O_6$, and the formula weight is 418. Chromium is present in the diet and in human tissues. The normal range of plasma chromium values is 0.1 to 2.1 μg/mL (Cerulli et al., 1998). The content of chromium in human liver has been reported at 5.4 to 470 η/g wet weight liver (~0.1–9 μM) (Versieck, 1985). The tolerable upper intake level for chromium is 25 μg/day (IOM, 2001). The estimated chromium content of

[1]This is a summary of a prototype monograph, prepared for the purpose of illustrating how a safety review of a dietary supplement ingredient might be prepared following the format described in this report. While it was prepared as a prototype using the processes described in the report, it was not conducted under the auspices of the Food and Drug Administration utilizing all the resources available to the agency. Thus some pertinent information not available to the Committee could be of importance in evaluating safety to determine if use of this dietary supplement ingredient would present an unreasonable risk of illness or injury. Also, the development and review of this prototype was conducted by individuals whose backgrounds are in general aspects of evaluating science and whose expertise is not necessarily focused specifically on this dietary ingredient, although significant additional assistance was provided by consultants with relevant expertise. Therefore, this prototype monograph, while extensive, does not represent an authoritative statement regarding the safety of this dietary supplement ingredient. The full prototype monograph and its data tables on chromium picolinate may be accessed at http://www.iom.edu/fnb.

the usual diet consumed in the United States is 15 μg/1,000 kcal (Anderson and Kozlovsky, 1985).

Picolinic acid, as an endogenous metabolite of tryptophan metabolism, is present in human tissues only in trace amounts (Rebello et al., 1982). Some picolinic acid is expected to be present in the diet in small amounts; however, this subject has not been studied extensively.

Chromium picolinate is widely included in dietary supplements, especially in multivitamin, multimineral products. These supplements are usually available in capsule or tablet form.

Typical amounts of chromium picolinate used in multivitamin, multimineral dietary supplements range from 50 to 400 μg/day. Specialty dietary supplements may contain much more chromium picolinate and may include other forms of both chromium and picolinate. Chromium picolinate is also readily available in single-ingredient preparations or in combination with a few ingredients.

A. Summary

This monograph summary considers the safety of chromium picolinate as well as Cr(III) and picolinic acid to the degree to which they are expected to impact the safety of chromium picolinate.

The human data regarding chromium picolinate safety was derived from 17 randomized, double-blind, placebo-controlled human clinical trials of oral chromium picolinate; 2 similar trials (confounded by the choice of subjects with gestational diabetes or publication in German); 3 crossover-design trials; 1 uncontrolled study in subjects with diabetes; 1 phase II study; 2 pilot studies; 1 questionnaire; 11 clinical case reports; 1 case series report; and 21 spontaneous adverse event reports to Special Nutrition/Adverse Event Monitoring System where chromium picolinate was the lone supplement reported. Data were also examined from adverse event reports in which two or more supplements containing chromium picolinate were ingested; all of these reports involved serious adverse events.

Animal and *in vitro* general toxicity data, as well as data addressing the questions raised by human data, were collected using literature searches. The quality and quantity of the data from *in vitro*, animal, and human experiments and studies is good and also reasonable. The benchmark for this conclusion is the quality and quantity of data for nutritional supplements in general. Data from questionable sources outside the widely accepted medical literature were included in footnotes to the data tables in the full monograph to indicate awareness of this data; however, little value was placed on this type of data.

No consistent, frequent adverse events were evident from the human data, although most of the human studies were not informative with regard to adverse effects of chromium picolinate that might manifest after long-term consumption. Similarly, no clear or distinct patterns were observed from the diverse congeries of literature.

Possible concerns arise from *in vitro* data that suggest Cr(III) increases oxidative stress and carcinogenesis (including carcinogenesis that may not be mediated by oxidative stress). However, data about such intracellular effects of Cr(III) (e.g., DNA fragmentation) are difficult to integrate into the evaluation of the safety of chromium picolinate as a dietary supplement; it is not clear whether intracellular Cr(III) concentrations sufficient to cause nuclear mutations and/or oxidative stress would result from chromium picolinate ingestion at doses found in the dietary supplements. Controversy concerning the relevance of *in vitro* studies to human health commonly evolves from a general skepticism about the physiologic relevance of high intracellular concentrations attained during *in vitro* studies. In the case of chromium picolinate, the controversy comes from a different source; a particular question arises about picolinate as a carrier of chromium into the cell and the subsequent release of Cr(III). At this time, there is insufficient experimental data to evaluate the long-term safety of chromium picolinate regarding carcinogenesis.

The human studies evaluated would not have detected carcinogenesis; only two of the studies might have detected oxidative stress if it did occur. These two studies examined measures indicative of oxidative stress and did not detect them; an 8-week study using 400 μg/day of Cr(III) failed to demonstrate oxidative damage to DNA (Kato et al., 1998), and a 12-week study using 924 μg/day Cr(III) failed to demonstrate a shift from protein-bound iron to the free (reactive) metal ion (Campbell et al., 1997). Additionally, animal studies provide some mitigation of the concern raised by *in vitro* studies; a 24-week study in female Sprague-Dawley rats with chromium picolinate (up to 100 μg Cr(III)/g diet) and lifespan studies in several strains of rats with chromium chloride (at 5–25 ppm Cr(III) in the drinking water) or chromium oxide (up to 5 percent w/w in bread dough) failed to demonstrate toxicity or carcinogenicity.

B. Conclusions and Recommendations About the Safety of the Ingredient Based on the Strength of the Scientific Evidence

Considering the totality of the data reviewed, there is no consistent evidence of reasonable expectation of harm from chromium picolinate. There is also not sufficient evidence to raise concern regarding the safety or toxicity of chromium picolinate when used in the intended manner for a length of time consistent with the published clinical data, that is, up to 1.6 mg of chromium picolinate/day (200 μg of Cr(III)/day) for 3 to 6 months.

This conclusion is consistent with the findings of the Agency for Toxic

Substances and Disease Registry in a recent toxicological profile for chromium (ATSDR, 2000).

C. Unresolved Issues and Uncertainties in the Available Data

There are some unresolved issues given the currently available data regarding the safety of chromium picolinate. However, at this time, the totality of the data does not indicate an urgent need for additional research studies or data gathering. An issue of concern is the lack of information on the long-term effects of chronic chromium picolinate at the recommended doses. Long-term effects might be addressed by determining if ingestion of chromium picolinate in the amount and duration typical of dietary supplements results in sufficient intracellular Cr(III) concentration to cause nuclear damage and/or oxidative stress.

The individual usage patterns of chromium picolinate are needed in a published format that is readily accepted by the scientific community. To know how many people take how much chromium and for how long is an important consideration in evaluating long-term safety.

Since there are studies in which adverse effects are not mentioned or in which the rate of subject withdrawal data is missing, it is advised that the authors of those studies be contacted and specifics be obtained.

D. Data Gaps and Future Research Recommended

There are no recommendations for future research at this time.

REFERENCES

Anderson RA, Kozlovsky AS. 1985. Chromium intake, absorption and excretion of subjects consuming self-selected diets. *Am J Clin Nutr* 41:1177–1183.

ATSDR (Agency for Toxic Substances and Disease Registry). 2000. *Toxicologial Profile for Chromium*. Atlanta: ATSDR.

Campbell WW, Beard JL, Joseph LJ, Davey SL, Evans WJ. 1997. Chromium picolinate supplementation and resistive training by older men: Effects on iron-status and hematologic indexes. *Am J Clin Nutr* 66:944–949.

Cerulli J, Grabe DW, Gauthier I, Malone M, McGoldrick MD. 1998. Chromium picolinate toxicity. *Ann Pharmacother* 32:428–431.

IOM (Institute of Medicine). 2001. *Dietary Reference Intakes for Vitamin A, Vitamin K, Arsenic, Boron, Chromium, Copper, Iodine, Iron, Manganese, Molybdenum, Nickel, Silicon, Vanadium, and Zinc*. Washington, DC: National Academy Press.

Kato I, Vogelman JH, Dilman V, Karkoszka J, Frenkel K, Durr NP, Orentreich N, Toniolo P. 1998. Effect of supplementation with chromium picolinate on antibody titers to 5-hydroxymethyl uracil. *Eur J Epidemiol* 14:621–626.

Rebello T, Lonnerdal B, Hurley LS. 1982. Picolinic acid in milk, pancreatic juice, and intestine: Inadequate for role in zinc absorption. *Am J Clin Nutr* 35:1–5.

Versieck J. 1985. Trace elements in human body fluids and tissues. *Crit Rev Clin Lab Sci* 22:97–184.

Appendix H

Saw Palmetto: Prototype Monograph Summary[1]

V. SUMMARY AND CONCLUSIONS

A. Summary

Saw palmetto is a dietary supplement with a long history of human use. Currently, it appears to be used primarily by men. The plant part typically used in dietary supplements is the fruit. A primary form of saw palmetto currently marketed is an *n*-hexane extract of the fruit, which is rich in lipids. Other forms include ethanol extracts of the fruit and powdered dried, ripe fruit. In addition to lipids, other known chemical components of

[1]This is a summary of a prototype monograph, prepared for the purpose of illustrating how a safety review of a dietary supplement ingredient might be prepared following the format described in this report. While it was prepared as a prototype using the processes described in the report, it was not conducted under the auspices of the Food and Drug Administration utilizing all the resources available to the agency. Thus some pertinent information not available to the Committee could be of importance in evaluating safety to determine if use of this dietary supplement ingredient would present an unreasonable risk of illness or injury. Also, the development and review of this prototype was conducted by individuals whose backgrounds are in general aspects of evaluating science and whose expertise is not necessarily focused specifically on this dietary ingredient, although significant additional assistance was provided by consultants with relevant expertise. Therefore, this prototype monograph, while extensive, does not represent an authoritative statement regarding the safety of this dietary supplement ingredient. The full prototype monograph and its data tables on saw palmetto may be accessed at http://www.iom.edu/fnb.

saw palmetto fruit include flavonoids, polyisoprenoids, and saccharides. The identity of the biologically active constituents has not been firmly established. Preparations of saw palmetto powdered fruit and saw palmetto extracts are typically analyzed for fatty acid content. Currently, the majority of saw palmetto is obtained from the southern coastal United States. It should be noted that the chemical profile of any plant may vary substantially if it is collected from a significantly different environment.

The typical daily amount ingested (usually by men with benign prostatic hyperplasia) is 320 mg of lipid/sterol extract of saw palmetto (LESP). The historical use of the plant was limited to whole fruit and teas; however, current widespread usage is primarily as the LESP. There are also blended products that include saw palmetto as one ingredient in a sometimes complex mixture of botanical or other ingredients. One such blend, PC-SPES, was found to be contaminated with the drug warfarin and was voluntarily withdrawn from the market in 2002. The safety/toxicity of blended products is not addressed in this prototype monograph, although the information about such combinations was considered to determine if it was relevant to the safety of saw palmetto.

The evidence regarding the safety of saw palmetto extracts was derived from nine randomized, double-blind, placebo-controlled clinical trials and three reference-controlled human clinical trials. It should be pointed out that these studies used a variety of preparations of saw palmetto fruit extracts. Numerous other studies have been conducted, but their usefulness was limited by publication in foreign languages, deficiencies in experimental design, or deficiencies in the published record. There has been one clinical case report of a serious adverse effect (hemorrhage during an operative procedure) possibly associated with saw palmetto consumption; however, the specific preparation or product and dosage were not reported and the symptoms could be consistent with a contaminated blended product, such as contamination by the anticoagulant warfarin. Although there have been four Special Nutrition/Adverse Event Monitoring System reports, there was no indication of clear causal relationships with saw palmetto. To date, there have been no reports of studies on drug interactions.

Some animal studies showed antiandrogenic effects on hyperplasia. These effects themselves were not considered to have serious implications to the safety of saw palmetto in older men, but they are consistent with saw palmetto being bioavailable and bioactive following oral ingestion and are consistent with saw palmetto's purported beneficial antiandrogenic effects in humans. Also consistent are *in vitro* studies demonstrating some biological effects such as inhibition of steroid 5-α-reductase and antagonism of α_1-adrenergic receptors.

Of the chemical constituents known to be present in saw palmetto fruit, none are recognized as toxic substances. Likewise, the plant family, Arecaceae, is not generally regarded as a toxic plant family.

Based on the limited *in vitro* studies to date, functionally related substances might include drugs that are inhibitors of steroid 5-α-reductase or antagonists of α_1-adrenergic receptors. In general, these drugs are contraindicated for women and children (GlaxoSmithKline, 2001; Thomson PDR, 2004). Pregnant women are even cautioned not to touch broken tablets containing inhibitors of steroid 5-α-reductase (GlaxoSmithKline, 2001; Thomson PDR, 2004). Concern with these drugs are that *in utero* effects of inhibiting testosterone synthesis or action can deleteriously affect the external genitalia and internal reproductive organs of a male fetus (Bowman et al., 2003; Clark et al., 1990, 1993; GlaxoSmithKline, 2001).

B. Conclusions and Recommendations About the Safety of the Ingredient Based on the Strength of the Scientific Evidence

At the present time, the weight of the scientific evidence does not suggest that the consumption of saw palmetto powdered fruit or fruit extracts poses a safety risk when consumed by men at the currently recommended doses. These conclusions are germane only to the fruit and fruit extracts presently used; introduction of new products involving different plant parts would warrant further scrutiny.

However, unlike for men, the reported adverse side effects for drugs that inhibit steroid 5-α-reductase or antagonize α_1-adrenergic receptors raise concern about women who may become pregnant while using saw palmetto. This concern is mitigated somewhat by the apparent popularity of saw palmetto with men rather than women, but as noted, saw palmetto use is not limited to men. It is not evident that the testosterone pathway effects raise concerns about the safe use of saw palmetto fruit or fruit extracts in men.

C. Unresolved Issues and Uncertainties in the Available Data

- Additional phytochemical analyses of the fruit and, especially, of the various fruit extracts (in which minor components would be expected to be concentrated) are needed in order to determine the presence of biologically active chemical components.
- *In vitro* reports of cytotoxicity in prostate cancer cell lines have not been extended to other cell types in order to ascertain whether there is broader cytotoxicity.

D. Data Gaps and Future Research Recommended

- Additional phytochemical analyses to identify the biologically active components should be a high priority. Once biologically active components are identified, further biological evaluation should be conducted. Safety concerns should be revisited upon identification of additional components.
- There is a need to establish the mechanism of action of saw palmetto preparations.
- There are insufficient data to conclude that there are no drug interactions between saw palmetto preparations and conventional prescription drugs.
- Studies to establish the effects of saw palmetto products on bleeding times could shed additional light on the possible causal relationship of saw palmetto to the single clinical case report of excessive bleeding during surgery.
- Studies could shed light on the possibility of detrimental effects on the fetus.

REFERENCES

Bowman CJ, Barlow NJ, Turner KJ, Wallace DG, Foster PMD. 2003. Effects of *in utero* exposure to finasteride on androgen-dependent reproductive development in the male rat. *Toxicol Sci* 74:393–406.

Clark RL, Antonello JM, Grossman SJ, Wise LD, Anderson C, Bagdon WJ, Prahalada S, MacDonald JS, Robertson RT. 1990. External genitalia abnormalities in male rats exposed *in utero* to finasteride, a 5 alpha-reductase inhibitor. *Teratology* 42:91–100.

Clark RL, Anderson CA, Prahalada S, Robertson RT, Lochry EA, Leonard YM, Stevens JL, Hoberman AM. 1993. Critical developmental periods for effects on male rat genitalia induced by finasteride, a 5 alpha-reductase inhibitor. *Toxicol Appl Pharmacol* 119:34–40.

GlaxoSmithKline. 2001. *Approval Package. Duagen (Dutasteride) Soft Gel Capsules. Pharmacology Reviews.* Online. Available at http://www.fda.gov/cder/foi/nda/2001/21319_Duagen.htm. Accessed January 8, 2003.

Thomson PDR. 2004. *Physicians' Desk Reference.* 58th ed. Montvale, NJ: Thomson PDR.

Appendix I

Shark Cartilage: Prototype Monograph Summary[1]

V. SUMMARY AND CONCLUSIONS

A. Summary

Shark cartilage is not a defined single product. Native shark cartilage is harvested as the tough elastic cartilage, or endoskeleton, of multiple species of shark and contains proteins, proteoglycans, glycosaminoglycans, minerals, carbohydrate, and lipid. Because of harvest conditions, preparations are often contaminated by other shark tissues (e.g., shark liver containing squalamine) and possibly by heavy metals (e.g., mercury) and bacterial and viral contaminants acquired during storage and/or processing.

---

[1]This is a summary of a prototype monograph prepared for the purpose of illustrating how a safety review of a dietary supplement ingredient might be prepared following the format described in this report. While it was prepared as a prototype using the processes described in the report, it was not conducted under the auspices of the Food and Drug Administration utilizing all the resources available to the agency. Thus some pertinent information not available to the Committee could be of importance in evaluating safety to determine if use of this dietary supplement ingredient would present an unreasonable risk of illness or injury. Also, the development and review of this prototype was conducted by individuals whose backgrounds are in general aspects of evaluating science and whose expertise is not necessarily focused specifically on this dietary ingredient, although significant additional assistance was provided by consultants with relevant expertise. Therefore, this prototype monograph, while extensive, does not represent an authoritative statement regarding the safety of this dietary supplement ingredient. The full prototype monograph and its data tables on shark cartilage may be accessed at http://www.iom.edu/fnb.

Several very different products are marketed as "shark cartilage," including aqueous extracts of the homogenized cartilage, and the processing of powdered shark cartilage preparations may include extensive washing, soaking, and/or bleaching. These processes may deplete the product of any readily water-extractable components. While one aqueous extract and a powdered shark cartilage preparation are presently being used in clinical trials to investigate its antitumor potential, information about the composition of this or any other product is not currently available in the public domain. In the absence of information about the specific composition of a shark cartilage product, it must be assumed that adverse effects seen in one product apply to all products labeled as shark cartilage.

Human data: Shark cartilage dietary supplements are taken for a variety of conditions. Case reports occasionally mention nonserious side effects such as nausea, vomiting, diarrhea, constipation, and flatulence, but it is unclear whether such effects are due to the supplement, palatability issues, or placebo effects. Serious adverse effects, such as hepatotoxicity, have been anecdotally reported, but specific susceptibility, confounding causes, or other contributing factors were not adequately assessed in the reports. Serious adverse effects have not been observed in clinical trials of specific shark cartilage preparations, but most of these studies are in progress. The studies published to date have not been randomized, double-blind, placebo-controlled trials.

Animal data: Animal toxicity studies have been conducted using various types and amounts of shark cartilage preparations and using various routes of administration and laboratory animal species. Details of these studies are not published or available to assess the adequacy of animal toxicity; however, information from summaries and abstracts of nonpublished data do not indicate overt toxicity.

In vitro ***data:*** Shark cartilage extracts have been shown to inhibit angiogenesis in cell culture experiments. Extracts specifically inhibit the proliferation of endothelial cells in culture media and inhibit the activities of vascular endothelial growth factor and basic fibroblast growth factor in accepted assays for angiogenesis. *In vitro* studies and other data also demonstrate that shark cartilage powder and extracts possess matrix metalloprotease inhibitors; inhibition of metalloproteinases inhibits angiogenesis. Antiangiogenesis activity of shark cartilage has been confirmed in chick embryonic chorioallantoic membrane (CAM), an accepted assay for angiogenesis. There are no published studies demonstrating antiangiogenic activity in whole animals using shark cartilage via the oral route.

Related substances: Related dietary supplements include bovine cartilage, chondroitin sulfate, and glucosamine. The safety of these substances was not thoroughly reviewed for this prototype monograph.

Since antiangiogenic activity has been suggested as the mechanism of action of shark cartilage preparations and *in vitro* studies have shown antiangiogenic potential, it is relevant to consider safety cautions in place for other compounds with antiangiogenic activity (i.e., functional relatedness as described in Chapter 6). Indeed, there is a potential for adverse side effects when angiogenesis is inhibited. For example, thalidomide, a known teratogen, has antiangiogenic activity. Clinical trials using other antiangiogenic agents have reported a wide variety of adverse effects, including neurotoxic effects.

Other information: Squalamine, a potential contaminant during processing, has been associated with reversible nonserious side effects (when administered by intravenous infusion to subjects with advanced-stage cancer).

B. Conclusions and Recommendations About the Safety of the Ingredient Based on the Strength of the Scientific Evidence

There is a substantial lack of safety data for shark cartilage both clinically and in animal toxicity studies, including a lack of any serious adverse event reports. In the context of the large numbers of individuals that have been exposed, the lack of serious acute adverse event reports may be indicative of no serious overt acute toxicity. However, chronic toxicity has not been systematically evaluated. Shark cartilage does not appear to be associated with any serious adverse events, even when taken chronically in gram quantities; however, nonserious side effects have been reported. Nonserious side effects, especially nausea and vomiting, may motivate the individual to discontinue consumption. It should be noted that most clinical trials involved critically ill individuals and thus these gastrointestinal disturbances may be associated with other clinical circumstances or treatments. The incidence of these nonserious side effects is in the range of side effects expected in a placebo group. Although the available evidence does not indicate sufficient evidence for concern about shark cartilage as a dietary supplement ingredient, there has not been a systematic and scientific safety evaluation of shark cartilage.

Antiangiogenesis: There is a body of evidence that some shark cartilage preparations, when tested *in vitro*, contain a substance that has antiangiogenic properties. A common assay used to demonstrate angiogenicity (i.e., chick embryonic CAM assay) has also been used to determine antiangiogenic activity with shark cartilage preparations. Since thalidomide, a known teratogenic agent, has antiangiogenic effects as one of its mechanisms, it is reasonable to have concerns that the long-term use of shark cartilage preparations could produce teratogenic effects. Antiangiogenic effects might contribute to abnormal fetal development and other physiological conditions (i.e., delayed tissue repair) in which angiogenesis is crucial to the formation of normal structures.

Neurotoxicity: Clinical trials are under way based on the presumption that shark cartilage has antiangiogenic activity *in vivo*. Based on limited animal and *in vitro* studies, there is no evidence to suggest neurotoxicity. Antiangiogenic agents, based on limited animal and *in vitro* studies, show no evidence that suggests neurologic toxicity. However, both peripheral and central nervous system toxicity have been reported in a review of short-term clinical studies. Adverse effects included central and peripheral neuropathies (e.g., sustained paralysis, cerebellar ataxia, spastic diplegia, sensory neuropathy, sedation, headache), with some toxicities resolving upon discontinuation of the antiangiogenic agent.

These clinical observations support a potential association between shark cartilage preparations with purported antiangiogenic activity and adverse neurological effects. It should be recognized that the subjects in the shark cartilage clinical trials had advanced cancer, other chronic disease, and/or were taking concurrent medications. Many angiogenic mediators can act as neurotrophic factors, and this bioactivity may contribute to neurological abnormalities. Additional studies are warranted to establish the neurotoxic risk from antiangiogenic agents.

C. Unresolved Issues and Uncertainties in the Available Data

It is very difficult to address the safety of this substance because of the lack of its characterization. There is no generally accepted standard composition of shark cartilage supplements. There are several different products labeled as shark cartilage, and composition differs among them. It is not known if composition changes by batch as well as by product, thereby potentially influencing safety. No active ingredient of shark cartilage preparations has been defined. Furthermore, the effect of processing during the preparation of different products on the bioactivity/bioavailability of the components of shark cartilage is unknown. At this time it cannot be determined whether any of the potential safety issues are relevant to specific shark cartilage preparations or to shark cartilage in general.

D. Data Gaps and Future Research Recommended

Although the available evidence does not indicate sufficient evidence for concern about shark cartilage as a dietary supplement ingredient, there has not been a systematic and scientific safety evaluation of it.

Clinical trials are under way with various preparations of shark cartilage, including clinical trials supported by the National Cancer Institute. These will provide data relevant to safety, and may provide insight into potential serious adverse effects. It is expected that more data will be generated within the next few years as the studies in progress unfold.

Other research needed:

- Characterization of shark cartilage products, including the identification and characterization of bioactive components.
- Analytical methods (chemical or bioactive assays) for standardization of products.
- Demonstration and quantification of bioavailability.
- Acute and chronic animal toxicological data that use currently accepted standards.
- Ongoing clinical trials that monitor side effects, evaluate safety concerns, and are designed to identify antiangiogenic activity associated with shark cartilage preparations.

Appendix J

Prototype Focused Monograph: Review of Liver-Related Risks for Chaparral[1]

I. DESCRIPTION OF THE INGREDIENT

A. Chaparral as a Dietary Supplement Ingredient

Chaparral is one name for an herbaceous woody shrub that grows in the southwestern region of the United States and the northern region of Mexico. It is also called creosote bush or greasewood. The common Spanish names are hediondilla, which means "little smelly one," because the bush has a strong odor similar to the smell of creosote (a distillate of coal/wood tar used as a wood preservative), and gobernadora, which means "governess," because the bushes can dominate an area by creating an ad-

[1]This is a focused monograph, prepared for the purpose of illustrating how a safety review of a dietary supplement ingredient might be prepared following the format for focused monographs described in this report. While it was prepared as a prototype using the processes described in the report, it was not conducted under the auspices of the Food and Drug Administration utilizing all the resources available to the agency. Thus some pertinent information not available to the Committee could be of importance in evaluating safety to determine if use of this dietary supplement ingredient would present an unreasonable risk of illness or injury. Also, the development and review of this prototype was conducted by individuals whose backgrounds are in general aspects of evaluating science and whose expertise is not necessarily focused specifically on this dietary ingredient, although significant additional assistance was provided by consultants with relevant expertise. Therefore, this prototype monograph, while extensive, does not represent an authoritative statement regarding the safety of this dietary supplement ingredient.

verse environment for the growth of other plants, resulting in a monoculture in some areas (Schultz and Floyd, 1999). One remarkable feature of the chaparral bush is the complex resinous coating on the leaves that serves as a chemical defense against grazing by herbivores and against attack by insects. The chemicals in the resin find their way into the desert soil surrounding the chaparral plant and discourage growth by other plant species, thus effectively reducing competition for water and nutrients (Mabry et al., 1977).

Chaparral is formally known as *Larrea tridentata* (Sessé and Moc. ex DC.) Coville (synonymous with *Larrea mexicana* Moric.) of Zygophyllaceae (McGuffin et al., 1997). Historically, the dry leaves, green stems, and fine twig tips of chaparral were used for various ailments. Since about 1969, these same plant components have been used as dietary supplements. Various forms have been available: dried plant material for making teas (water extracts), aqueous-alcoholic extracts or tinctures, and tablets or capsules containing ground, dried plant material. During the past 10 years, chaparral products have not been as readily available as in the past; however, each of these forms is currently available in the U.S. marketplace in varying degrees.

B. Individual Components

Table A contains a list of the components of primary interest in chaparral (i.e., present in leaves, stems, and twigs). Some components of chaparral are common in other plants and are widespread in the human diet. The major components of the resinous coating of chaparral are lignans (Mabry et al. 1977; Sakakibara et al. 1976) which can comprise up to 80 percent of some extracts of chaparral, such as methanol extracts of green leaves or green stems (Hyder, 2001). Lignans are low-molecular-weight plant products made up of phenylpropanoid dimers or trimers. Mature chaparral leaves contain lower amounts of lignans than new leaves (Gisvold and Thaker, 1974). The major lignan in chaparral is nordihydroguaiaretic acid (NDGA) (Downum et al., 1988), which is a derivative of guaiaretic acid and is a catechol having two hydroxyl groups on each of the two phenol rings. NDGA comprises approximately 10 percent of the dry leaf weight, but may be as much as 15 percent in some instances (Obermeyer et al., 1995). NDGA comprises approximately 50 percent of the phenolic resin extracted from the external surface of the leaves (Botkin and Duisberg, 1949; Mabry et al., 1977; Sakakibara et al., 1976). Chaparral also contains guaiaretic acid and other substituted guaiaretic acid derivatives (Table A). Other lignans in chaparral are classified as furanoid lignans and 1 aryl tetralin lignans. The latter are structurally related to podophyllotoxins.

Chaparral contains flavonoids as non-water-soluble aglycones, as water-soluble glycosides, and as sulfated flavonoids (Mabry et al., 1977). Chaparral also contains triterpenes, including sapogenins (Mabry et al., 1977). The aglycone forms of the flavonoids and triterpenes are listed in Table A. Chaparral contains volatile oils, wax esters, sterols, and other hydrocarbons (Mabry et al., 1977; Waller and Gisvold, 1945).

Although a number of the known components of chaparral exhibit cytotoxic activity under various conditions, these effects are judged to be weak and require high concentrations of the substance, and thus would extrapolate to the ingestion of large amounts of chaparral in order to exhibit potential toxic activity in humans. Additionally, many of these components are present in the diet from other sources.

C. Description of Dietary Supplement Preparations and Amounts Ingested in Ordinary Use

Chaparral is sold in several forms, one of which is the dried, broken leaves, green stems, and fine twig tips that can be brewed as a tea (i.e., an aqueous extract). An example of the modern preparation of chaparral tea would be to steep 7 to 8 g of crumbled dried leaves, stems, and twigs in one quart of hot water. In ordinary use as a water extract, chaparral might be consumed in the amount of 1 to 3 cups of chaparral tea per day for a period of 2 to 3 weeks (Micromedex, 2002).

Another form of chaparral is a tincture or aqueous alcohol extract. The ordinary use of such an extract might be 20 to 30 drops per day for a period of 2 to 3 weeks (Micromedex, 2002).

Chaparral is also available as a dried leaf powder (frequently sold in capsule or tablet form). Typical suggested uses of such capsules or tablets would be one to two 500-mg capsules or tablets per day for 2 to 3 weeks.

Chaparral is also available as a component of various botanical mixtures sold as tinctures and as loose leaves, stems, and twigs for teas. Chaparral dried leaf capsules are also available in combination with silymarin (a flavanolignan complex from milk thistle), vitamin C, or other antioxidants.

II. INFORMATION RELEVANT TO LIVER CONCERNS

A. Human Use Information and Safety Data

1. Historical use

Chaparral has been used for many centuries for a variety of medicinal purposes (Heron and Yarnell, 2001). Native populations in the southwestern United States have used chaparral tea for decades without published evidence of toxicity. Most processing of chaparral used in American Indian cultures involved aqueous extracts, such as hot water teas (Heron and Yarnell, 2001). A tea has very little NDGA (a constituent of concern, see below) compared with an alcoholic extract or the powdered dry leaf because NDGA is poorly soluble in water (Obermeyer et al., 1995). Pima Indians used the tea orally as a diuretic, emetic, or expectorant, and topically as an antiseptic or poultice (Mabry et al., 1977). In many American Indian cultures, chaparral tea has been used to mitigate colds, bronchitis, and other breathing problems; for menstrual cramps; and for numerous intestinal problems. It has also been applied topically for painful joints, skin infections, snakebites, burns, and allergies (Mabry et al., 1977; Moerman, 1998). The leaves have been used both as a decoction in a bath or as an external poultice for rheumatism and arthritis, as well as for scratches, wounds, and bruises (Moerman, 1998). There are a few reports of the use of chaparral extracts by southwest native healers in the management of type 2 diabetes (Gowri et al., 2000). In the medical literature there is a paucity of reports involving the ingestion of chaparral capsules or tablets, except for those resulting in adverse effects (described below).

2. Adverse effects

The clinical data suggest a pattern of hepatotoxicity. This pattern is discussed in more detail below. One difficulty in evaluating the clinical data on chaparral is that in most of the cases, the chaparral preparation ingested was not described in any detail. Additionally, the product purity and quality were not reported.

Clinical trial data: Table B provides a summary of a small clinical trial that was conducted among 59 terminal cancer patients to examine the effect of NDGA and chaparral tea on tumor growth. Thirty-six patients consumed chaparral tea (16–24 oz/d) while 23 patients consumed NDGA (250–3,000 mg/day). Selected blood tests and urinalysis were repeated at 2 to 4 week intervals. An analysis of the 45 patients who were treated for at least 4 weeks suggested that there were no hematological or chemical abnormalities that could be attributed to the treatment. Patients reported minor adverse effects as described in Table B. Of the 59 treated patients, no pattern of hepatotoxicity was reported following consumption of either chaparral tea or NDGA by the terminally ill cancer patients. The reasons why 14 subjects dropped out were not reported.

Clinical case reports: Table C-1 summarizes clinical case reports of patients who took chaparral without the added complication of additional ingredients. Careful inspection of Table C-1 reveals 9 cases of well-diagnosed hepatotoxicity (Cases #1–9) and 6 cases of suspected or probable hepatotoxicity (Cases #10–15). The cases are arranged in order of apparent severity with the most severe case, which required a liver transplant, presented as Case #1. Many of these patients ingested chaparral in capsule or tablet form (Cases #1–3, 5–11). Most of the chaparral products were unidentified as to whether they contained dried plant material or extracts. The listed amount of chaparral ingested ranged from 0.3 to 6 g/day; however, this information was not included in all case reports. The duration of chaparral use (which is not indicated in 2 of the cases) ranged from 20 days to "many years." It is notable that Case #15 was the only patient known to use chaparral tea: 4 bags daily for 1.5 years. The product used by this patient was examined using microscopic and chromatographic analysis and was correctly identified as *Larrea tridentata* with no evidence of biochemical or biological contamination (Sheikh et al., 1997). The severity of the liver damage in these case reports does not seem to correlate directly with either the amount of chaparral consumed or the duration of use. There are five cases with documented recovery from liver damage after cessation of chaparral use (Cases #2, 5, 8, 9, 10). There is one case (#8) documenting a return of jaundice following resumption of chaparral ingestion.

Table C-2 summarizes the clinical case reports of patients who took chaparral in combination with other supplements or ingredients, primarily other botanicals. The six cases of hepatotoxicity found in Table C-2 are difficult to evaluate because of the confounding factor of possible adverse effects due to these other substances. These cases include well-documented hepatotoxicity (Cases #17–20) but the cause of the liver damage is difficult to interpret. Two cases returned to normal after cessation of chaparral (Cases #18, 22). There are also reports (Cases #25–29 and Series A) of subjects taking an aqueous alcoholic extract (90 percent ethanol) as 8 to 10 percent of a formula with other herbs, ingesting a total of 30 to 240 mL over a period of 40 days to 5 months, with no indication of liver damage according to liver function tests.

Adverse event reports to Special Nutrition/Adverse Event Monitoring System (SN/AEMS): Table D presents the available information on cases reported in the SN/AEMS. The 18 reports include 12 cases indicating varying degrees of liver damage. (These 12 cases are included among the patients in Table C-1.) It should be noted that in the SN/AEMS reports there is no indication of whether a causal relationship exists between the adverse event and chaparral ingestion.

3. Interactions

There are no known interactions with chaparral.

4. Consequences of unusually large intake or chronic cumulative use

There may be adverse effects associated with consumption of excessively large amounts of chaparral (Heron and Yarnell, 2001). This type of overuse is typically related to encapsulated chaparral products.

B. Animal Studies

Animal studies on chaparral: There were no animal studies identified that showed liver toxicity as the result of chaparral administration. In studies with rats, significant toxic effects were demonstrated following administration of chaparral; however, the nature of the toxicity was not documented (Nakazato et al., 1998; Ulreich et al., 1997). The ethanol:water tincture of chaparral administered to the rats was lethal in the relatively large amounts administered in these studies. In all, there is evidence of considerable toxic effects from four different animal models: using rats (Konno et al., 1987; Nakazato et al., 1998; Ulreich et al., 1997), hamsters (Granados and Cardenas, 1994), chickens (Zamora, 1984), and insects (Mabry et al., 1977) with relatively high exposures to chaparral. In considering all of the animal studies (Table E), the evidence evaluating any aspects of the safety of chaparral in animal studies is minimal.

Acute studies on NDGA in animals: The evidence evaluating the safety of NDGA, a major component of chaparral, is more substantial but is still incomplete (Table E). NDGA administered by gavage to rats and mice was reported to have an LD_{50} of > 4 g/kg body weight. NDGA was somewhat more toxic in guinea pigs, with an LD_{50} of 0.8 g/kg body weight. Thus, the LD_{50} is less than 100× a typical human intake.

Chronic studies on NDGA in animals: Chronic studies on the safety of NDGA are limited to toxicity studies conducted primarily in small rodents (Table E). Rats fed NDGA at 0.5 percent of their diet exhibited massive hemorrhages and multiple renal cysts in experiments reported only in abstract (Cranston et al., 1947) and reviews (Lehman et al., 1951). Strong evidence has been published that NDGA fed to rats at high doses (1 or 2 percent of the diet) clearly leads to various pathological changes. In various rat models, growth inhibition and structural changes in or near the kidney have been shown to develop within 2 to 6 months (Cranston et al., 1947; Gardner et al., 1986, 1987; Lehman et al., 1951). Renal and mesenteric cysts form within 6 to 12 months of NDGA feeding (Goodman et al., 1970; Grice et al., 1968; Lehman et al., 1951). By 18 months of feeding 1 percent NDGA (Grice et al., 1968) or 6 months of feeding 2 percent NDGA (Evan and Gardner, 1979), the development of renal and mesenteric cysts is profound. The renal cysts contained degenerating tubular cells and the renal damage was predominantly in the proximal convoluted tubules. Biochemical analysis showed no free NDGA in the lymph nodes or kidney extracts; only the orthoquinone metabolite of NDGA could be detected (Grice et al., 1968).

In complementary studies, single dose administration of 250 mg of NDGA into the small intestine of rats revealed formation of the orthoquinone metabolite at the region of the ileocecal junction (Grice et al., 1968).

Studies using other species and/or other routes of administration verify the toxicity of NDGA (Giri and Hollinger, 1996; Hsu et al., 2001; Madrigal-Bujaidar et al., 1998; Mikuni et al., 1998; Telford et al., 1962).

Other observations: Pretreatment of rats with NDGA (50 mg/kg body weight, by gavage) significantly aggravated indomethacin-induced gastric ulcers (Cho and Ogle, 1987). Treatment of rats with NDGA (10 μg/kg body weight, by intravenous administration) worsened ischemia-reperfusion injury to liver (Okboy et al., 1992).

C. *In Vitro* Studies

Investigations on the *in vitro* effects of chaparral and NDGA on a variety of chemical and biological systems are summarized in Tables F-1 and F-2. While a few studies involved extracts of chaparral, most focused on the effects of NDGA, and a few considered the effects of other lignans with structural similarities to NDGA.

Some cytochrome P450 oxidations are inhibited by NDGA *in vitro* (Agarwal et al., 1991; Capdevila et al., 1988).

D. Liver-Related Information About Related Substances

Studies on taxonomically related substances: Five species of *Larrea* are recognized: the bifolate species, *L. tridentata* (native to the southwestern United States and northern Mexico), *L. divaricata* (native to northwestern Argentina and parts of Peru), and *L. cuneifolia* (native to Argentina), plus two multifolate species that grow at high altitudes, *L. nitida* (native to certain parts of South America, especially Argentina) and *L. ameghinoi* (native to a few parts of South America) (Brinker, 1993–1994). No useful safety data were found on *L. cuneifolia*, *L. nitida*, or *L. ameghinoi*. The toxicity of *L. divaricata*, a South American species that is taxonomically related to *L. tridentata*, has been studied to a very limited extent. A water extract of the dried leaves was injected into mice intraperitoneally and the LD_{50} was found to be 10 g/kg body weight for males and 4 g/kg for females (Anesini et al., 1997).

Substances related to the individual components of chaparral: Table G contains a list of substances that were considered as structurally, taxonomically, or functionally related to the components of chaparral (present in leaves, stems, and twigs). Known toxicities of these related substances were considered in evaluating the potential toxicity of chaparral. For comparison, Table A contains a listing of the known components of chaparral with the chemical structures of those that may be relevant to the safety of chaparral. In Table G it should be noted that larreantin is a potential hepatotoxin and is known to be present in the root of *L. tridentata* (Luo et al., 1988). Several mechanisms were considered whereby it might be possible that chaparral products could contain larreantin. First, chaparral root might be included with the other plant material (leaves, stems, and twigs). Second, under certain environmental conditions, a component of the root of a plant might physiologically be present in the leaves. Third, the presence of trace amounts of larreantin in the leaves, stems, or twigs could have been undetected. Although each of these mechanisms is possible, it seems unlikely that larreantin is present in chaparral preparations in significant amounts.

Functionally related substances: It was reported that NDGA is metabolized to an orthoquinone derivative (De Smet, 1993; Grice et al., 1968), which could be further metabolized by conjugation to glutathione. Because hepatic levels of glutathione are often limiting, drugs undergoing glutathione conjugation could interact negatively with the quinone derivative of NDGA by both substances drawing on glutathione reserves in the liver, leading to glutathione depletion (Slattery et al., 1987).

Knowledge about chemical structures of chaparral components: As stated above, NDGA is metabolized to an orthoquinone derivative (De Smet, 1993; Grice et al., 1968). Acetaminophen is also a quinone, but one that is understood to be cytotoxic and to cause substantial liver problems. Large doses of acetaminophen cause centrilobular hepatic necrosis (Hojo et al., 2000). The current understanding is that the hepatotoxicity of acetaminophen is due to cytochrome P450-dependent formation of N-acetyl para-(benzo)quinone imine (NAPQI) in the centrilobular region of the liver (Harman et al., 1991; Hojo et al., 2000; Holme et al., 1984).

By extrapolation, the site of chaparral toxicity might be expected to reflect the site of metabolism of NDGA to the quinone. NAPQI causes mitochondrial damage, including inhibition of oxidative phosphorylation (Andersson et al., 1990; Fujimura et al., 1995; Moore et al., 1985). Likewise, NDGA causes inhibition of the mitochondrial electron transport chain. Thus there are some similarities between NAPQI toxicity and NDGA toxicity that can be used to hypothesize a mechanism of hepatotoxicity based on the formation of a NDGA quinone. Acetaminophen-induced toxicity is also seen in the kidney, another site of metabolism of the drug to NAPQI. Therefore, one might hypothesize that chaparral ingestion would lead to toxicity in the kidney also if chaparral toxicity is related to NDGA metabolism to a toxic quinone, which is purely theoretical. Indeed, renal toxicity of NDGA is evident in animal studies (Table E).

III. OTHER RELEVANT INFORMATION

A. Sources

Chaparral grows as a wild desert shrub. It is an evergreen bush that grows in arid regions and can reach a height of 9 feet (Brinker, 1993–1994). The identification of the plant used as *L. tridentata* is very important to the safety of the chaparral product.

Misnaming and species identification: There may be some instances of substitution of another plant product for *L. tridentata*. *L. divaricata* has been commonly confused with *L. tridentata*. The two species are very similar in appearance (Brinker, 1993-1994), but originate from distinct locations. The major source of confusion is the misnaming of the two species, even in published reports of clinical or experimental data (Gisvold, 1947; Smart et al., 1970).

Contaminants and adulterants: Adulteration has not been reported.

Processing issues: As described in the human use information section, most processing of chaparral used in American Indian cultures involved aqueous extracts, such as hot water teas (Heron and Yarnell, 2001). A tea has very little NDGA compared with an alcoholic extract or the powdered dry leaf because NDGA is poorly soluble in water (Obermeyer et al., 1995).

The extraction liquid generally used to make a tincture of chaparral has a high percent of ethanol (up to 95 percent, v/v) so that the extract will contain phenolic compounds, such as NDGA and flavonoids. The amount of solvent-extractable natural products does not change considerably regardless of whether fresh or dried leaves are used in processing (Mabry et al., 1977). The solvent used does make a considerable difference in the quantity of individual components. Diethyl ether gives a high yield, as compared with 85 percent aqueous methanol, which also extracts considerable chlorophyll (Mabry et al., 1977).

Analytic issues: Analytical methods have been published for the determination of a number of components of chaparral. These methods include gas liquid chromatography, high pressure liquid chromatography, and mass spectrometric analysis of lignans (Gonzalez-Coloma et al., 1988; Obermeyer et al., 1995; Valentine et al., 1984), and the ammonium molybdate spectrophotometric assay for NDGA (Duisberg et al., 1949). Pharmacokinetic analysis of NDGA administered to mice used a method with a limit of detection of 0.5 μg/mL plasma or serum (Lambert et al., 2001).

B. Conditions of Use Suggested or Recommended in Labeling or Other Marketing Material

Common popular uses: Chaparral has had numerous ethnomedicinal, homeopathic, and folk medicine uses. Homeopathic medicine has used chaparral tea in the treatment of colds, cold sores, coughs, bronchitis, viral infections, urinary tract infections, indigestion, heartburn, abdominal cramps, enteritis, dysentery, parasites, dysmenorrhea, menstrual cramps, premenstrual syndrome, neuritis, and sciatica (Heron and Yarnell, 2001; Mabry et al., 1977). Chaparral has been used as an abortifacient and as a means to increase fertility (Heron and Yarnell, 2001). Chaparral products have been described as having a beneficial impact on liver metabolic functions (Heron and Yarnell, 2001).

In folk medicine, chaparral has been used for leukemia and many different types of cancers. It has been suggested that chaparral contains immune-stimulating polysaccharides and that NDGA may have some antitumor properties. From conventional medical sources there is anecdotal and *in vitro* evidence of cytotoxic activity with varying toxicity depending on the concentration of NDGA.

Currently chaparral is marketed to consumers for arthritis, rheumatism, and bursitis; as an antioxidant; for immune function; for various cancers, such as melanomas, leukemia, breast cancer, ovarian cancer, and Kaposi's sarcoma; as a blood and liver cleanser; as a diuretic; for colds and the flu; for herpes family viruses including herpes simplex, herpes zoster, cytomegalovirus, and Epstein-Barr; and for acne and skin disorders.

C. Liver-Related Cautions Noted

Cautions provided in labeling or other marketing material: A review of chaparral product labels and Internet marketing materials indicates that many (but not all) provide cautions to consumers to seek advice from health care providers before using the product if they have a history of liver or kidney disease or currently have digestive problems and to avoid using if pregnant or nursing. One caution indicated that the chaparral product was not intended for long-term use. Two informational websites that did not sell chaparral products suggested that people consuming chaparral tea should drink 3 cups a day for a maximum of 2 weeks unless under the care of a physician or health practitioner experienced in the use of botanical medicines. At least three informational websites that did not sell products cautioned against the use of chaparral capsules since several adverse event reports were associated with this form.

Cautions issued by manufacturing associations: In 1994 the American Herbal Products Association (AHPA) commissioned a review. Four case studies were examined and it was concluded that:

> . . . since the patients were ingesting chaparral during the time each developed acute hepatitis, most likely of a hepatocellular nature, it is reasonable to conclude a relationship exists between the ingestion and the disease. However, no clinical data were found in the medical records to indicate that chaparral is inherently a hepatic toxin. Moreover, each patient had a medical history not incompatible with prior liver disease. A fair conclusion is [that] the disease in each patient was the result of an individual idiosyncratic reaction to the drug [botanical product], possibly the result of an autoimmunologic reaction, which given the quantity of chaparral ingested in this country, must be exceedingly rare (AHPA, 2002).

Following the Food and Drug Administration (FDA) warning issued in 1992 (see Section IIIE, below), many manufacturers voluntarily removed most products containing this botanical (FDA, 1993). In 1995 AHPA recommended that if member companies chose to sell chaparral, all consumer labeling contain the following informational language:

> Seek advice from a health care practitioner before use if you have had, or may have had, liver disease. Discontinue use if nausea, fever, fatigue or jaundice (e.g., dark urine, yellow discoloration of the eyes) should occur (APHA, 2002).

D. Usage Patterns

Prevalence of use in the general population: According to a survey conducted by the Herb Research Foundation from 1973 to 1993, at least 200 tons of chaparral was sold in the U.S. market (Blumenthal, 1993). This would be equivalent to 500 million doses at 500 mg/dose. No current data are available; there has been no recent tracking of sales data.

Knowledge of use by particular groups: There are no published surveys in the literature that provide knowledge about the use of chaparral by specific groups. However, anecdotal reports suggest that indigenous American Indian groups in the southwestern United States and Hispanics may use chaparral, primarily as an aqueous extract (tea).

E. Information on Regulatory Actions

FDA actions: In late August and early September 1992, FDA and the Centers for Disease Control and Prevention (CDC) were informed of two cases in which individuals consuming chaparral over several weeks experienced severe jaundice and abdominal pain. These cases, and the potential link between acute nonviral hepatitis and chaparral, were discussed in an issue of *Morbidity and Mortality Weekly Report* (CDC, 1992).

In a press release issued in December 1992, the FDA Commissioner conveyed a public advisory against the purchase or consumption of chaparral because it was associated with acute toxic hepatitis (FDA, 1992). FDA advised chaparral users to stop taking chaparral immediately and to consult a physician if a user had a history of liver disease or was not feeling well (FDA, 1992). Subsequent warnings were issued (CFSAN, 1993).

The major lignan in chaparral is NDGA, a potent antioxidant. Beginning in 1943, NDGA (at 0.02 percent, w/w) was used as an antioxidant in many foods (Mabry et al., 1977). In 1968 NDGA lost its status as a generally recognized as safe ingredient. FDA then required removal of NDGA from most foods. The U.S. Department of Agriculture oversees the safety of meats and meat products; at this time, it allows use of NDGA as an antioxidant in lard, animal shortening, and other products that are susceptible to the development of rancidity.

Other relevant regulatory actions: Canadian regulations do not allow chaparral as a nonmedicinal ingredient for oral-use products (McGuffin et al., 1997). The current edition of the German Commission E monographs does not mention chaparral (Blumenthal, 1998).

F. Available Information on Physiological and Biochemical Aspects

Very little is known about the digestion, absorption, distribution, metabolism, and excretion of some chaparral components (triterpenes). Other components have been well characterized (i.e., fatty acids and other hydrocarbons).

There is one pharmacokinetic study on NDGA. In female mice, NDGA was administered i.v. at 50 mg/kg to yield a primary half-life of 30 min and a secondary half-life of 135 minutes, with the peak plasma concentration C_{max} being 15 μg/mL (Lambert et al., 2001). It has been reported that a major metabolite of NDGA is the orthoquinone derivative (De Smet, 1993; Grice et al., 1968).

G. Supplementary Information

No information applicable to liver concerns.

IV. TABLES ON CHAPARRAL*

Table A	Chaparral: Individual Components
Table B	Chaparral: Summary of Adverse Effects in a Clinical Trial
Table C-1	Chaparral: Summary of Clinical Case Reports
Table C-2	Summary of Clinical Case Reports and a Case Series Report with Chaparral Used in Combination
Table D	Chaparral: Summary of Adverse Event Reports
Table E	NDGA: Summary of Animal Studies
Table F-1	Chaparral: Summary of *In Vitro* Studies
Table F-2	NDGA: Summary of *In Vitro* Studies
Table G	Chaparral: Related Substances that Might Suggest Risk

V. SUMMARY AND CONCLUSIONS

A. Summary

Reports of chaparral toxicity are inconsistent. Reportedly native populations in the southwestern United States have used chaparral tea for decades without evidence of toxicity. In addition, a clinical study looking at chaparral tea and NDGA in advanced, incurable cancer patients showed no evidence of hepatotoxicity. Limitations of this study included a lack of detail on those who did not complete the trial (25 percent of the subjects). This evidence is somewhat inconsistent with other information on chaparral use, as follows.

There are nine reported cases of definite hepatotoxicity temporally related to chaparral use as a single known agent; there are an additional six cases of possible hepatotoxicity. Five of the cases exhibited documented recovery after cessation of chaparral use and one case exhibited abnormal liver function upon rechallenge. One patient required an orthotopic liver transplant but had major confounding variables, such as hepatitis C and prior drug and ethanol abuse. In all the other cases, liver function tests became significantly abnormal with clinically evident jaundice that reversed upon discontinuation of chaparral use. In at least three cases of chaparral-associated hepatotoxicity, the patient had prior history of alcohol abuse or underlying liver disease and may represent a vulnerable population.

In determining causation, one looks for a dose-response relationship.

*Tables appear at the end of this appendix.

The amount of chaparral ingested ranged from 0.3 to 6 g/day over periods ranging from 20 days to "many years." The absence of pharmacokinetic data or even characterization of the formulations ingested made it difficult to determine actual dose in the various case reports. Thus there was no apparent dose-response relationship, although evidence of toxicity was clearly reflected in abnormal liver function tests.

Another important factor in determining causation is characterization of the product responsible for the adverse effect. In most of the reported cases, the product ingested by the subject was simply described as chaparral capsules or tablets. This description does not reveal whether the contents of the capsule or tablet were dried, ground plant material or dried extract. Further, without examination of the quality of the product, contamination or adulteration cannot be ruled out.

Only in 1 out of the 15 case reports of chaparral-associated hepatotoxicity was it reported that a chaparral tea had been ingested. This is important because chaparral tea contains very little NDGA or other lipophilic compounds as compared with other preparations, such as a dried extract prepared with an organic solvent. If NDGA is the causal agent, the content of NDGA in various preparations becomes an important variable in determining causality.

Animal studies evaluating chaparral did not show hepatotoxicity. Animal studies evaluating NDGA did not exhibit hepatotoxicity, but did exhibit renal proximal tubular damage and cyst formation. In other studies, rodents exhibited both renal and hepatic toxicity in response to the toxic quinone imine from acetaminophen; this involves proximal tubular damage, but not cyst formation. A plausible mechanism in both hepatotoxicity and nephrotoxicity is the cytochrome P450-dependent metabolism of NDGA to a toxic quinone with failure to remove this reactive metabolite by conjugation if glutathione is limiting. The link between the nephrotoxicity of NDGA in animals and the hepatotoxicity of chaparral in humans is not definite, but similar links have been shown with structurally related chemicals, such as the quinone of acetaminophen.

While the human data strongly suggest an association between chaparral consumption and hepatotoxicity, a number of confounding factors also require consideration. The temporal clustering of the majority of the hepatotoxicity cases (1992–1993) provides some suggestion of a localized contamination problem. Inadequate characterization of the preparations used by individual patients does not allow determination of possible product contamination during harvesting/processing or natural alterations in composition of chaparral plants due to environmental factors. If typical chaparral preparations contained hepatotoxic principles, it is possible that many more reports of human hepatotoxicity during the period of significant chaparral use (1970–1992) would have emerged. Pre-existing liver disease, including excessive alcohol use, hepatitis, or chronic acetaminophen use, could possibly have predisposed some of the individuals to hepatotoxicity. Such possibilities are hypothetical, but the quality of the data provided in the case reports is inadequate to rule out such possibilities.

B. Conclusions and Recommendations About Liver Concerns

Conclusions (concerns and caveats): **The available literature raises concern for hepatic toxicity. The reasons for concern about hepatotoxicity and possibly related nephrotoxicity can be summarized as case reports showing a pattern of hepatotoxicity, nephrotoxicity in rats given NDGA, and *in vitro* studies showing that NDGA exhibited cytotoxic activity. The consistency and biological plausibility of these observations is strengthened by knowledge of NDGA structure and knowledge about mechanisms of quinone toxicity.**

While the human data strongly suggest an association between chaparral consumption and hepatotoxicity, a number of confounding factors also require consideration. There was a clinical study (published in 1970) in which serum glutamic-oxaloacetic transaminase (SGOT), a marker of liver damage, was evaluated; this was an uncontrolled, poorly designed study, yet no elevation in SGOT was reported. However, the subjects were critically ill cancer patients and 15 of the subjects (25 percent of the total) were removed from the study. At the time of this study, there was no awareness of a possible relationship between chaparral ingestion and hepatotoxicity; these individuals could have been removed from the study because elevations in SGOT were used to indicate a measure of general health and appropriateness, a possible criteria to remain in the study.

The temporal clustering of the majority of the hepatotoxicity cases (1992–1993) provides some suggestion of localized contamination or a variation in constituent concentration, perhaps due to inadequate characterization or lack of standardization. It is unfortunate that animal studies were not conducted at the time this cluster of hepatotoxic events was reported. During a period of 20 years (1973–1993), 200 tons of chaparral was sold on the U.S. market, equivalent to 500 million doses at 500 mg/dose. If typical chaparral preparations contained hepatotoxic principles, it is possible that many more reports of human hepatotoxicity during the period of significant chaparral use (1970–1992) would have emerged. Traditional uses of chaparral tea by native populations have not revealed reports of hepatotoxicity. Pre-existing liver disease, including excessive alcohol use, hepatitis, or chronic acetaminophen use, may have predisposed some of the individuals to hepatotoxicity. Since the quality of the data provided in the case reports is inadequate to rule them out, such possibilities remain hypothetical.

The evidence for toxicity of chaparral in humans is supported by a similar toxicity observed in animal studies using NDGA. Classic toxicity studies with NDGA were conducted in several species, and toxicity of NDGA was demonstrated over a range of doses; this is a common finding in toxicity studies using different animal species (Ashby, 2002). Of the animal studies reported, only two identified hepatic effects following administration of NDGA to rats or mice; the one mouse study used intraperitoneal administration of NDGA and is confounded by coadministration of endotoxin, a known hepatotoxin. Thus only minimal hepatotoxicity was exhibited in animals treated with NDGA. However, if toxicity of a compound is related to the site of its metabolism, hepatotoxicity would be expected because liver is the major site of xenobiotic metabolism. Instead, nephrotoxicity was the major toxicity found in rats treated with NDGA; this nephrotoxicity is discussed in detail below (Kacew, 2001).

Of the 15 reported cases of chaparral-associated hepatotoxicity, only 1 was associated with ingestion of chaparral tea, whereas 11 cases were associated with ingestion of capsules or tablets containing chaparral. If NDGA contributes to the toxicity, it is important to note that NDGA and other nonpolar compounds, including lignans, appear to be minimal in a water extract/tea in contrast to an alcoholic extract (Obermeyer et al., 1995). This differential extraction of lignans by water versus alcohol extraction (Obermeyer et al., 1995) is explained by the lipophilic character of lignans. Therefore, alcoholic extracts of leaf or other aerial plant parts would contain larger amounts of NDGA and other lipophilic compounds than a water extract/tea.

NDGA can be expected to be a substrate for cytochrome P450-dependent quinone formation based on its chemical structure, as well as on evidence discussed by Obermeyer et al. (1995). A plausible mechanism of cytotoxicity of NDGA is the cytochrome P450-dependent metabolism to a toxic quinone and failure to remove this reactive metabolite by conjugation if glutathione is limiting. The link between the nephrotoxicity of NDGA in animals and hepatotoxicity of chaparral in humans is based on the fact that both the renal proximal tubules and the liver are major sites of xenobiotic metabolism. A parallel finding has also been demonstrated in rodents; both renal and hepatic toxicity develop in response to the toxic quinone imine from acetaminophen.

Summary of the conclusions: **Although substantial limitations exist in the available information, concerns about the hepatotoxicity of chaparral remain based on the weight of the evidence discussed above. This is especially applicable for certain groups, including those with pre-existing hepatic conditions, those taking drugs that affect liver function, and those with current or prior alcohol abuse. There is more concern with ingestion of**

chaparral preparations containing leaves/stems or alcoholic extracts than with the ingestion of aqueous extracts (i.e., teas) because of the higher content of NDGA and other lipophilic compounds in the former preparations.

C. Data Gaps and Future Research Recommended

Detailed toxicity studies in animals are needed to explore the possible dose-response relationship in the development of hepatotoxicity and nephrotoxicity as the result of chaparral ingestion. In animal studies, pair feeding should be included in the experimental protocol due to possible aversion to the chow if NDGA has been added (Goodman et al., 1970). Ideally, studies should compare the different preparations of chaparral (i.e., powdered leaf, alcoholic extract, and water extract).

The differences in the chemical composition of the various preparations of chaparral need to be explored. The literature shows that a preponderance of toxicities were associated with preparations other than tea; hepatotoxicity was not reported in a clinical trial of cancer patients drinking chaparral tea. This suggests there that there are differences in the bioavailability of the various components of chaparral that result from differences in the chemical composition of the preparations. These differences need to be explored in detail.

In all further research, it is important to carry out careful product characterization. A qualified taxonomist should identify the plant material, and a botanical sample should be retained in an herbarium for future reference. It is important to carefully describe the plant part utilized. As an example, newer leaves should be distinguished from older leaves because newer leaves contain a higher proportion of the NDGA-containing resin. Chaparral roots contain a quinone not reported to be present in the aerial parts of the plants and, thus, roots should be carefully excluded. The plant material should be chemically profiled, including a quantitative determination of NDGA and other lignans. As a quality measure, there should be an analysis of metals since chaparral plants concentrate metals from the soil (Gardea-Torresdey et al., 2001). Furthermore, when reporting human experience with ingesting chaparral, the formulation is important to note. The formulation can best be critically evaluated if the manufacturer, date, and lot number are reported.

VI. LITERATURE SEARCH STRATEGY

This prototype focused monograph was prepared by excluding information not possibly related to hepatotoxicity after conducting a literature search for the full prototype monograph. This was probably a more effective approach, although more time consuming, than initially limiting searches to liver information because information not about liver toxicity *per se*, but possibly related to liver toxicity, could be identified.

To prepare the chaparral monograph, the databases indicated below were searched using the terms [chaparral] OR [Larrea tridentata] (in any field). In the AGRICOLA database, it was necessary to limit the search to exclude other meanings of the word "chaparral." These searches were conducted in April 2002 and yielded approximately 125 citations (excluding duplicate citations brought up by the various databases). The databases were independently searched for the entire genus *Larrea*, and articles pertaining to the North American plant were investigated to confirm that all articles that actually reported on *L. tridentata* were considered. Citations for many references that predate the electronic databases were collected from among the reference sections of the literature reviewed. Because the number of published articles on this topic are limited, an effort was made to collect abstracts representing research in this area. In August 2002, the databases were searched again for more recent articles and a few citations were added. A literature search on NDGA was also conducted in April 2002 and yielded approximately 325 citations (excluding duplicate citations brought up by the various databases). As NDGA is commonly used as a reagent, the search parameters were limited as follows: [nordihydroguaiaretic acid] OR [NDGA] (in title field) for most databases; [nordihydroguaiaretic acid] OR [NDGA] (in any field) for TOXLINE and AGRICOLA.

Electronic searches were conducted using the following databases: PubMed (1966–2002, TOXLINE Core inclusive), TOXLINE (TOXLINE Core and TOXLINE Special), EMBASE (1980–2002), and AGRICOLA (1979–2002). It should be noted that EMBASE contains a considerable amount of foreign literature and AGRICOLA contains a considerable amount of the veterinary literature. WorldCat, EMB/Cochrane Reviews, IBIDS, BEAST, and Dissertation Abstracts were used to a limited extent. NAPRALERT was used for natural products. Patents were accessed using the website of the U.S. Patent and Trademark Office. Information on the SN/AEMS and regulatory actions taken by FDA were obtained from the FDA website. Information on regulatory actions by the Federal Trade Commission (FTC) was obtained from the FTC website. It is highly recommended that Chemical Abstracts also be used, although this database was not used for the prototype monographs due to the limitations of time and resources. In the database search, no restriction was placed on language or type of publication. However, the ability to interpret non-English-language publications was limited. The foreign language literature was included when it was deemed important in order to be complete. The majority of the literature cited is drawn from primary research sources, followed by secondary sources as appropriate.

VII. LITERATURE CITED

ACS (American Cancer Society). 1970. *Unproven Methods of Cancer Treatment: Chaparral Tea*. New York: ACS.

Adlercreutz H, Bannwart C, Wahala K, Makela T, Brunow G, Hase T, Arosemena PJ, Kellis JT Jr, Vickery LE. 1993. Inhibition of human aromatase by mammalian lignans and isoflavonoid phytoestrogens. *J Steroid Biochem Mol Biol* 44:147–153.

Afifi FU, Al-Khalil S, Abdul-Haq BK, Mahasneh A, Al-Eisawi DM, Sharaf M, Wong LK, Schiff PL Jr. 1991. Antifungal flavonoids from *Varthemia iphionoides*. *Phytother Res* 5:173–175.

Agarwal R, Wang ZY, Bik DP, Mukhtar H. 1991. Nordihydroguaiaretic acid, an inhibitor of lipoxygenase, also inhibits cytochrome P-450-mediated monooxygenase activity in rat epidermal and hepatic microsomes. *Drug Metab Dispos* 19:620–624.

AHPA (American Herbal Products Association). 2002. *Code of Ethics and Business Conduct*. Silver Spring, MD: AHPA.

Alderman S, Kailas S, Goldfarb S, Singaram C, Malone DG. 1994. Cholestatic hepatitis after ingestion of chaparral leaf: Confirmation by endoscopic retrograde cholangiopancreatography and liver biopsy. *J Clin Gastroenterol* 19:242–247.

Andersson BS, Rundgren M, Nelson SD, Harder S. 1990. N-acetyl-p-benzoquinone imine-induced changes in the energy metabolism in hepatocytes. *Chem Biol Interact* 75:201–211.

Anesini C, Boccio J, Cremaschi G, Genaro A, Zubillaga M, Borda LS, Borda ES. 1997. *In vivo* antitumoural activity and acute toxicity study of *Larrea divaricata* Cav. extract. *Phytother Res* 11:521–523.

Ashby J. 2002. Scientific issues associated with the validation of *in vitro* and *in vivo* methods for assessing endocrine disrupting chemicals. *Toxicology* 181–182:389–397.

Banskota AH, Tezuka Y, Tran KQ, Tanaka K, Saiki I, Kadota S. 2000. Methyl quadrangularates A-D and related triterpenes from *Combretum quadrangulare*. *Chem Pharm Bull (Tokyo)* 48:496–504.

Batchelor WB, Heathcote J, Wanless IR. 1995. Chaparral-induced hepatic injury. *Am J Gastroenterol* 90:831–833.

Bernhard HO, Thiele K. 1981. Additional flavonoids from the leaves of *Larrea tridentata*. *Planta Med* 41:100–103.

Bhuvaneswaran C, Dakshinamurti K. 1972. Inhibition of electron and energy transfer in rat liver mitochondria by nordihydroguaiaretic acid. *Biochemistry (Mosc)* 11:85–91.

Biswal SS, Datta K, Shaw SD, Feng X, Robertson JD, Kehrer JP. 2000. Glutathione oxidation and mitochondrial depolarization as mechanisms of nordihydroguaiaretic acid-induced apoptosis in lipoxy-genase-deficient FL5.12 cells. *Toxicol Sci* 53:77–83.

Blalock JE, Archer DL, Johnson HM. 1981. Anticellular and immunosuppressive activities of food-borne phenolic compounds. *Proc Soc Exp Biol Med* 167:391–393.

Blumenthal M. 1993. Herb industry and FDA issue chaparral warning. *Herbalgram* 28:38–39.

Blumenthal M. ed. 1998. *Therapeutic Guide to Herbal Medicines. The Complete German Commission E Monographs*. Austin, TX: American Botanical Council.

Bohnstedt CFMTJ. 1979. The volatile constituents of the genus *Larrea* (Zygophyllaceae). *Rev Latinoamer Quim* 10:128–131.

Botkin C, Duisberg P. 1949. The Nordihydroguaiaretic Acid Content of the Creosote Bush. Bulletin 349. Las Cruces, NM: Agricultural Experiment Station, New Mexico College of Agriculture and Mechanic Arts.

Brinker F. 1993. *The Chaparral Handbook*. Portland, OR: Eclectic Medical Publications.

Brinker F. 1993–1994. *Larrea tridentata* (DC) Coville (chaparral or creosote bush*). Br J Phytother* 3:10–29.

Burba JV, Becking GC. 1969. Effect of the antioxidant nordihydroguaiaretic acid on the *in vitro* activity of catecholo-methyl transferase. *Arch Int Pharmacodyn Ther* 180:323–330.

Burk D, Woods M. 1963. Hydrogen peroxide, catalase, glutathione peroxidase, quinones, NDGA, and phosphopyridine nucleotides in relation to X-ray action on cancer cells. *Rad Res Suppl* 3:212–246.

Capdevila J, Gil L, Orellana M, Marnett LJ, Mason JI, Yadagiri P, Falck JR. 1988. Inhibitors of cytochrome P-450-dependent arachidonic acid metabolism. *Arch Biochem Biophys* 261:257–263.

CDC (Centers for Disease Control and Prevention). 1992. Chaparral-induced toxic hepatitis—California and Texas, 1992. *Morb Mortal Wkly Rep* 41:812–814.

CFSAN (Center for Food Safety and Applied Nutrition). 1993. *Illnesses and Injuries Associated with the Use of Selected Dietary Supplements.* Online. Available at http://www.cfsan.fda.gov/~dms/dsill.html. Accessed August 26, 2002.

Chae YH, Ho DK, Cassady JM, Cook VM, Marcus CB, Baird WM. 1992. Effects of synthetic and naturally occurring flavonoids on metabolic activation of benzo[a]pyrene in hamster embryo cell cultures. *Chem Biol Interact* 82:181–193.

Chang J, Skowronek MD, Cherney ML, Lewis AJ. 1984. Differential effects of putative lipoxygenase inhibitors on arachidonic acid metabolism in cell-free and intact cell preparations. *Inflammation* 8:143–155.

Chirikdjian JJ. 1973. Flavonoide von *Larrea tridentata. Zeitschrift Für Naturforschung [C]* 28C:32–35.

Chirikdjian JJ. 1974. Isolation of kumatakenine and 5,4'-dihydroxy-3,7,3'-trimethoxiflavone from *Larrea tridentata. Pharmazie* 29:292–293.

Cho CH, Ogle CW. 1987. Potentiation of indomethacinduced gastric ulcers in rats by nordihydroguaiaretic acid (NDGA), an inhibitor of lipoxygenase. *Asia Pacif J Pharmacol* 2:49–52.

Clark F, Reed R. 1992. Chaparral-induced toxic hepatitis—California and Texas, 1992. *J Am Med Assoc* 268:3295–3298.

Cranston E, Jensen MJ, Moren A, Brey T, Bell ET, Bieter RN. 1947. The acute and chronic toxicity of nordihydroguaiaretic acid. *Fed Proc* 6:318–319. Abstract.

Dahlgren C. 1991. Effect of different inhibitors on the intracellularly and extracellularly generated chemiluminescence induced by formylmethionyl-leucyl-phenylalanine in polymorphonuclear leukocytes. Cellular response in the presence of mannitol, benzoate, taurine, indomethacin and NDGA. *J Biolumin Chemilumin* 6:29–34.

Damayanthi Y, Lown JW. 1998. Podophyllotoxins: Current status and recent developments. *Curr Med Chem* 5:205–552.

De Smet PAGM. ed. 1993. *Adverse Effects of Herbal Drugs*. Vol. 2. Berlin: Springer-Verlag. Pp. 231–240.

Downum KR, Dole J, Rodriguez E. 1988. Nordihydroguaiaretic acid: Inter- and intrapopulational variation in the Sonoran Desert creosote bush (*Larrea tridentata*, Zygophyllaceae). *Biochem Syst Ecol* 16:551–555.

Duisberg PC, Shires LB, Botkin CW. 1949. Determination of NDGA in the leaf of *Larrea divericata. Anal Chem* 21:1393–1396.

Evan AP, Gardner KD Jr. 1979. Nephron obstruction in nordihydroguaiaretic acid-induced renal cystic disease. *Kidney Int* 15:7–19.

FDA (Food and Drug Administration). 1992. *FDA Advice to Chaparral Users*. Online. Available at http://www.fda.gov/bbs/topics/ANSWERS/ANS00456.html. Accessed July 1, 2004.

FDA. 1993. *Dietary Supplements: Making Sure Hype Doesn't Overwhelm Science*. Online. Available at http://www.fda.gov/bbs/topics/CONSUMER/CON00259.html. Accessed August 26, 2002.

Fernandez S, Hurtado LM, Hernandez F. 1979. Fungicidal components of creosote bush resin. In: Geissbuhler H, ed. *Advances in Pesticide Science*. Vol. 2. New York: Pergamon Press. Pp. 315–355.

Ferrandiz ML, Ramachandran Nair AG, Alcaraz MJ. 1990. Inhibition of sheep platelet arachidonate metabolism by flavonoids from Spanish and Indian medicinal herbs. *Pharmazie* 45:206–208.

Fronczek FR, Caballero P, Fischer NH, Fernandez S, Hernandez E, Hurtado LM. 1987. The molecular structure of 3'-demethoxynorisoguaiacin triacetate from creosote bush (*Larrea tridentata*). *J Natural Prod* 50:497–499.

Fujii K, Jaffe H, Bishop Y, Arnold E, Mackintosh D, Epstein SS. 1970. Structure-activity relations for methylenedioxyphenyl and related compounds on hepatic microsomal enzyme function, as measured by prolongation of hexobarbital narcosis and zoxazolamine paralysis in mice. *Toxicol Appl Pharmacol* 16:482–494.

Fujimura H, Kawasaki N, Tanimoto T, Sasaki H, Suzuki T. 1995. Effects of acetaminophen on the ultra-structure of isolated rat hepatocytes. *Exp Toxicol Pathol* 47:345–351.

Gardea-Torresdey JL, Arteaga S, Tiemann KJ, Chianelli R, Pingitore N, Mackay W. 2001. Absorption of copper (II) by creosote bush (*Larrea tridentata*): Use of atomic and x-ray absorption spectroscopy. *Environ Toxicol Chem* 20:2572–2579.

Gardner KD Jr, Evan AP, Reed WP. 1986. Accelerated renal cyst development in deconditioned germ-free rats. *Kidney Int* 29:1116–1123.

Gardner KD Jr, Reed WP, Evan AP, Zedalis J, Hylarides MD, Leon AA. 1987. Endotoxin provocation of experimental renal cystic disease. *Kidney Int* 32:329–334.

Giri SN, Hollinger MA. 1996. Effect of nordihydroguaiaretic acid and ibuprofen on bleomycin and hyperoxia-induced changes in lung superoxide dismutase, prostaglandins and lethality. *Arch Toxicol* 70:271–276.

Gisvold O. 1947. A preliminary survey of the occurrence of nordihydroguaiaretic acid in *Larrea divaricata*. *J Am Pharm Assoc* 37:194–196.

Gisvold O, Thaker E. 1974. Lignans from *Larrea divaricata*. *J Pharm Sci* 63:P1905–P1907.

Gnabre J, Huang RCC, Bates RB, Burns JJ, Calderea S, Malcomson ME, McClure KJ. 1995. Characterization of anti-HIV lignans from *Larrea tridentata*. *Tetrahedron* 51:12203–12210.

Gonzalez-Coloma A, Wisdom CS, Undel PW. 1988. Ozone impact on the antioxidant nordihydroguaiaretic acid content in the external leaf resin of *Larrea tridentata*. *Biochem Syst Ecol* 16:59–64.

Goodman T, Grice HC, Becking GC, Salem FA. 1970. A cystic nephropathy induced by nordihydroguaiaretic acid in the rat. Light and electron microscopic investigations. *Lab Invest* 23:93–107.

Gordon DW, Rosenthal G, Hart J, Sirota R, Baker AL. 1995. Chaparral ingestion. The broadening spectrum of liver injury caused by herbal medications. *J Am Med Assoc* 273:489–490.

Gowri MS, Reaven GM, Azhar S. 1998. Effect of Masoprocol on glucose transport and lipolysis by isolated rat adipocytes. *J Investig Med* 46:144A. Abstract.

Gowri MS, Azhar RK, Kraemer FB, Reaven GM, Azhar S. 2000. Masoprocol decreases rat lipolytic activity by decreasing the phosphorylation of HSL. *Am J Physiol* 279:E593–E600.

Granados H, Cardenas R. 1994. Biliary calculi in the golden hamster. The prophylactic action of the creosote bush (*Larrea tridentata*) in pigmented cholelithiasis produced by vitamin A. *Rev Gastroenterol México* 59:31–35.

Grant KL, Boyer LV, Erdman BE. 1998. Chaparral-induced hepatotoxicity. *Integr Med* 1:83–87.

Grice HC, Becking G, Goodman T. 1968. Toxic properties of nordihydroguaiaretic acid. *Food Cosmet Toxicol* 6:155–161.

Habermehl G, Christ B. 1974. Die freien steroide in *Larrea divaricata*. *Phytochemistry* 13:1293–1294.

Habermehl G, Moeller H. 1974. Isolation and structure of larreagenin A. *Justus Liebigs Ann Chem.* 1-6:169–175.

Harman AW, Kyle ME, Serroni A, Farber JL. 1991. The killing of cultured hepatocytes by N-acetyl-p-benzoquinone imine (NAPQI) as a model of the cytotoxicity of acetaminophen. *Biochem Pharmacol* 41:1111–1117.

Heiser RW, Cheng CC, Pardini RS. 1977. Inhibition of mitochondrial electron transport by partially demethylated dihydroguaiaretic acid. *Pharmacol Res Commun* 9:917–926.

Heron S, Yarnell E. 2001. The safety of low-dose *Larrea tridentata* (DC) Coville (creosote bush or chaparral): A retrospective clinical study. *J Altern Complement Med* 7:175–185.

Hojo M, Hanioka K, Miyata M, Yamazoe Y. 2000. Hepatotoxicity of acetaminophen and N-acetyl-p-benzoquinone imine and enhancement by fructose. *Xenobiotica* 30:933–991.

Holme JA, Dahlin DC, Nelson SD, Dybing E. 1984. Cytotoxic effects of N-acetyl-p-benzoquinone imine, a common arylating intermediate of paracetamol and N-hydroxyparacetamol. *Biochem Pharmacol* 33:401–406.

Hsu BR, Juang JH, Fu SH, Kuo CH, Lu WT. 2001. Reduction in primary nonfunction of syngeneic islet transplants with nordihydroguaiaretic acid, a lipoxygenase inhibitor. *Cell Transplant* 10:255–262.

Hyder PW. 2001. *Total Phenolics, Condensed Tannins, and Nordihydroguaiaretic Acid (NDGA) as Potential Allelopathic Compounds in Creosote Bush and Tarbush in the Northern Chihuahuan Desert.* Las Cruces, NM: New Mexico State University. Dissertation.

Jaeschke H, Gores GJ, Cederbaum AI, Hinson JA, Pessayre D, Lemasters JJ. 2002. Mechanisms of hepatotoxicity. *Toxicol Sci* 65:166–176.

Kacew S. 2001. Confounding factors in toxicity testing. *Toxicology* 160:87–96.

Kamitani H, Geller M, Eling T. 1998. Expression of 15-lipoxygenase by human colorectal carcinoma Caco-2 cells during apoptosis and cell differentiation. *J Biol Chem* 273:21569–21577.

Katz M, Saibil F. 1990. Herbal hepatitis: Subacute hepatic necrosis secondary to chaparral leaf. *J Clin Gastroenterol* 12:203–206.

Kellett GL, Barker ED, Beach NL, Dempster JA. 1993. Effect of nordihydroguaiaretic acid on glucose absorption, metabolism and (Na++K+)-ATPase activity in rat jejunum. *Biochem Pharmacol* 45:1932–1935.

Klaassen CD, ed. 1995. *Casarett and Doull's Toxicology. The Basic Science of Poisons.* 5th ed. New York: McGraw-Hill.

Konno C, Martin A, Ma B-X, Lu Z-Z, Xue H-Z, Erdelmeier CAJ, Nuzzo NA, Soejarta DD, Cordell GA, Waller DP, Fong HHS. 1987. Search for fertility regulating agents from *Larrea tridentata*. Proceedings: The First Princess Chulabhorn Science Congress 1987, International Congress on Natural Products. 2:328–337.

Konno C, Xue HZ, Lu ZZ, Ma BX, Erdelmeier CAJ, Che CT, Cordell GA, Soejarto DD, Waller DP, Fong HHS. 1989. 1-Aryl tetralin lignans from *Larrea tridentata. J Natural Prod* 52:1113–1117.

Konno C, Lu ZZ, Xue HZ, Erdelmeier CA, Meksuriyen D, Che CT, Cordell GA, Soejarto DD, Waller DP, Fong HH. 1990. Furanoid lignans from *Larrea tridentata. J Natural Prod* 53:396–406.

Korn SJ, Horn R. 1990. Nordihydroguaiaretic acid inhibits voltage-activated Ca2+ currents independently of lipoxygenase inhibition. *Mol Pharmacol* 38:524–530.

Kozubik A, Hofmanova J, Hola J, Netikova J. 1993. The effect of nordihydroguaiaretic acid, an inhibitor of prostaglandin and leukotriene biosynthesis, on hematopoiesis of gamma-irradiated mice. *Exp Hematol* 21:138–142.

Lambert JD, Meyers RO, Timmermann BN, Dorr RT. 2001. Pharmacokinetic analysis by high-performance liquid chromatography of intravenous nordihydroguaiaretic acid in the mouse. *J Chromatogr B Biomed Sci Appl* 754:85–90.

Lehman AJ, Fitzhugh OG, Nelson AA, Woodard G. 1951. The pharmacological evaluation of antioxidants. *Adv Food Res* 3:197–208.

Lopez-Lazaro M, Martin-Cordero C, Ayuso MJ. 1999. Flavonoids of *Retama sphaerocarpa. Planta Med* 65:777–778.

Luo Z, Meksuriyen D, Erdelmeier CAJ, Fong HHS, Cordell GA. 1988. Larreantin, a novel, cytotoxic naphthoquinone from *Larrea tridentata. J Org Chem* 53:2183–2185.

Luther H, Jordanov D, Ludwig P, Schewe T. 1991. Inhibition of rabbit erythroid 15-lipoxygenase and sheep vesicular gland prostaglandin H synthase by gallic esters. *Pharmazie* 46:134–136.

Mabry TJ, Hunkiker JH, DiFeo DR. 1977. *Creosote Bush: Biology and Chemistry of Larrea in New World Deserts.* Stroudsburg, PA: Dowden, Hutchinson & Ross.

Madrigal-Bujaidar E, Diaz Barriga S, Cassani M, Molina D, Ponce G. 1998. *In vivo* and *in vitro* induction of sister-chromatid exchanges by nordihydroguaiaretic acid. *Mutat Res* 412:139–144.

Maldonado Z, Hoeneisen M, Silva M. 1993. Constituents of *Haplopappus bezanillanus* and *H. hirtellus. Bol Soc Chil Quim* 38: 43–48.

McGuffin M, Hobbs C, Upton R, Goldberg A, eds. 1997. *American Herbal Products Association's Botanical Safety Handbook.* Boca Raton, FL: CRC Press.

Micromedex (Micromedex Thomson Healthcare). 2002. *Chaparral.* Online. Available at http://www.cooperfitness.com/content/Support/Pharmaceutical/AltMed/Detail.asp?DocID=1489. Accessed August 26, 2002.

Mikuni M, Yoshida M, Hellberg P, Peterson CA, Edwin SS, Brännström M, Peterson CM. 1998. The lipoxygenase inhibitor, nordihydroguaiaretic acid, inhibits ovulation and reduces leukotriene and prostaglandin levels in the rat ovary. *Biol Reprod* 58:1211–1216.

Miles DH, Chittawong V, Hedin PA, Kokpol U. 1993. Potential agrochemicals from leaves of *Wedelia biflora. Phytochemistry* 32:1427–1429.

Moerman DE. 1998. *Native American Ethnobotany.* Portland, OR: Timber Press.

Moore M, Thor H, Moore G, Nelson S, Moldeus P, Orrenius S. 1985. The toxicity of acetaminophen and N-acetyl-p-benzoquinone imine in isolated hepatocytes is associated with thiol depletion and increased cytosolic Ca2+. *J Biol Chem* 260:13035–13040.

Moridani MY, Galati G, O'Brien PJ. 2002. Comparative quantitative structure toxicity relationships for flavonoids evaluated in isolated rat hepatocytes and HeLa tumor cells. *Chem Biol Interact* 139:251–264.

Mufti NA, Shuler ML. 1996. Possible role of arachidonic acid in stress-induced cytochrome P450IA1 activity. *Biotechnol Prog* 12:847–854.

Nagano N, Imaizumi Y, Hirano M, Watanabe M. 1996. Opening of Ca(2+)-dependent K+ channels by nordihydroguaiaretic acid in porcine coronary arterial smooth muscle cells. *Jpn J Pharmacol* 70:281–284.

Nakayama T. 1994. Suppression of hydroperoxide-induced cytotoxicity by polyphenols. *Cancer Res* 54:1991s–1993s.

Nakazato PZ, Ulreich JB, Boles JL, Patel MR, Rorie CJ, Fisher RL, Brendel K. 1998. Nephrotoxicity and hepatotoxicity of chaparral (*Larrea tridentata*) in rats and humans. *Toxicologist* 37:287. Abstract.

Njoku CJ, Hopp DC, Alali F, Asuzu IU, McLaughlin JL. 1997. Dihydroguaiaretic acid: A bioactive component of the stem bark of *Pycnanthus angolensis*. *Planta Med* 63:580–581.

Noro T, Oda Y, Miyase T, Ueno A, Fukushima S. 1983. Inhibitors of xanthine oxidase from the flowers and buds of *Daphne genkwa*. *Chem Pharm Bull (Tokyo)* 31(11):3984-3987.

Obermeyer WR, Musser SM, Betz JM, Casey RE, Pohland AE, Page SW. 1995. Chemical studies of phytoestrogens and related compounds in dietary supplements: Flax and chaparral. *Proc Soc Exp Biol Med* 208:6–12.

Okboy N, Yegen C, Aktan AO, Dosluoglu HH, Sav A, Yalin R, Ercan S. 1992. The effect of iloprost and NDGA in ischemia reperfusion injury in rat liver. *Prostaglandins Leukot Essent Fatty Acids* 47:291–295.

Palacios P, Gutkind G, Rondina RV, de Torres R, Coussio JD. 1983. Genus *Baccharis*. II. Antimicrobial activity of *B. crispa* and *B. notosergila*. *Planta Med* 49:128.

Pardini RS, Heidker JC, Fletcher DC. 1970. Inhibition of mitochondrial electron transport by nordihydroguaiaretic acid (NDGA). *Biochem Pharmacol* 19:2695–2699.

Pardini RS, Kim CH, Biagini R, Morris RJ, Fletcher DC. 1973. Inhibition of mitochondrial electron transport systems by norisoguaiacin. *Biochem Pharmacol* 22:1921–1925.

Parry EW. 1993. Cycloheximide or nordihydroguaiaretic acid protects mice against the lethal and hepatocytolytic effects of a combined challenge with D-galactosamine and bacterial endotoxin. *J Comp Pathol* 108:185–190.

Pavani M, Fones E, Oksenberg D, Garcia M, Hernandez C, Cordano G, Munoz S, Mancilla J, Guerrero A, Ferreira J. 1994. Inhibition of tumoral cell respiration and growth by nordihydroguaiaretic acid. *Biochem Pharmacol* 48:1935–1942.

Reed MJ, Meszaros K, Entes LJ, Claypool MD, Pinkett J, Reaven GM. 1998. Metabolic effects of masoprocol in a rodent model of non-insulin-dependent diabetes mellitus. *J Investig Med* 46:144A. Abstract.

Reed MJ, Meszaros K, Entes LJ, Claypool MD, Pinkett JG, Brignetti D, Luo J, Khandwala A, Reaven GM. 1999. Effect of masoprocol on carbohydrate and lipid metabolism in a rat model of type II diabetes. *Diabetologia* 42:102–106.

Robison TW, Sevanian A, Forman HJ. 1990. Inhibition of arachidonic acid release by nordihydroguaiaretic acid and its antioxidant action in rat alveolar macrophages and Chinese hamster lung fibroblasts. *Toxicol Appl Pharmacol* 105:113–122.

Sakakibara M, Mabry TJ. 1975. A new 8-hydroxyflavonol from *Larrea tridentata*. *Phytochemistry* 14:2097–2098.

Sakakibara M, Timmermann BN, Nakatani N, Waldrum H, Mabry TJ. 1975. New 8-hydroxyflavonols from *Larrea tridentata*. *Phytochemistry* 14:849–851.

Sakakibara M, DiFeo D Jr, Nakatani N, Timmerman B, Mabry TJ. 1976. Flavonoid methyl ethers on the external leaf surface of *Larrea tridentata* and *L. divaricata*. *Phytochemistry* 15:727–731.

Sapienza PP, Ikeda GJ, Obermeyer WR. 1997. *In vitro* effect of chaparral on xenobiotic metabolizing enzymes in rat liver. Online, FDA 1997 Science Forum (Poster Abstract):J9. Abstract.

Schegg KM, Welch W Jr. 1984. The effect of nordihydroguaiaretic acid and related lignans on formyltetrahydrofolate synthetase and carboxylesterase. *Biochim Biophys Acta* 788:167–180.

Schultz JC, Floyd T. 1999. An immigrant to the Southwest, the creosote bush is a desert survivor that dominates the landscape and engineers biodiversity. *Natural History* 108:24–29.

Seufferlein T, Seckl MJ, Schwarz E, Beil M, Wichert G, Baust H, Luhrs H, Schmid RM, Adler G. 2002. Mechanisms of nordihydroguaiaretic acid-induced growth inhibition and apoptosis in human cancer cells. *Br J Cancer* 86:1188–1196.

Shad JA, Chinn CG, Brann OS. 1999. Acute hepatitis after ingestion of herbs. *South Med J* 92:1095–1097.

Sheikh NM, Philen RM, Love LA. 1997. Chaparral-associated hepatotoxicity. *Arch Intern Med* 157:913–919.

Shen YC, Chen CY, Chen YJ, Kuo YH, Chie CTLYM. 1997. Bioactive lignans and taxoids from the roots of formosan *Taxus mairei*. *Chin Pharm J (Taipei)* 49:285–296.

Shi L, Pardini RS. 1995. Effect of NDGA on beef heart mitochondria and EMT6 mouse mammary carcinoma cells. *Res Commun Mol Pathol Pharmacol* 90:235–254.

Slattery JT, Wilson JM, Kalhorn TF, Nelson SD. 1987. Dose-dependent pharmacokinetics of acetaminophen: Evidence of glutathione depletion in humans. *Clin Pharmacol Ther* 41:413–418.

Smart CR, Hogle HH, Vogel H, Broom AD, Bartholomew D. 1970. Clinical experience with nordihydroguaiaretic acid—"Chaparrel tea" in the treatment of cancer. *Rocky Mt Med J* 67:39–43.

Smith AY, Feddersen RM, Gardner KD Jr, Davis CJ Jr. 1994. Cystic renal cell carcinoma and acquired renal cystic disease associated with consumption of chaparral tea: A case report. *J Urol* 152:2089–2091.

Smith BC, Desmond PV. 1993. Acute hepatitis induced by ingestion of the herbal medication chaparral. *Aust NZ J Med* 23:526.

Stetler-Stevenson WG, Krutzsch HC, Liotta LA. 1992. TIMP-2: Identification and characterization of a new member of the metalloproteinase inhibitor family. *Matrix Suppl* 1:299–306.

Su W, Tseng LL, Lin MC, Chang HJ, Lee KC, Chou KJ, Lo YK, Cheng JS, Chang HT, Wang JL, Liu CP, Chen WC, Jan CR. 2002. Effect of nordihydroguaiaretic acid on intracellular Ca^{2+} concentrations in C6 glioma cells. *Neurochem Int* 40:249–254.

Tang DG, Honn KV. 1997. Apoptosis of W256 carcinosarcoma cells of the monocytoid origin induced by NDGA involves lipid peroxidation and depletion of GSH: Role of 12-lipoxygenase in regulating tumor cell survival. *J Cell Physiol* 172:155–170.

Telford IR, Woodruff CS, Linford RH. 1962. Fetal resorption in the rat as influenced by certain antioxidants. *Am J Anat* 110:29–36.

Ulreich JB, Okafor JM, Chavez RC, Le T, Maveddat M, Boles JL, Zavala JL, Stringer SK, Young CJ, Nakazato PZ. 1997. Hepatotoxicity of chaparral in Fischer 344 rats. *Toxicologist* 36:228. Abstract.

Valentine JL, McKenzie L, Kovarik F. 1984. Gas chromatographic determination of nordihydroguaiaretic acid in *Larrea divaricata*. *Anal Lett* 17:1617–1626.

Van der Merwe MJ, Jenkins K, Theron E, van der Walt BJ. 1993. Interaction of the dicatechols rooperol and nordihydroguaiaretic acid with oxidative systems in the human blood. A structure-activity relationship. *Biochem Pharmacol* 45:303–311.

Vedovato M, Salvatorelli G, Daniele C, De Paoli Vitali E. 1994. Changes in human epithelial kidney cells induced by nordihydroguaiaretic acid *in vitro*. *Cytobios* 78:19–22.

von Ardenne M, Chaplain R, Reitnauer P. 1969. *In vitro* measurements of damage to cancer with a good substrate supply, following combined attack by NDGA and 40'C hyperthermia, with and without irradiation at a dose of 1000 r. *Arch Geschwulstforsch* 34:1–12.

Wagenknecht B, Schulz JB, Gulbins E, Weller M. 1998. Crm-A, bcl-2 and NDGA inhibit CD95L-induced apoptosis of malignant glioma cells at the level of caspase 8 processing. *Cell Death Differ* 5:894–900.

Waller CW, Gisvold O. 1945. A phytochemical investigation of *Larrea divaricata* Cav. *J Am Pharm Assoc Sci Ed* 34:78–81.

Weidenborner M, Hindorf H, Jha HC, Tsotsonos P, Egge H. 1989. Antifungal activity of isoflavonoids against storage fungi of the genus *Aspergillus*. *Phytochemistry* 28:3317–3319.

Whitman S, Gezginci M, Timmermann BN, Holman TR. 2002. Structure-activity relationship studies of nordihydroguaiaretic acid inhibitors toward soybean, 12-human, and 15-human lipoxygenase. *J Med Chem* 45:2659–2661.

Xue HZ, Lu ZZ, Konno C, Soejarto DD, Cordell GA, Fong HHS, Hodgson W. 1988. 3-Beta-(3,4-dihydroxycinnamoyl)-erythrodiol and 3-beta-(4-hydroxycinnamoyl)-erythrodiol from *Larrea tridentata*. *Phytochemistry* 27:233–235.

Yamamoto S, Nakadate T, Nakaki T, Ishii K, Kato R. 1982. Prevention of glucose-induced insulin secretion by lipoxygenase inhibitor. *Eur J Pharmacol* 78:225–227.

Yamamura H, Sakamoto K, Ohya S, Muraki K, Imaizumi Y. 2002. Mechanisms underlying the activation of large conductance Ca2+-activated K+ channels by nordihydroguaiaretic acid. *Jpn J Pharmacol* 89:53–63.

Zamora JM. 1984. *Cytotoxic, Antimicrobial and Phytochemical Properties of Larrea tridentata Cav*. Auburn, AL: Auburn University. Dissertation.

Zamora JM, Mora EC, Parish EJ. 1992. A comparison of the cytotoxicity of nordihydroguaiaretic acid and its derivatives. *J Tenn Acad Sci* 67:77–80.

TABLE A Chaparral: Individual Components

Substance	Structure	Safety Issues
Lignans, nordihydroguaiaretic acid (NDGA), and other substituted guaiaretic acid derivatives		
NDGA (Duisberg et al., 1949; Waller and Gisvold, 1945) Present in all parts of *Larrea tridentata,* including leaves, stems and twigs at 5–15% of the dry leaf weight (Mabry et al., 1977)	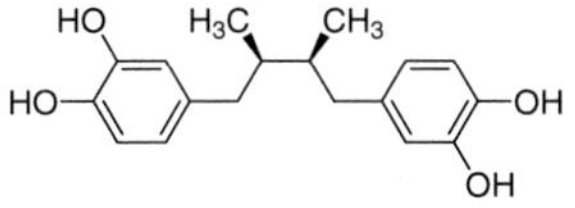	Animal studies: see Table E for safety issues from animal studies with NDGA *In vitro* study: see Table F-2 for safety issues from *in vitro* studies with NDGA
Dihydroguaiaretic acid (Obermeyer et al., 1995) Partially demethylated dihydroguaiaretic acid is also present (Gisvold and Thaker, 1974)	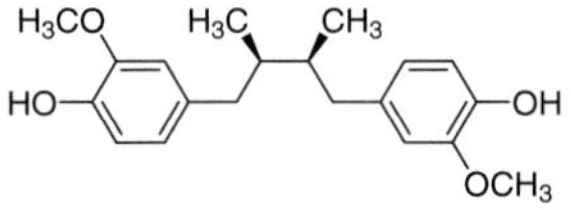	*In vitro* study: weak cytotoxic activity (IC_{50} 1–3 μg/mL) (Njoku et al., 1997) *In vitro* study: weak cytotoxic activity (10 μg/mL) and (Gisvold and Thaker, 1974)
Guaiaretic acid (Obermeyer et al., 1995)	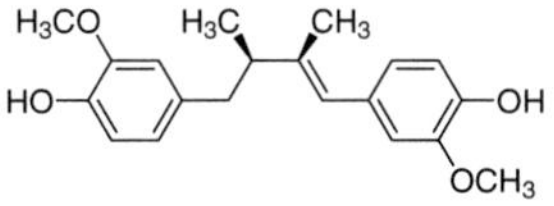	No data suggestive of toxicity are available
Secoisolariciresinol (Obermeyer et al., 1995) Present in the stems of *L. tridentata* (Konno et al., 1990)	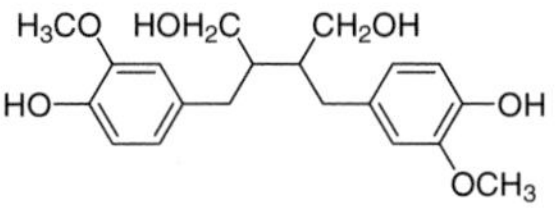	*In vitro* study: weak cytotoxic activity (IC_{50} 0.6–8.3 μg/mL) (Shen et al., 1997); see Table F-2
Lignans, furanoid		
Larreatricin (Konno et al., 1987) Present in the stems of *L. tridentata* (Konno et al., 1990) in trace amounts (0.001% of dry leaf weight)	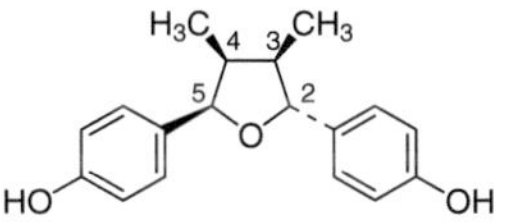	No data suggestive of toxicity are available
4-*epi*-Larreatricin (Konno et al., 1987) Present in the leaves, twigs and stems of *L. tridentata* (Konno et al., 1990) in trace amounts (up to 0.0003% of dry leaf weight)	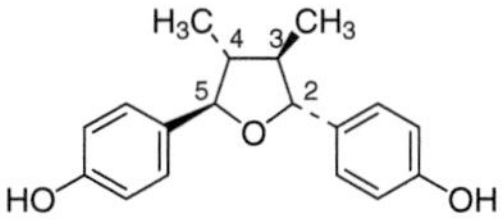	No data suggestive of toxicity are available

continued

TABLE A Continued

Substance	Structure	Safety Issues
3″-Hydroxy-4-*epi*-larreatricin (Konno et al., 1987) Present in the leaves and twigs of *L. tridentata* (Konno et al., 1990) in trace amounts (0.0008% of dry leaf weight)	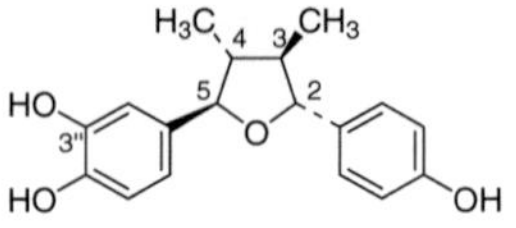	No data suggestive of toxicity are available
3′, 3″-Dimethoxy-larreatricin (Konno et al., 1987) Present in the stems of *L. tridentata* (Konno et al., 1990) in trace amounts (0.0002% of dry leaf weight)	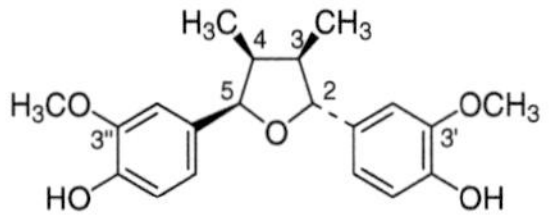	No data suggestive of toxicity are available
3,4-Dehydrolarreatricin (Konno et al., 1987) Present in the stems of *L. tridentata* (Konno et al., 1990) in trace amounts (up to 0.0002% of dry leaf weight)	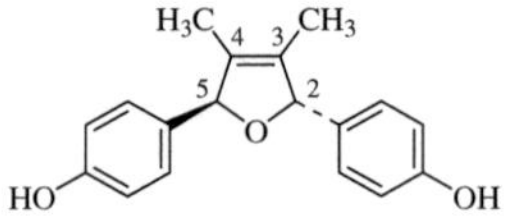	No data suggestive of toxicity are available
Larreatridenticin (Konno et al., 1987) Present in the stems of *L. tridentata* in trace amounts (0.00008% of dry leaf weight) (Konno et al., 1987)	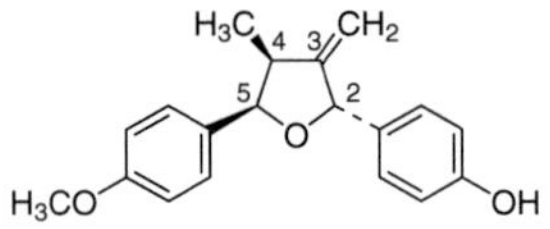	No data suggestive of toxicity are available

Lignans, 1-aryl tetralin

All of the 1-aryl tetralin lignans are structurally related to podophyllotoxins (Damayanthi and Lown, 1998)

Substance	Structure	Safety Issues
Isoguaiacin (Konno et al., 1987) Present in the stems of *L. tridentata* (Konno et al., 1990) in trace amounts (0.00002% of dry leaf weight)	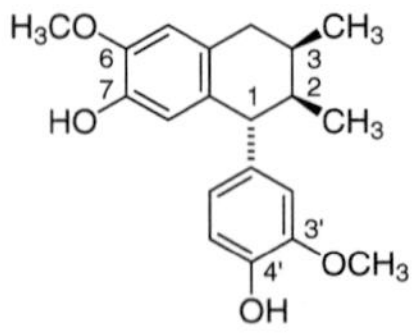	No data suggestive of toxicity are available

TABLE A Continued

Substance	Structure	Safety Issues
6-O-Demethylisoguaiacin Norisoguaiacin, R1=OCH_3, R2=OH (Gisvold and Thaker, 1974) Present in the stems of *L. tridentata* (Konno et al., 1990) at 0.003% of the dry leaf weight	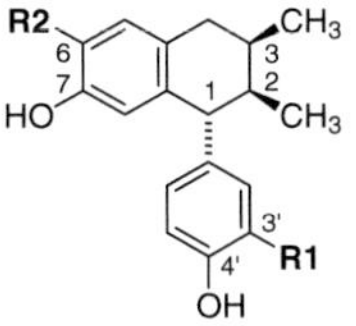	*In vitro* study: inhibited electron transport (0.2 μM, rat liver mitochondria) (63 μM, bovine heart mitochondria) (Pardini et al., 1973) *In vitro* study: weak cytotoxicity (100 μg/mL) (Gisvold and Thaker, 1974) *In vitro* study: inhibited carboxylesterase (30 μM) and formyltetrahydrofolate synthetase (350 μM) (Schegg and Welch, 1984)
3′ Demethoxyisoguaiacin R1=H, R2=OCH_3 (Gisvold and Thaker, 1974)		No data suggestive of toxicity are available
3′ Demethoxy-6-O-demethylisoguaiacin 3′ Demethoxynorisoguaiacin, nor-3′-demethoxyisoguaiacin, NDI, R1=H, R2=OH (Fronczek et al., 1987) Present in the twigs (Konno et al., 1990) and leaves (Fronczek et al., 1987) of *L. tridentata* (Konno et al., 1989) in trace amounts (up to 0.005%)		No data suggestive of hepatotoxicity are available
6-3′-Di-O-demethylisoguaiacin 3′-Hydroxynorisoguaiacin, R1=OH, R2=OH (Konno et al., 1987) Present in leaves and twigs of *L. tridentata* (Konno et al., 1989) at 0.004% of the dry leaf weight		No data suggestive of toxicity are available
Flavonoids (present as aglycones and glycosides) Flavonoids are widespread in the human diet and no toxicities have been associated with them		
Apigenin (Sakakibara et al., 1976)	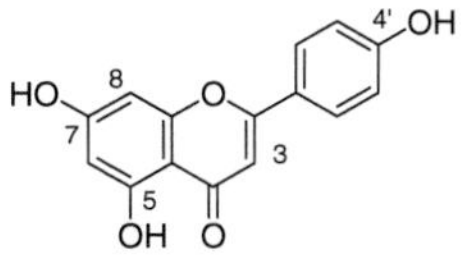	*In vitro* study: weak cytotoxic activity (0.8 mg/disc) (Palacios et al., 1983)

continued

TABLE A Continued

Substance	Structure	Safety Issues
		In vitro study: weak cytotoxic activity (25 μg/mL) (Chae et al., 1992) *In vitro* study: inhibitor of CYP 1A1 (IC_{50} 16 μg/mL) (Chae et al., 1992)
Apigenin 7-methyl ether Genkwanin (Sakakibara et al., 1976)	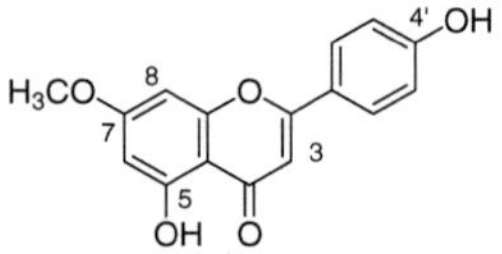	*In vitro* study: weak cytotoxicity (0.4 mg/disc) (Palacios et al., 1983) *In vitro* study: inhibitor of MAO (Noro et al., 1983) and CYP 1A1 (IC_{50} > 50 μg/mL) (Chae et al., 1992)
Gossypetin 3,7-dimethyl ether R1=CH_3, R2=CH_3, R3=H, R4=H (Sakakibara and Mabry, 1975) Present in leaves of *L. tridentata* (Sakakibara et al., 1976)	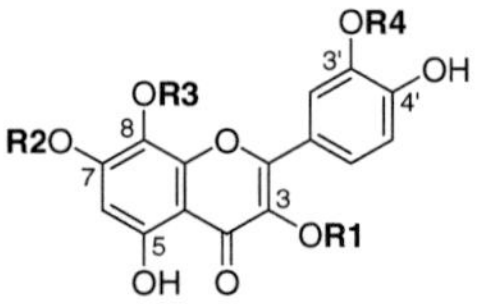	No data suggestive of toxicity are available
Gossypetin 3,7,3′-trimethylether 5,8,4′-Trihydroxy-3,7,3′-trimethoxyflavone, R1=CH_3, R2=CH_3, R3=H, R4=CH_3 (Sakakibara et al., 1975) Present in leaves of *L. tridentata* (Sakakibara et al., 1976)		No data suggestive of toxicity are available
Gossypetin 3,7,8,3′-tetramethyl ether Ternatin, R1=CH_3, R2=CH_3, R3=CH_3, R4=CH_3 Present in leaves of *L. tridentata* (Bernhard and Thiele, 1981)		No data suggestive of toxicity are available

TABLE A Continued

Substance	Structure	Safety Issues
Herbacetin 3,7-dimethyl ether 8-Hydroxy-kaempferol, R1=CH_3, R2=CH_3, R3=H, R4=H (Sakakibara et al., 1975) Present in leaves of *L. tridentata* (Sakakibara et al., 1976)	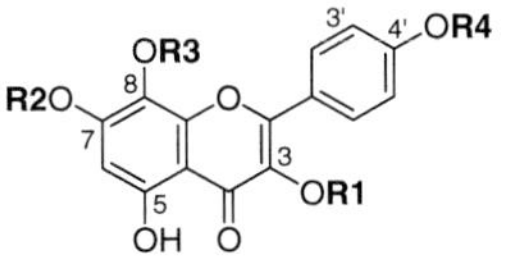	No data suggestive of toxicity are available
Herbacetin 3,7,8-trimethyl ether R1=CH_3, R2=CH_3, R3=CH_3, R4=H Present in leaves of *L. tridentata* (Bernhard and Thiele, 1981)		No data suggestive of toxicity are available
Herbacetin 3,7,4′-trimethyl ether R1=CH_3, R2=CH_3, R3=H, R4=CH_3 (Fernandez et al., 1979)		No data suggestive of toxicity are available
Kaempferol (Chirikdjian, 1973; Sakakibara et al., 1976)	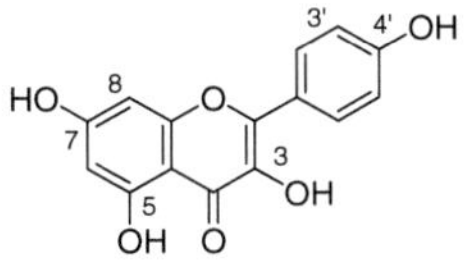	*In vitro* study: weak cytotoxic activity (18 µg/mL) (Chae et al., 1992) *In vitro* study: inhibitor of CYP 1A1 (IC_{50} 14 µg/mL) (Chae et al., 1992)
Kaempferol 3-methyl ether Isokaempferide, R1=CH_3, R2=H, R3=H (Chirikdjian, 1973; Sakakibara et al., 1976)	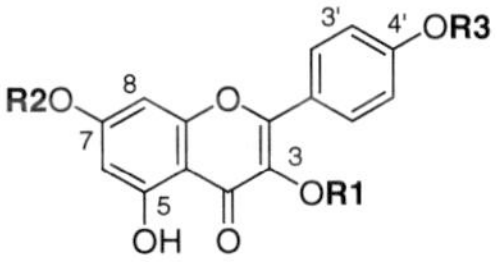	*In vitro* study: cytotoxicity (IC_{50} 5 µM (Banskota et al., 2000)
Kaempferol 7-methyl ether Rhamnocitrin, R1=H, R2=CH_3, R3=H (Sakakibara et al., 1976)		No data suggestive of toxicity are available
Kaempferol 3,7-dimethyl ether Kumatakenin, R1=CH_3, R2=CH_3, R3=H (Sakakibara et al., 1976)		*In vitro* study: weak cytotoxicity (300 µg/agar plate*)* (Afifi et al., 1991)

continued

TABLE A Continued

Substance	Structure	Safety Issues
Kaempferol 3,4′-dimethyl ether R1=CH_3, R2=H, R3=CH_3 (Mabry et al., 1977)		No data suggestive of toxicity are available
Luteolin 3′-methyl ether Chrysoeriol, R1=H, R2=CH_3 (Sakakibara et al., 1976)	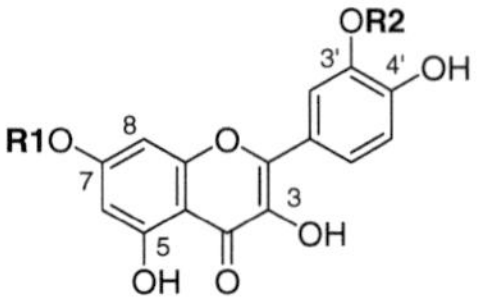	No data relative to safety are available
Luteolin 7,3′-dimethyl ether Velutin, R1=CH_3, R2=CH_3 (Sakakibara et al., 1976)		No data suggestive of toxicity are available
Quercetin (Chirikdjian, 1973) Some investigators have not been able to identify quercetin as a component of *L. tridentata* (Mabry et al., 1977)	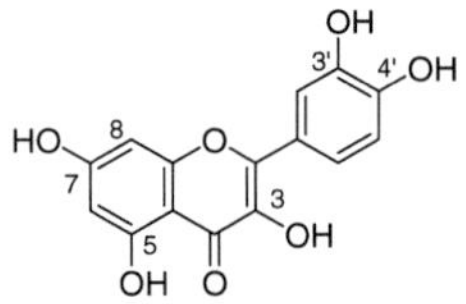	No data suggestive of hepatotoxicity are available
Quercetin 3-methyl ether R1=CH_3, R2=H, R3=H, R4=H (Chirikdjian, 1973) Some investigators have not been able to identify quercetin 3-methyl ether as a component of *L. tridentata* (Mabry et al., 1977)	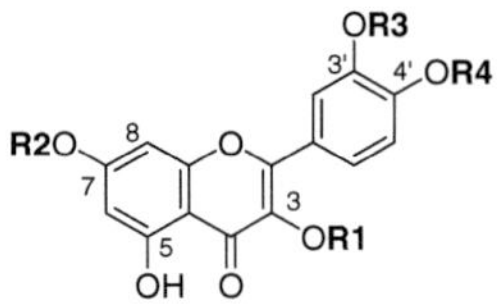	No data suggestive of toxicity are available
Quercetin 3′-methyl ether Isorhamnetin, R1=H, R2=H, R3=CH_3, R4=H (Chirikdjian, 1973; Sakakibara et al., 1976)		No data suggestive of toxicity are available
Quercetin 3,7-dimethyl ether Kumatakenine, R1=CH_3, R2=CH_3, R3=H, R4=H (Chirikdjian, 1974; Sakakibara et al., 1976)		No data suggestive of toxicity are available
Quercetin 3,3′-dimethyl ether R1=CH_3, R2=H, R3=CH_3, R4=H (Sakakibara et al., 1976)		No data suggestive of toxicity are available

TABLE A Continued

Substance	Structure	Safety Issues
Quercetin 7,3′-dimethyl ether Rhamnazin, R1=H, R2=CH_3, R3=CH_3, R4=H (Sakakibara et al., 1976)		*In vitro* study: weak cytotoxicity (50% growth inhibition at 4–30 μg/mL) (Lopez-Lazaro et al., 1999; Miles et al., 1993)
Quercetin 3,7,3′-trimethyl ether R1=CH_3, R2=CH_3, R3=CH_3, R4=H (Sakakibara et al., 1976)		No data suggestive of toxicity are available
Quercetin 3,7,4′-trimethyl ether Ayanin, R1=CH_3, R2=CH_3, R3=H, R4=CH_3 (Gnabre et al., 1995)		No data suggestive of toxicity are available
Quercetin 7,3′,4′-trimethyl ether R1=H, R2=CH_3, R3=CH_3, R4=CH_3 (Korn and Horn, 1990)		No data suggestive of toxicity are available
Quercetin 3,7,3′,4′-tetramethyl ether Retusine, R1=CH_3, R2=CH_3, R3=CH_3, R4=CH_3 (Sakakibara et al., 1976)		*In vitro* study: weak cytotoxicity (50–200 μM) (Weidenborner et al., 1989)
Dihydromyricetin 3′,5′-dimethyl ether Dihydrosyringetin (Sakakibara et al., 1976)	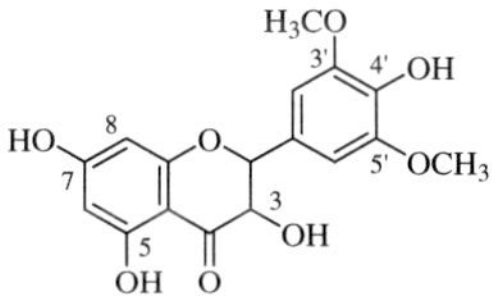	No data suggestive of toxicity are available
5,4′-Dihydroxy-3,7,3′-trimethoxyflavone (Chirikdjian, 1974)	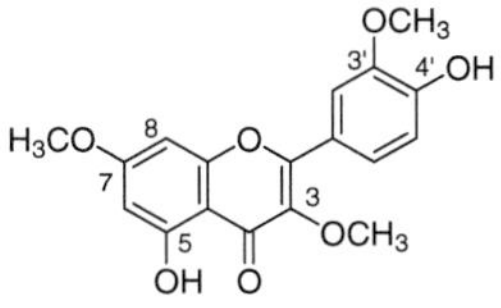	*In vitro* study: cytotoxicity (IC_{50} 5 μM) (Banskota et al., 2000; Maldonado et al., 1993)

continued

TABLE A Continued

Substance	Structure	Safety Issues
Triterpenes (present as aglycones and glycosides, which are also called saponins)		
3β-(4-Hydroxycinnamoyl)-erythrodiol (Konno et al., 1987) Present in the stems of *L. tridentata* (Xue et al., 1988)	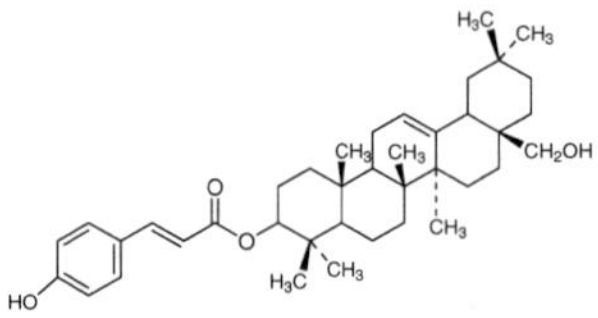	No data suggestive of toxicity are available
3β-(3,4-Dihydroxycinnamoyl)-erythrodiol (Konno et al., 1987) Present in the stems of *L. tridentata* (Xue et al., 1988)	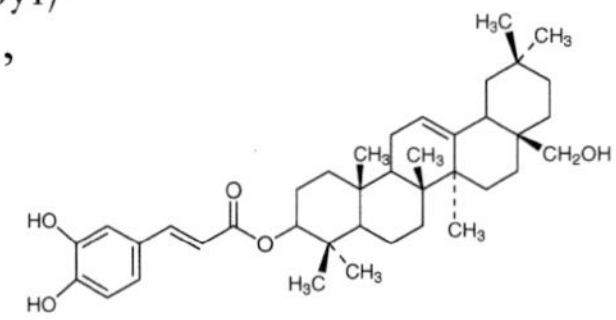	No data suggestive of toxicity are available
Triterpenes: sapogenins		
Larreagenin A Present in the leaves of *L. tridentata* (Habermehl and Moeller, 1974)	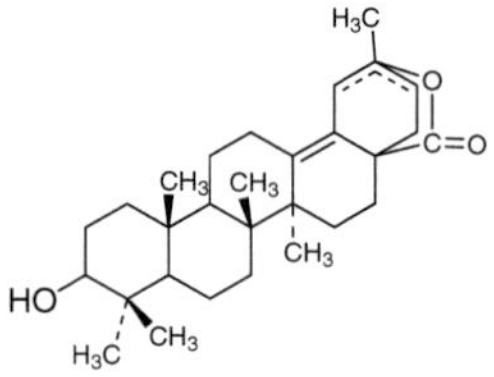	No data suggestive of toxicity are available
Larreic acid Present in the leaves of *L. tridentata* (Habermehl and Moeller, 1974)	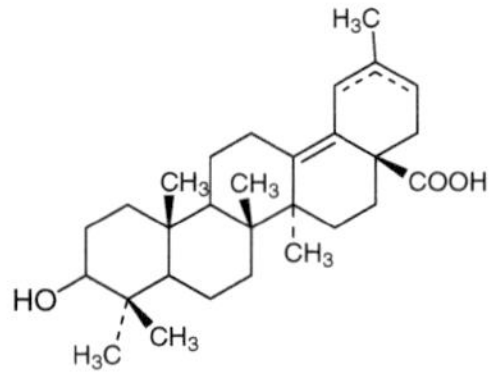	No data suggestive of toxicity are available
Other components		

Volatile oils (0.1–0.2% of fresh leaf weight by steam distillation) (Mabry et al., 1977)

Monoterpene hydrocarbons: camphene, Δ-3-carene, limonene, α-pinene; traces of α-fenchene, β-ocimene, β-pinene (Bohnstedt, 1979; Mabry et al., 1977)

Oxygenated monoterpene: borneol, bornyl acetate, camphor, *p*-cymene, linalool; traces of copaene, 2-rossalene (Bohnstedt, 1979; Mabry et al., 1977)

Sesquiterpene hydrocarbons: α-bergamotene, calamenene, cuparene, α-curcumene, edulane, β-santalene (Bohnstedt, 1979)

Oxygenated sesquiterpenes: α-agarofuran, β-eudesmol, γ-eudesmol, farnesol (Bohnstedt, 1979)

Aromatic hydrocarbons: benzaldehyde, benzyl acetate, benzyl butanate, 1,2-dihydro-1,5,8-trimethyl-naphthalene, ethyl benzoate, *o*-methyl anisate, methyl naphthalene; traces of acetophenone (Bohnstedt, 1979)

TABLE A Continued

Substance	Structure	Safety Issues
Wax esters (found on the external surface of leaves and stems; 0.1% w/w of fresh leaf weight by steam distillation): alkyl esters (C48–C56), fatty acids (C48–C56) (Bohnstedt, 1979; Mabry et al., 1977; Waller and Gisvold, 1945)		
Sterols: campesterol, β-sitosterol, stigmasterol, cholesterol (Habermehl and Christ, 1974; Konno et al., 1987; Xue et al., 1988)		
2-Ketones (probably contribute to the odor of *L. tridentata*): 2-dodecanone, 2-undecanone, 2-tridecanone; traces of 2-tetradecanone, 2-pentadecanone, 3-hexanone, 2-heptanone, 2-nonanone (Bohnstedt, 1979; Brinker, 1993–1994; Mabry et al., 1977)		
Vinyl ketones (probably contribute to odor of chaparral of *L. tridentata*): 1-hexen-3-one, 1-octen-3-one; traces of 1-hepten-3-one (Bohnstedt, 1979; Brinker, 1993–1994; Mabry et al., 1977)		
Fatty alcohols (C22–C32) (Bohnstedt, 1979)		
Other hydrocarbons: *n*-tridecane, *n*-tetradecane; traces of 3-methylbutanal, 3-hexanol, hexanal, 3-hexen-1-yl acetate, isobutyric acid (Bohnstedt, 1979; Brinker, 1993–1994; Mabry et al., 1977)		

NOTE: IC_{50} = Concentration at which the response has decreased to 50% of the original response, CYP = cytochrome P450, MAO = monoamine oxidase.

TABLE B Chaparral: Summary of Adverse Effects in a Clinical Trial

Study Design	Subjects	Parameters Monitored	Supplement	Adverse Effects and Related Findings
Smart et al., 1970[a] 36 subjects in chaparral tea group; 23 subjects in NDGA group; no control group	Condition: advanced incurable malignancy Age: unknown Male/Female: unknown Concurrent medications: at least one subject continued treatment with 5-fluorouracil Pre-existing medical conditions: none mentioned beyond malignancy	Parameters monitored: Regression vs. nonregression Hemoglobin, white blood cell count, BUN, SGOT, and urinalysis (before trial and at 2–4 wk intervals in the majority of subjects) Subjective improvement Duration was not stated but most subjects (≥ 45 out of the total 59 subjects) were treated for ≥ 4 wk	Chaparral tea group: Number of subjects: 36 Dose: chaparral tea, 16–24 oz/d Route: oral Frequency: 1×/d Duration: unknown NDGA group: Number of subjects: 23 Dose: NDGA, 250–3,000 mg/d Route: oral Frequency: 1×/d Duration: unknown	Combined groups: Adverse effects: fever (1 subject) In a significant number of subjects, there appeared to be stimulation of tumor growth No clinical laboratory abnormalities were observed that could be attributed to chaparral tea or NDGA Total of 14 subjects (25%) withdrew before 4 wk and were not evaluated

NOTE: NDGA = nordihydroguaiaretic acid, BUN = blood urea nitrogen, SGOT = serum glutamic-oxaloacetic transaminase.

[a] This study was evaluated as published with additional information and quotes from one of the authors published by the American Cancer Society (ACS, 1970).

TABLE C-1 FOLLOWS

TABLE C-1 Chaparral: Summary of Clinical Case Reports

Category/Case/Reference[a]	Number of Subjects[b]	Date
Case #1 Sheikh et al., 1997	1*	
Case #2 Clark and Reed, 1992; Sheikh et al., 1997	1*	7/92
Case #3 Sheikh et al., 1997	1*	10/92
Case #4 Sheikh et al., 1997	1*	1/93
Case #5 Clark and Reed, 1992; Sheikh et al., 1997	1*	7/92
Case #6 Sheikh et al., 1997	1*	3/93

Subject/Supplement	Adverse Effects[c] and Related Findings
38-year-old female (Sheikh's patient no. 10) Chaparral capsules, 400 mg/d taken as a nutritional supplement for many Subject history: drug abuse, previous alcohol use and previous hepatitis C infection	Diagnosis: chaparral-induced toxic liver damage or "chaparral may have potentiated or exacerbated the underlying liver disease in this individual" (Sheikh et al., 1997) Subject had elevated aminotransferase levels and joint stiffness of the right hand; eventually required a liver transplant
41-year-old female (Clark's patient no. 2 and Sheikh's patient no. 2) Chaparral (259 mg/d as tablets for 11 wk) taken for a skin condition; estimated cumulative dose of 68–96 g (Sheikh et al., 1997) Concurrent drugs or herbals: none	Diagnosis: chaparral-induced toxic liver damage (Clark and Reed, 1992; Sheikh et al., 1997) Subject presented with jaundice and abdominal pain of 4 wk duration; discontinued chaparral use and returned to normal within several months
44-year-old female (Sheikh's patient no. 5) Chaparral capsules, 2,400 mg/d for 10 d then 800 mg/d for 10 d, taken for allergies and fatigue; estimated cumulative dose of 24.8 g (per Sheikh et al., 1997; actual estimated cumulative dose would be 32 g)	Diagnosis: chaparral-induced toxic liver damage (Sheikh et al., 1997) Subject had fatigue, jaundice, dark urine, nausea, abdominal pain, and diarrhea; recovered within 7 wk
60-year-old female (Sheikh's patient no. 6) Single-ingredient chaparral product	Diagnosis: chaparral-induced toxic liver damage (Sheikh et al., 1997) Subject had symptoms of cholecystitis and elevated aminotransferase levels; recovered within 7 wk
42-year-old male (Clark's patient no. 1 and Sheikh's patient no. 1) Chaparral (3× 500 mg capsules/d for 6 wk); supplement promoted as "free radical scavenger"; estimated cumulative dose of 96 g (Sheikh et al., 1997)	Diagnosis: hepatic dysfunction secondary to chaparral ingestion (Clark and Reed, 1992; Sheikh et al., 1997) Subject presented with scleral icterus and diffuse jaundice; returned to normal within 1 mo; history of alcohol use
25-year-old male (Sheikh's patient no. 8) Chaparral, 3,840 mg/d for 2–3 wk, then 5,760 mg/d for 10 wk, capsules; taken for asthma; estimated cumulative dose of 70–114 g (Sheikh et al., 1997)	Diagnosis: chaparral-induced toxic liver damage (Sheikh et al., 1997) Subject had fatigue, jaundice, and dark urine; recovered within 2 wk

continued

TABLE C-1 Continued

Category/Case/Reference[a]	Number of Subjects[b]	Date
Case #7 Sheikh et al., 1997	1*	3/93
Case #8 Batchelor et al., 1995	1	4/89
Case #9 Katz and Saibil, 1990	1	
Case #10 Batchelor et al., 1995	1	Fall/89

Subject/Supplement	Adverse Effects[c] and Related Findings
57-year-old female (Sheikh's patient no. 7) Chaparral, 480 mg/d for 8 wk, capsule; estimated cumulative dose of 24 g (Sheikh et al., 1997) Patient history: past use of conjugated estrogen (possible hepatotoxin with persistent effects but deemed unlikely in this case)	Diagnosis: chaparral-induced toxic liver damage confirmed by liver biopsy (Sheikh et al., 1997) Subject had fatigue, jaundice, abdominal pain, light stools, and pruritus; recovered within 1 wk
71-year-old male (Batchelor's patient no. 1) Chaparral leaf as tablets Concomitant medication: none Patient history: concomitant and long-term alcohol use (14 oz wine/d) Subject-elected rechallenge: symptoms recurred upon restarting chaparral without alcohol	Diagnosis: jaundice and possible toxic liver damage (Batchelor et al., 1995) Subject presented with a 2-wk history of flu-like illness, ascites, and jaundice Symptoms resolved within 2 mo after cessation of chaparral and alcohol intake; restarted chaparral without alcohol and within 1 mo symptoms of liver damage recurred Subject was readmitted with jaundice, ascites, scleral icterus, and nausea; liver biopsy showed diffuse necrosis with inflammation, portal tract expansion, mild cholestasis, and mild fibrous septation; after 3 mo, symptoms again resolved and a repeat biopsy indicated marked improvement
33-year-old female "Chaparral leaf" (15 tablets/d for 3–4 mo, then various amounts), symptoms waxed and waned with variation in dose	Diagnosis: drug-induced hepatotoxicity due to ingestion of chaparral leaf (Katz and Saibil, 1990) Subject presented with jaundice, ascites, abdominal pain, fatigue, scleral icterus, anorexia, and pedal edema due to subacute hepatic necrosis; responded to diuretic therapy Subject workup was negative except for use of chaparral; the most common causes of hepatitis were ruled out, including an autoimmune response Subject recovered with cessation of chaparral intake
43-year-old female (Batchelor's patient no. 2) Chaparral leaf (≥ 3 tablets/d) for 6 wk, taken for relief from chronic tension headaches	Diagnosis: subacute chaparral-induced liver damage (Batchelor et al., 1995) Subject presented with a 2-wk history of flu-like illness and jaundice; recovered within 4 mo

continued

TABLE C-1 Continued

Category/Case/Reference[a]	Number of Subjects[b]	Date
Case #11 Sheikh et al., 1997	1*	5/93
Case #12 Sheikh et al., 1997	1*	1/93
Case #13 Sheikh et al., 1997	1*	
Case #14 Sheikh et al., 1997	1*	
Case #15 Sheikh et al., 1997	1*	

[a] The numbering of cases is consistent with that used in the full prototype monograph for chaparral, which included a Case #16 and a Case #24. These two cases are not included here because they do not address hepatotoxicity, the subject of the focused monograph.

[b] Many of the subjects included in Tables C-1 and C-2 as case reports are also included in

Subject/Supplement	Adverse Effects[c] and Related Findings
Concomitant medication: aspirin Patient history: infrequent alcohol use	
36-year-old female (Sheikh's patient no. 16) Chaparral as capsules, taken for 1 y; taken to gain energy Concurrent medication: naproxen sodium and ketorolac trimethamine	Diagnosis: possible subacute liver damage (Sheikh et al., 1997) Subject experienced nausea and abdominal pain with elevated bilirubin, but other clinical labs were within normal limits; recovered within 3 wk
63-year-old male (Sheikh's patient no. 14) Chaparral taken for 8 wk for degenerative arthritis of the knees Patient history: alcohol use	Diagnosis: subacute liver damage (Sheikh et al., 1997) Subject was asymptomatic, with transient (< 1 wk) elevated bilirubin and aminotransferase levels
57-year-old female (Sheikh's patient no. 11) Chaparral taken for 4 wk	Diagnosis: hepatotoxicity (Sheikh et al., 1997) Subject had jaundice and abnormal liver enzyme tests for 1 wk but refused follow-up; information is incomplete
54-year-old female (Sheikh's patient no. 12) Chaparral, 1,600 mg/day for 2.8 wk taken as a "cleanser"; estimated cumulative dose of 38 g (Sheikh et al., 1997)	Diagnosis: consistent with chaparral-associated liver damage (Sheikh et al., 1997) Subject had jaundice and abdominal pain; recovered within 6 wk; information is incomplete
39-year-old female (Sheikh's patient no. 13) Chaparral tea, 4 bags of single-ingredient chaparral tea daily for approximately 1.5 y (78 wk) taken for weight loss	Diagnosis: consistent with chaparral-associated liver damage (Sheikh et al., 1997) Subject had jaundice and abdominal pain; recovered within 1 wk; information is incomplete

Table D as Special Nutrition Adverse Event Monitoring System reports and are identified with an asterisk. Some cases that do not have an asterisk may also be included in more than one table. However, verification of duplicate cases was not possible given the available data.

[c] The clinical cases are arranged in decreasing order of apparent severity of the adverse effects.

TABLE C-2 Summary of Clinical Case Reports and a Case Series Report with Chaparral Used in Combination

Category/Case/Reference[a]	Number of Subjects[b]	Date
Liver toxicity		
Case #17 Gordon et al., 1995; Sheikh et al., 1997	1*	
Case #18 Smith and Desmond, 1993	1	
Case #19 Grant et al., 1998	1	

Subject/Supplement	Adverse Effects[c] and Related Findings
59/60-year-old-female (Gordon's patient and Sheikh's patient no. 4) Chaparral (1.8 g/d as capsules) over previous 10–12 mo; 3 wk before admission, increased capsules to 3–5 g/d; estimated cumulative dose of 108 g (Sheikh et al., 1997) Concurrent medications: diltiazem HCl, atenolol, enteric-coated aspirin, nitroglycerin patch, and occasional acetaminophen Concurrent botanicals: garlic powder, nettle, chickweed tea	Diagnosis: liver failure due to chaparral-induced toxic liver damage (Gordon et al., 1995; Sheikh et al., 1997) Subject presented with severe jaundice due to liver damage (including ascites, collapsed liver nodules with some regeneration, acute hepatitis, hepatocyte ballooning, portal inflammation, marked proliferation of bile ducts) Subject required a liver transplant and also experienced secondary renal failure requiring kidney transplant
36-year-old female Chaparral (2 capsules/d for 8 wk prior to onset of symptoms) Patient history: hepatitis A at age 7 Concurrent herbals: Numerous, but not specified	Diagnosis: severe acute toxic liver damage following ingestion of chaparral confirmed by liver biopsy (Smith and Desmond, 1993) Subject presented with a 5-wk history of anorexia, nausea, and malaise, and a 3-wk history of dark urine, icterus, and pruritus Subject discontinued chaparral use and recovered within 4 mo This is the only report from Australia
27-year-old male Chaparral "leaf" (capsules—Arizona Natural; 1,500–2,500 mg/d for 10–12 mo), taken to "prevent illness," label recommended 1,000 mg/d Patient history: occasional binge alcohol use in past few years; ceased smoking 4 yr earlier; denied illegal drug use; no prior transfusions Concurrent medication: none Concurrent supplement use: numerous, including *Echinacea purpurea* root plus another form of *Echinacea* (in 2 different preparations), goldenseal root, slippery elm bark (in 2 different preparations), mullein leaf, yerba santa leaf, ginger root, *Capsicum annum* (in 2 different preparations)	Diagnosis: toxic liver damage confirmed by liver biopsy (Grant et al., 1998) Subject presented with nausea, vomiting, diarrhea, and abdominal pain; subject had jaundice; liver enzyme tests were elevated and continued to increase over 3 wk until admitted to hospital and chaparral intake ceased Infectious hepatitis was ruled out (tested for A, B, C, and E) Biopsy showed hepatocellular injury with necrosis and periportal inflammation Liver transplant was considered until subject began to improve 3 wk later; condition stabilized

continued

TABLE C-2 Continued

Category/Case/Reference[a]	Number of Subjects[b]	Date
Case #20 Sheikh et al., 1997	1*	7/92
Case #21 Alderman et al., 1994	1	7/92
Case #22 Sheikh et al., 1997	1*	
Case #23 Shad et al., 1999	1	

Subject/Supplement	Adverse Effects[c] and Related Findings
45-year-old female (Sheikh's patient no. 3 and probably Alderman's patient) Chaparral, 1,440 mg/d as capsules for 2 wk then 1,920 mg/d for 8 wk; took chaparral as "general cleansing tonic"; estimated cumulative dose of 102 g (Sheikh et al., 1997) Patient history: concurrent alcohol use, obese, hypertension Concurrent medications: clonidine HCl, lovastatin (possible hepatotoxin, but unlikely in this case) Concurrent supplements: niacinamide, multivitamin tablets, magnesium, lecithin, passionflower, valerian, hops, and dandelion extract	Diagnosis: chaparral-induced toxic liver damage confirmed by liver biopsy (Sheikh et al., 1997) (See Alderman et al., 1994) Subject presented with jaundice, fatigue, nausea, vomiting, abdominal pain, bouts of diarrhea, and constipation
45-year-old female (probably Sheikh's patient no. 3) Chaparral tablets, 160 mg/d for previous 2–3 mo, taken to "relieve the craving for alcohol" Patient history: prior alcohol abuse until 2–3 mo prior to diagnosis Concurrent prescription drugs: clonidine, also lovastatin during part of the time Concurrent herbals: passionflower, valerium, hops; dandelion extract for a short period	Diagnosis: cholestatic hepatitis, possibly chaparral induced Alderman et al., 1994) (See Sheikh et al., 1997) Subject presented with jaundice without other symptoms; biopsy suggested cholangiolitic hepatitis due to drug treatment Subject recovered after treatment with prednisone
33-year-old female (Sheikh's patient no. 9) Chaparral, multi-ingredient product for 5–6 mo Concurrent medication: off and on use of acetaminophen (a possible hepatotoxin, but this effect is unlikely in this case) Concurrent supplements: liver oil, 1×/wk	Diagnosis: chaparral-induced toxic liver damage (Sheikh et al., 1997) Subject presented with fatigue, jaundice, dark urine, nausea, vomiting, and abdominal pain Subject recovered within 4 wk after discontinuation of chaparral-containing product
69-year-old male Chaparral, multi-ingredient herbal product (21 ingredients) (14 tablets/d, 6 wk)	Diagnosis: possible chaparral-induced toxic liver damage (Shad et al., 1999) Subject presented with jaundice Subject recovered within 8 wk after discontinuation of the chaparral-containing product

continued

TABLE C-2 Continued

Category/Case/Reference[a]	Number of Subjects[b]	Date
Other toxicity		
Case #25 Heron and Yarnell, 2001	1	6/97
Case #26 Heron and Yarnell, 2001	1	5/97
Cancer[e]		
Case #27 Heron and Yarnell, 2001	1	8/98
No *toxicity reported*		
Case #28 Heron and Yarnell, 2001	1	5/97

Subject/Supplement	Adverse Effects[c] and Related Findings
49-year-old female (Heron's patient no. 1) Multiherb tincture containing 8% chaparral,[d] ≤ 32 mL taken over 3.5 mo; proposed as a treatment for allergies Concurrent drug use: estrogens, progesterone, fluticasone nasal spray Concurrent herbals use: numerous	Subject reported dizziness when 10 mL was taken at one time General clinical history and physical examination findings were unremarkable; clinical lab tests were virtually unchanged, including serum liver enzymes, BUN, creatinine, glucose, electrolytes, bilirubin, iron ferritin, lipoproteins, and CBC; no elevations in liver function tests that would have indicated liver damage (Heron and Yarnell, 2001)
52-year-old female (Heron's patient no. 2) Multiherb tincture containing 8% chaparral, ≤ 240 mL taken over 5 mo; proposed as a treatment for respiratory symptoms of allergies Concurrent medications: loratidine, clonazepam, zolpidem, valproic acid, thyroid hormone Concomitant botanicals use: numerous	No elevations in liver function tests that would have indicated liver damage; changes in clinical laboratory values were likely related to concurrent medications; subject had chronic low WBC and platelet counts and low HDL cholesterol; TSH was high necessitating change in medication dose (Heron and Yarnell, 2001)
53-year-old male (Heron's patient no. 3) Multiherb tincture containing 7% chaparral, ≤ 34 mL taken over 40 d; proposed as treatment for painful axillary lymphadenopathy, which was later diagnosed as malignant melanoma, 5 mL, 1×/d Recurrence: 5 combined mL tincture, 3×/d plus topical chaparral in castor oil	Clinical lab tests included serum liver enzymes, BUN, creatinine, glucose, electrolytes, bilirubin, iron ferritin, lipoproteins, and CBC No elevations in blood levels of hepatic enzymes that would indicate liver damage Subject's clinical laboratory values did change in a manner consistent with the eventual diagnosis of malignant melanoma; the disease had metastasized (Heron and Yarnell, 2001)
51-year-old female (Heron's patient no. 4) Multiherb tinctures containing 10% chaparral, 5 mL, 3×/d, ≤ 138 mL taken over 3–4 mo; proposed as aid in weight-loss program	General clinical history and physical examination findings were unremarkable; clinical lab tests were virtually unchanged, including serum liver enzymes, BUN, creatinine, glucose, electrolytes, bilirubin, iron ferritin, lipoproteins, and CBC

continued

TABLE C-2 Continued

Category/Case/Reference[a]	Number of Subjects[b]	Date
Case #29 Heron and Yarnell, 2001	1	4/97
Case Series A Heron and Yarnell, 2001	8	

NOTE: Numbering of cases is continued from Table C-1. BUN = blood urea nitrogen, CBC = complete blood cell count, WBC = white blood cell count, HDL = high-density lipoprotein, TSH = thyroid-stimulating hormone.

[a] The numbering of cases is consistent with that used in the full prototype monograph for chaparral, which included a Case #16 and a Case #24. These two cases are not included here because they do not address hepatotoxicity, the subject of the focused monograph.

[b] Many of the subjects included in Tables C-1 and C-2 as case reports are also included in Table D as Special Nutrition Adverse Event Monitoring System reports and are identified with an asterisk. It was apparent that Case #16 was reported in two publications. Cases #18 and #19 appear to be the same subject, but this could not be confirmed based on the information reported. Some cases that do not have an asterisk may also be included in more than one table. However, verification of duplicate cases was not possible given the available data.

Subject/Supplement	Adverse Effects[c] and Related Findings
Concomitant use of botanicals: numerous	No elevations in liver function tests that would have indicated liver damage and (Heron and Yarnell, 2001)
Female (Heron's patient no. 5) Multiherb tincture containing 10% chaparral, ≤ 215 mL taken intermittently over 14 mo; proposed as treatment for recurrent dental infections	No elevations in liver function tests that would have indicated liver damage and (Heron and Yarnell, 2001)
Multiherb tincture containing chaparral, ≤ 30 mL ingested	No elevations in liver function tests that would have indicated liver damage and Heron and Yarnell, 2001)

[c] The clinical cases are arranged in decreasing order of apparent severity of the adverse effects.

[d] In the initial extraction, fresh (not dried) leaves and flowers of *Larrea tridentata* were lightly ground in ethanol:water (90:10) at 1:2.5 (w/v). (Heron and Yarnell, 2001).

[e] One other case report involving cancer exists (Smith et al., 1994), but it was omitted from this table for the following reasons. The cause and effect relationship between the subject's intake of chaparral and the development of cancer was not well documented. The subject (a 56-year-old female) used chaparral tea (3–4 cups/d) for 3 mo during the 1.5-y period prior to the diagnosis of cystic renal cell carcinoma. The subject also used taheebo tea (5–6 cups/d) for 6 mo almost 20 y earlier. Taheebo tea is reported to contain quinones. The date of the onset of the malignancy is unknown. In this report the correlation between the subject's cancer and the consumption of chaparral tea seems to have been made on the basis of the known effects of nordihydroguaiaretic acid (the major lignan in chaparral) in causing multiple renal cysts in rats. Thus there is no evidence that the subject's renal cancer was the result of consumption of chaparral.

TABLE D Chaparral: Summary of Adverse Event Reports from the Special Nutritionals Adverse Event Monitoring System (SN/AEMS)[a]

Category	Number of Subjects	Supplement	Adverse Events
Hepatic	1	Chaparral	Hepatitis (nonviral), nausea, fever
	1	Chaparral	Severe liver problems, kidney failure
	1	Chaparral	Severe hepatic injury with bile duct narrowing and cholestasis
	1	Chaparral	Acute toxic hepatitis, jaundice, abdominal pain, pruritus, dark urine
	1	Chaparral	Hepatitis
	1	Chaparral	Hepatitis
	1	Chaparral	Hepatitis, jaundice
	1	Chaparral	Jaundice, cholangitis, colitis, nausea, vomiting
	1	Chaparral	Jaundice, nausea
	1	Chaparral	Jaundice
	1	Chaparral (or chaparral-containing product, unspecified)	Jaundice
	1	Chaparral	Chaparral toxicity (likely hepatic involvement)
	1	Chaparral	Coma, liver damage

NOTE: There were reports in this monitoring system of five additional subjects who took chaparral along with other dietary supplements. These subjects were not considered in this analysis due to the unclear association between the adverse events and the use of chaparral as a result of the concomitant use of multiple dietary supplements. However, it should be noted that these five additional adverse events involved two deaths, two cases of hepatitis, and tachycardia with loss of vision in one eye.

[a] The Food and Drug Administration's SN/AMES is currently in the process of being updated to track and analyze adverse event reports related to dietary supplements. The information contained in this monograph was obtained from the system prior to August 29, 2002, when the database was withdrawn from the Internet.

TABLE E Nordihydroguaiaretic Acid (NDGA): Summary of Animal Studies

Species/Study Design	Results and Conclusions
Acute toxicity studies, gavage or oral administration	
Toxicity Data	Species / LD_{50} / Route Rat / 5.5 g/kg / Gavage (Lehman et al., 1951) Mouse / 4 g/kg / Gavage (Lehman et al., 1951) Mouse / 0.1–0.8 g/kg / i.p. (Fujii et al., 1970; Kozubik et al., 1993; Madrigal-Bujaidar et al., 1998) Guinea pig / 0.8 g/kg / Gavage (Lehman et al., 1951)
Rats (male, S/D), NDGA (single dose at 25 or 50 mg/kg body weight, gavage), ± indomethacin (20 mg/kg body weight, gavage), animals were sacrificed 4 hr later	NDGA enhanced indomethacin-induced mast cell degranulation in gastric mucosa NDGA increased prostanoid activity in gastric glandular mucosa With NDGA pretreatment, indomethacin-induced lesions in the gastric mucosa were more severe; this is a possible cytotoxic effect (Cho and Ogle, 1987)
Acute toxicity studies, other routes of administration	
Rats (Wistar Albino), NDGA (1 dose at 10 µg/kg body weight, i.v.)	In a model of ischemia reperfusion injury to the liver, rats were given NDGA 5 min before reperfusion (± iloprost, 25 µg/kg i.v., given just before warm ischemia) By histopathologic examination, liver damage was more extensive in the rats treated with NDGA compared with the control (saline-injected) animals (Okboy et al., 1992)
Mice (female, CD1), NDGA (50 mg/kg body weight, i.v.)	Pharmacokinetic analysis (using M_4NDGA as a standard): Peak plasma concentration = 14 µg/mL Exposure (AUC) = 248 µg/mL/min Clearance = 202 mL/(min/kg) Volume of distribution = 3.4 L/kg Half-life in 1st compartment = 30 min Half-life in 2nd compartment = 135 min NDGA appears to follow a 2-compartment pharmacokinetic model (Lambert et al., 2001)
Mice (male, CBA), NDGA (2 doses, 2-h apart, 50 mg/kg body weight, i.p.)	At 2 wk after treatments (NDGA, galactosamine, and endotoxin), histological examination of liver showed small foci of necrosis adjacent to areas of infiltration of inflammatory cells; some of this hepatic damage was due to endotoxin administration (Parry, 1993)

continued

TABLE E Continued

Species/Study Design	Results and Conclusions
Chronic toxicity studies, gavage or oral administration	
Rats (male, S/D), fed NDGA (2% of the diet, 0.4 g NDGA/d), up to 6 wk	With NDGA treatment, renal lesions (interstitial and tubular, but not glomerular) were observed as follows: infiltration of inflammatory cells, tubular cell proliferation or necrosis, cyst formation. The timeline for the appearance of the renal lesions and the severity varied with the germ-free/conventional (i.e., contaminated) state of the animal. Specifically, after deconditioning (removal from germ-free environment), lesions appeared more rapidly (within 1 wk) and cyst formation was more severe than in rats housed conventionally from birth (Gardner et al., 1986)
Rats (male, S/D), fed NDGA (2% of the diet), 3 wk	With NDGA treatment loss of body weight and development of renal lesions were striking, but only when animals we also fed endotoxin-containing bacteria or were injected with endotoxin; renal lesions were not characteristic of classic endotoxin treatment Animals treated with endotoxin alone (without NDGA in the diet) did not develop renal lesions (Gardner et al., 1987)
Rats (male, Wistar), fed NDGA (2% of the diet), ≤ 99 d	Widespread lesions in the kidney: hydropic changes in tubular epithelial cells, tubular necrosis, proliferation of lysosomes in number and size, invasion by macrophages (Goodman et al., 1970)
Rats (male, S/D), fed NDGA (2% of the diet), 1–24 wk	With NDGA treatment, glomerular filtration rate was decreased as compared with controls Early during NDGA exposure, tiny polyps developed along the outer medullary segments of the collecting tubules in the kidney; this likely leads to partial nephron obstruction At 2 mo of NDGA exposure, kidneys were infiltrated by polymorphonuclear leukocytes and macrophages; basement membrane thickening, fibrosis, tubular atrophy, and eventually proximal tubular cell necrosis characterized adjacent to these infiltrate areas By 6 mo of NDGA exposure, cysts were found throughout the kidneys (Evan and Gardner, 1979)
Rats (male and female, Wistar), fed NDGA (0.5% or 1% of the diet), 74 wk	In 32 out of 33 rats given NDGA, there were cysts of the mesenteric lymph nodes at the ileocecal junction; in one rat the cystic nodes were invaded by a malignant reticulum cell sarcoma Mean body weight was lower in NDGA group vs. control group (Grice et al., 1968)

TABLE E Continued

Species/Study Design	Results and Conclusions
Rats (male), fed NDGA (0.5% of the diet), 2 y	Growth inhibition was seen with NDGA at 0.5% of the diet after 6 mo Massive cecal hemorrhages with single and multiple cysts in the mesentery near the cecum were seen (Lehman et al., 1951)
Rats (male), fed NDGA (0.5% of the diet), 2 y	Inflammatory cecal lesions and slight cystic enlargement of paracaecal lymph nodes were seen Growth inhibition at 6 mo of NDGA feeding (Lehman et al., 1951)
Rats (female), fed NDGA (1% of the diet), 6 mo	Growth inhibition at 6 mo of NDGA feeding (Lehman et al., 1951)
Rats, fed NDGA (0.5% of the diet)	No effect on food intake, kidneys, liver, or spleen Cranston et al., 1947)
Rats, fed NDGA (0.1, 0.5, or 1% of the diet)	Some animals developed cysts in mesentery at 0.5% and 1.0% NDGA (Cranston et al., 1947)

NOTE: Acute toxicity studies are defined as a single administration or exposure for less than 24 h; chronic toxicity studies are defined as repeated administration or exposure for 1 mo or longer, combining what some authors call subchronic and chronic (Klassen, 1995). i.p. = intraperitoneally, S/D = Sprague-Dawley, iv = intravenously, AUC = area under the curve.

TABLE F-1 Chaparral: Summary of *In Vitro* Studies

Substance	Study Design	Results and Conclusions
Inhibition of enzymes		
Chaparral, methanol extract	Enzyme assays using rat (male and female, Sprague-Dawley) liver microsomes incubated with 0.1–100 µg chaparral extract/mL	At 10 µg/mL the chaparral extract inhibited glutathione S-transferase At 100 µg/mL the chaparral extract also inhibited aminopyrine N-demethylase (various cytochrome P450 forms), aniline hydroxylase (cytochrome P450 2E1), and UDP-glucuronyl transferase The activity of NADPH-cytochrome c reductase was increased by the larger amounts of the extract (Sapienza et al., 1997)

TABLE F-2 Nordihydroguaiaretic Acid (NDGA): Summary of *In Vitro* Studies

Substance	Study Design	Results and Conclusions
Apoptosis		
NDGA, 25 μM	Cells in culture: SW 850 (human pancreatic cancer cell line) C4-I (human cervical cancer cell line)	NDGA induced apoptosis within 3 hr reaching maximum in 12–16 hr Seufferlein et al., 2002)
NDGA, 10 μM, 4–18 h	Cells in culture: FL5.12 cells (mouse hematopoietic/ lymphocytic cell line, lipoxygenase-deficient)	NDGA induced apoptosis and greatly increased caspase-3-like activity (Biswal et al., 2000)
NDGA, IC_{50} 5 μM	Cells in culture: Walker-256 cells (rat epithelial carcinoma cell line, LLC-WRC 256 cells)	NDGA induced apoptosis (Tang and Honn, 1997)
NDGA, 25 μM	Cells in culture: MTLN-3 cells (rat tumor cell line) RBL cells (rat tumor cell line)	NDGA induced apoptosis (Tang and Honn, 1997)
NDGA, 25 μM	Cells in culture: A431 cells (human epithelial carcinoma cell line) HEH cells HL-60 cells (human myeloblastic cell line) U937 cells (human monocytes cell line)	NDGA induced apoptosis in some human cell lines
NDGA	Cells in culture: PC-3 cells (human cell line) 1-IL cells (human cell line) DU145 cells (human cell line) WB35 cells (human cell line) WM983A cells (human cell line) neoT cells (human cell line) MCF-7 cells (human epithelial adenocarcinoma cell line) MCF-10A cells (human mammary epithelial cell line) HT-1080 cells (human epithelial fibrosarcoma cell line)	NDGA (25–35 μM) did not induce apoptosis in other human cells (Tang and Honn, 1997)
NDGA, 30 μM	Cells in culture: LN-18 cells (human malignant glioma cell line)	NDGA inhibited mediated by CD95 receptor apoptosis (Wagenknecht et al., 1998)

continued

TABLE F-2 Continued

Substance	Study Design	Results and Conclusions
Cytotoxicity		
NDGA, LC_{50} 200 μM	Cells in culture: EMT6 cells (mouse mammary carcinoma cell line)	NDGA caused slight cytotoxic activity in EMT6 tumor cells, likely related to depletion of sulfhydryl groups (Shi and Pardini, 1995)
NDGA, LD_{50} 9–20 μg/mL	Cells in culture: Vero cells (African green monkey kidney epithelial cell line) Hep-2 cells (HeLa epithelial cell line)	NDGA had weak cytotoxic activity (Zamora et al., 1992)
NDGA, 25–250 μM, ≤ 72 hr	Cells in culture: 786A cells (sarcoma cell line), IC_{50} 0.24 mM TA3 cells (mammary cell line), IC_{50} 0.21 mM	NDGA had weak cytotoxic activity Addition of NDGA (250 μM) decreased cellular respiration and ATP concentration within 1 hr (Pavani et al., 1994)
NDGA	In cell suspensions: NDGA inhibited aerobic and anaerobic glycolysis and respiration	NDGA had cytotoxic activity (Burk and Woods, 1963)
NDGA	Cells in culture: WISH cells (human HeLa cell line)	NDGA decreased viability (ID_{50} 100 μg/mL) Blalock et al., 1981)
NDGA	Cells in culture: Mouse L cells	NDGA decreased viability (ID_{50} 100 μg/mL) (Blalock et al., 1981)
NDGA	Cells in culture: Ehrlich ascites cells	NDGA sensitized cells to X-ray irradiation (1,000 r) (von Ardenne et al., 1969) *These data were published in German. Summary is based on the English abstract*
NDGA, 150–600 mM	Tissue slices: Rat liver slices (male, Fisher 344)	During incubation of precision-cut rat liver slices with NDGA, cell viability decreased by several indicators (decreased content of potassium, LDH, and glycogen) Ethanol was also cytotoxic and the total effect was additive (Ulreich et al., 1997)

TABLE F-2 Continued

Substance	Study Design	Results and Conclusions
NDGA, 150–600 mM	Tissue slices: Rat kidney slices	During incubation of precision-cut rat kidney slices with NDGA, cell viability decreased by two indicators (decreased content of potassium and LDH) (Nakazato et al., 1998)
NDGA, 150–600 mM	Tissue slices: Human liver slices Human kidney slices	During incubation of precision-cut human liver or kidney slices with NDGA, cell viability decreased by two indicators (decreased content of potassium and LDH) Cytotoxicity was dose-dependent (Nakazato et al., 1998)
NDGA, LD_{50} 150 µM	Isolated cells: Rat hepatocytes	During a 2-hr incubation with NDGA or 21 different flavonoids and polyphenols, NDGA was one of the most cytotoxic, behind galangin and chrysin (Moridani et al., 2002)
Inhibition of cellular processes		
NDGA, K_i 140 µM	Isolated jejunal loops from rats (female Wistar), using luminal perfusion	NDGA inhibited intestinal glucose absorption, glucose utilization, and lactate production (Kellett et al., 1993)
NDGA, 30 µM	Cells in culture: 3T3-4 cells	NDGA enhanced glucose transport and metabolism (± insulin) (Reed et al., 1998, 1999).
NDGA, 30 µM	Isolated rat adipocytes	NDGA enhanced glucose transport 2-fold (± 100 pM insulin) (Reed et al., 1998, 1999)
NDGA	Isolated rat pancreatic islets	NDGA inhibited insulin secretion induced by glucose (Yamamoto et al., 1982)

continued

TABLE F-2 Continued

Substance	Study Design	Results and Conclusions
NDGA, 100 μM	Tissue culture: Isolated mouse pancreatic islets in culture for 1–2 wk	NDGA in the culture media reduced insulin secretion induced by glucose (20 mM) even though the total insulin content of islets was equivalent in control and NDGA-treated cultures (Hsu et al., 2001)
NDGA, 30 μM	Isolated rat adipocytes	NDGA inhibited lipolysis in response to isoproterenol or 8-chlorophenyltheo cAMP (Gowri et al., 1998)
NDGA, 50 μM	Isolated rat adipocytes	NDGA reduced lipolytic activity induced by isoproterenol and decreased the phosphorylated form of hormone-sensitive lipase (Gowri et al., 1998)
NDGA	Cells in culture: SW 850 (human pancreatic cancer cell line) C4-I (human cervical cancer cell line)	NDGA inhibited anchorage-dependent proliferation (data not shown) After incubation with NDGA for 8 hr, cells began to detach from tissue culture dish Incubation of cells with NDGA (25 μM) inhibited expression of cyclin D1 (while expression of cyclin E was unchanged) Incubation of cells with NDGA (25 μM) resulted in disruption of the cytoskeleton (actin stress fibers but not the circumferential actin filament network) Incubation of cells with NDGA (25 μM) activated stress-activated MAP kinases (JNK1/2 and $p38^{mapk}$ but not ERK1/2) (Seufferlein et al., 2002)

TABLE F-2 Continued

Substance	Study Design	Results and Conclusions
NDGA, 15–30 µM	Cells in culture in soft agar: SW 850 (human pancreatic cancer cell line) C4-I (human cervical cancer cell line)	NDGA inhibited colony formation in response to 0.5% or 10% fetal bovine serum, thought to represent anchorage-independent growth (Seufferlein et al., 2002)
		NDGA inhibited anchorage-dependent proliferation (data not shown) (Seufferlein et al., 2002)
		After incubation with NDGA for 8 hr, cells began to detach from tissue culture dish
NDGA, 10 µM	Cells in culture: HEK293 cells (human embryonic cell line) Porcine coronary arterial smooth muscle cells)	NDGA at 10 µM activates the Ca^{2+}-dependent K^+ channel, releasing Ca^{2+} (Yamamura et al., 2002)
NDGA, > 10 µM	Cells in culture: HEK293 cells (human embryonic cell line) Porcine coronary arterial smooth muscle cells)	NDGA at > 10 µM quickly causes a large increase the intracellular concentration of Ca^{2+} (Yamamura et al., 2002)
NDGA, 5–100 µM	Cells in culture: Rat C6 glioma cells	NDGA increased the concentration of intracellular Ca^{2+} (Su et al., 2002)
NDGA, 1–100 µM	Isolated porcine coronary artery smooth muscle cells (inside-out and outside-in patches)	NDGA opens the Ca^{2+}-dependent K^+ channel, except in the presence of very low cytosolic Ca^{2+} concentrations (Nagano et al., 1996)
NDGA, 100 µM	Bovine heart mitochondria	NDGA inhibited mitochondrial electron transport (by inhibition of NADH-coenzyme Q reductase and succinate coenzyme Q reductase) (Pardini et al., 1970)
NDGA	Beef heart mitochondria	NDGA reduced microsomal electron transport by inhibiting succinate cytochrome c reductase (Shi and Pardini, 1995)

continued

TABLE F-2 Continued

Substance	Study Design	Results and Conclusions
NDGA, IC_{50} 15 ηmoles/mg mitochondrial	Rat liver mitochondria	NDGA inhibited mitochondrial electron transport (Bhuvaneswaran and Dakshinamurti, 1972)
Inhibition of enzymes		
NDGA	Rat epidermal and hepatic microsomal cytochrome P-450	NDGA inhibited aryl hydrocarbon hydroxylase (CYP 1A and 1B) and inhibited 7-ethoxy-resorufin O-demethylase (CYP 1A) activities (Agarwal et al., 1991)
NDGA, 100 μM	Cells in culture: Hep-G-2 cells	NDGA inhibited cytochrome 1A1 induction (hydrodynamic stress-induced) (Mufti and Shuler, 1996)
NDGA	Rat liver homogenate (IC_{50} 6 μM) Human liver homogenate Human placenta homogenate	NDGA inhibited catechol O-methyl transferase and (Burba and Becking, 1969)
NDGA, K_i 125 μM	Isolated jejunal loops from rats (female Wistar), luminal perfusion	NDGA inhibited ($Mg^{2+}/Na^+/K^+$)-ATPase and (Na^+/K^+)-ATPase in jejunum (Kellett et al., 1993)
NDGA	Various enzyme sources	NDGA inhibited carboxylesterase (2 μM) and inhibited formyltetrahydrofolate synthetase (ED_{50} 100 μM) (Schegg and Welch, 1984)
NDGA, 100 μM	Microsomes	NDGA inhibited cyclooxygenase (Van der Merwe et al., 1993)
NDGA, IC_{50} 1 μM	Rat platelets	NDGA inhibited platelet cyclooxygenase (Ferrandiz et al., 1990)
NDGA, IC_{50} 1–42 μM	Intact cells and cell-free preparations	NDGA inhibited 5-lipoxygenase activity (peritoneal neutrophils from female Wistar rats, IC_{50} 2–4 μM); inhibited 15-lipoxygenase activity (isolated from soybean, IC_{50} 4 μM); and inhibited

TABLE F-2 Continued

Substance	Study Design	Results and Conclusions
		cyclooxygenase activity (peritoneal macrophages from male CD-1 mice, IC_{50} 1–42 μM) (Chang et al., 1984).
NDGA, IC_{50} 0.2 μM	Soybean lipoxygenase	NDGA inhibited lipoxygenase (Whitman et al., 2002)
NDGA, IC_{50} 5 μM	Human platelet 12-lipoxygenase	NDGA inhibited human 12-lipoxygenase (Whitman et al., 2002).
NDGA, IC_{50} 0.1 μM	Human reticulocyte 15-lipoxygenase	NDGA inhibited human 15-lipoxygenase (Whitman et al., 2002)
NDGA, IC_{50} 10 μM	Cells in culture: Caco-2 (human colon epithelial cell line)	NDGA (10 μM) inhibited 15-lipoxygenase activity without inhibiting cyclooxygenase activity (data not shown) (Kamitani et al., 1998)
NDGA, IC_{50} 0.3 μM	Rabbit erythroid 15-lipoxygenase	NDGA inhibited 15-lipoxygenase (Luther et al., 1991)
NDGA, IC_{50} 180 μM	Sheep vesicular gland prostaglandin H synthase	NDGA inhibited prostaglandin H synthase (Luther et al., 1991)
NDGA, 10 μM	Rat alveolar macrophages and Chinese hamster lung fibroblasts	NDGA inhibited phospholipase A_2 (Robison et al., 1990)
NDGA, IC_{50} 11 μM	Human aromatase: Placental microsomes Choriocarcinoma cell line JEG-3	NDGA inhibited human aromatase (estrogen synthetase) (Adlercreutz et al., 1993)
NDGA, K_i 94 μM	Rabbit skeletal muscle enzyme	NDGA inhibited phosphofructokinase (Kellett et al., 1993)
NDGA, IC_{50} 41 μM	Rat liver microsomes	NDGA inhibited aryl hydrocarbon hydroxylase (Agarwal et al., 1991)
Other		
NDGA, 10 ηM	Cells in culture: Human renal tubular cells (epithelial cells)	NDGA increased the incorporation of hydroxyproline, a component of basement membrane (Vedovato et al., 1994)

continued

TABLE F-2 Continued

Substance	Study Design	Results and Conclusions
NDGA, 10 μM	Chemiluminescence was used to indicate production of oxidative metabolites from polymorphonuclear leukocytes interacting with formyl-methionyl-leucyl-phenylalanine.	NDGA acted as antioxidant that eliminates extracellular and intracellular production of oxidative metabolites (Dahlgren, 1991)
NDGA	Cells in culture: Chinese hamster V79 cells	NDGA reduced cytotoxicity of H_2O_2 (Nakayama, 1994)
Derivatives of NDGA (also present in chaparral)		
3′-*O*-Methyl NDGA, ID_{50} 41 ηmol/mg mitochondrial protein	Beef heart mitochondria	3′-*O*-Methyl NDGA inhibited mitochondrial electron transport (by inhibition of succinoxidase and NADH-oxidase) (Heiser et al., 1977)
Meso-dihydro-guiaretic acid	Rat liver microsomes	Inhibited aminopyrene N-demethylase activity (various CYP forms) (Stetler-Stevenson et al., 1992)
Secoisolariciresinol	Cells in culture: P-388 (mouse lymphocyte leukemia cell line) IC_{50} 8.3 μg/mL (23 μM) KB-16 (human nasopharyngcal carcinoma cell line) IC_{50} 0.8 μg/mL (2.2 μM) A-549 (human lung adenocarcinoma cell line) IC_{50} 1.4 μg/mL (3.9 μM) HT-29 (human colon adenocarcinoma cell line) IC_{50} 0.6 μg/mL (1.7 μM)	Weak cytotoxic activity (Shen et al., 1997)

NOTE: LC_{50} = concentration that is lethal to 50 percent of the organisms exposed, LD_{50} = dose that is lethal to 50 percent of the organisms exposed, ID_{50} = dose at which the response has decreased to 50 percent of the original response, LDH = lactate dehydrogenase, CYP = cytochrome P450, ED_{50} = dose required to produce a specified effect in 50 percent of the test organisms exposed, CD-1 = a strain of mice.

TABLE G Chaparral: Related Substances That Might Suggest Risk

Study Design	Structure	Results and Conclusions
Lignan: substituted guaiaretic acid derivative		
Tetra-O-methylnordihydroguaiaretic acid, synthetic (Lambert et al., 2001)	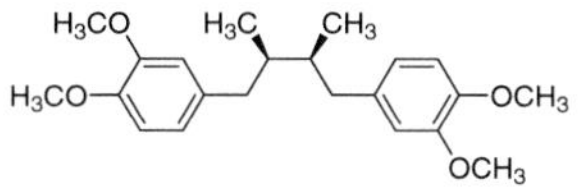	No data suggestive of toxicity are available
Naphthoquinone		
Larreantin Present in the roots of *L. tridentate* (Luo et al., 1988); not known to be present in the aerial parts of *L. tridentata*, but a possible component	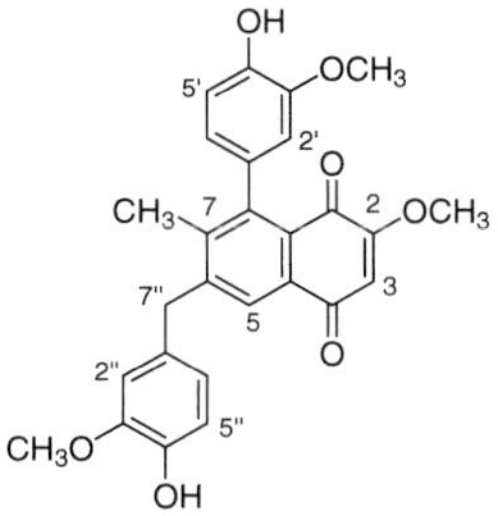	*In vitro* study: weak cytotoxic activity Potential hepatotoxin: in general, quinones are reactive species and readily form adducts with cellular macromolecules and thus can cause cellular damage; naphthoquinones are lipophilic and readily react with membrane-bound macromolecules (e.g., membrane bound enzymes such as the cytochrome P450s) as well as cytosolic molecules (e.g., glutathione) Another mechanism by which quinones cause cellular damage is by increasing the oxidative stress of the cell as the quinone/semiquinone pair repeatedly cycle, generating oxygen radicals or other intracellular radicals with each cycle (Jaeschke et al., 2002)

NOTE: Only the substances considered to be relevant to the risk of chaparral as a dietary supplement are included in the table. "Functionally related" substances may exhibit an activity that chaparral exhibits, based on *in vitro* or other data; they are not listed here because they have a similar chemical composition.

Appendix K

Prototype Focused Monograph: Review of Antiandrogenic Risks of Saw Palmetto Ingestion by Women[1]

I. DESCRIPTION OF THE INGREDIENT

A. Saw Palmetto as a Dietary Supplement Ingredient

Saw palmetto refers to *Serenoa repens* (W. Bartram) Small (Family: Arecaceae). An alternative name for the Arecaceae family is Palmae or Palmaceae. This plant is also known as (1) *Serenoa serrulatum* Schultes, (2) *Serenoa serrulata* (Michaux) Nichols, and (3) *Sabal serrulata* (Michaux) Nutall ex Schultes.

The medicinal part of saw palmetto is the fruit, which is about the size of a berry and is sometimes referred to as a "saw palmetto berry," although it is a single seed drupe. The fruit is rich in carbohydrates and lipid components. The dried ripe fruit is typically the part of the plant used for dietary supplements.

[1]This is a focused monograph, prepared for the purpose of illustrating how a safety review of a dietary supplement ingredient might be prepared following the format for focused monographs described in this report. While it was prepared as a prototype using the processes described in the report, it was not conducted under the auspices of the Food and Drug Administration utilizing all the resources available to the agency. Thus some pertinent information not available to the Committee could be of importance in evaluating safety to determine if use of this dietary supplement ingredient would present an unreasonable risk of illness or injury. Also, the development and review of this prototype was conducted by individuals whose backgrounds are in general aspects of evaluating science and whose expertise is not necessarily focused specifically on this dietary ingredient, although significant additional assistance was provided by consultants with relevant expertise. Therefore, this prototype monograph, while extensive, does not represent an authoritative statement regarding the safety of this dietary supplement ingredient.

B. Individual Components

Table A contains a list of the known components in extracts of saw palmetto fruit. Some components are common in many other plants and are widespread in the human diet. The components of extracts of saw palmetto fruit are commonly categorized as hexane extractable (i.e., phytosterols, phenolic components, free fatty acids, ethyl esters of fatty acids, and other lipid components), ethanol extractable (i.e., polyprenoids, flavonoid components, phenolic glycosides, and fatty alcohols), or water soluble (i.e., commonly found sugars and unique high-molecular-weight acidic polysaccharides). A hexane extract of saw palmetto fruit is the preparation that has been used most commonly in clinical trials. The hexane extract of saw palmetto fruit is unusual for a plant extract in that is has a very high content of medium-chain fatty acids and a high proportion of fatty acids present as ethyl esters.

C. Description of Dietary Supplement Preparations and Amounts Ingested in Ordinary Use

Saw palmetto is sold in several forms with lipid/sterol and "oily" extracts of the dried fruit being the most common forms on the market. A lipid/sterol extract of saw palmetto fruit (LESP) can be prepared by extraction with *n* hexane (100 percent), extraction with ethanol (70–95 percent, w/w), or by supercritical fluid extraction with liquid carbon dioxide. LESPs are somewhat quantifiable or standardized by total fatty acid content (usually 70–95 percent, w/w) or other components (USP, 2000). LESPs are commonly sold as capsules or tablets of a dried powder of the extract and in blended preparations where the powdered extract is combined with other ingredients, typically other powdered botanical extracts. Other forms of saw palmetto that may be available include powdered dried fruit (usually available in capsule or tablet form), dried whole fruit or preparations of the fruit (used in making a tea or water extract), tinctures (extracts made with aqueous ethanol as the solvent), and other liquid extracts.

In numerous clinical trials, the typical dose of saw palmetto for a subject with symptomatic benign prostatic hyperplasia (BPH)[2] was 320 mg

---

[2]BPH is a nonmalignant enlargement of the prostate from excessive proliferation, which causes nodules of the prostate gland to enlarge around the urethra, eventually limiting urinary flow from the bladder. Throughout life, dihydrotestosterone (DHT) directly stimulates the growth of the epithelial and stromal cells of the prostate. In aging men, the prostate is more responsive to androgen stimulation and the gland increases in size, causing urinary symptoms. Symptoms include difficulty in starting or stopping urine flow, a need to urinate frequently (especially at night), and a feeling of urgency-to-urinate. Urinary tract infections and urinary obstruction are common.

of LESP per day in 1 to 3 divided doses taken orally (or rectally in a few trials). The duration of ingestion of LESP varied from several weeks to several years.

II. SAFETY INFORMATION

A. Human Safety Data

1. Historical use

Historical use of saw palmetto for symptoms of BPH has been common in Asia and in native cultures in North America for centuries (Lowe, 2001; Wilt et al., 1998). Of the 30 plants known to have been used historically in phytotherapy for symptoms of BPH, saw palmetto has been the most widely used (Wilt et al., 1998). Historical uses were limited to saw palmetto in the form of the whole fruit, teas, aqueous extracts, and tinctures. They did not include lipid/sterol extracts of saw palmetto fruit such as those available in the current market.

In American Indian cultures, specifically in Florida, saw palmetto fruit was considered useful as a diuretic, sedative, aphrodisiac, nutritional tonic (due to the high oil content of the fruit), and to create a soothing vapor used as an expectorant. As American and European cultures learned about American Indian phytotherapy, the saw palmetto fruit came to be used to improve sexual vigor; to increase sperm production; as a mild diuretic; to relieve urinary difficulty, such as urgency-to-urinate and nocturnal enuresis in both men and women; and to improve urogenital disorders in women, such as ovarian enlargement and dysmenorrhea (Gennaro, 2000; Wilt et al., 1998).

Typically, the dried, ripe fruit is used for medicinal purposes. At times, the fresh fruit may be used; the safety of this practice has not been evaluated.

2. Adverse effects

Clinical trials: The clinical data for saw palmetto is primarily generated on male subjects. The one trial in women is in Table B, but there is no indication that pregnant women were included in this trial.

Spontaneous adverse event reports: Spontaneous reports related to possible effects *in utero* did not exist.

3. Interactions

Not applicable to the focus of this monograph.

B. Animal Studies

Animal studies: Only minimal classical animal toxicity data are available (Barsanti et al., 2000). These studies did not assess possible effects *in utero* or in offspring.

Table E summarizes information available from animal experiments related to antiandrogenic activity. In summary, in some model systems, antiandrogenic activity (specifically inhibition of hormonally or chemically induced prostate hyperplasia) can be demonstrated for extracts of saw palmetto fruit. In other model systems, no antiandrogenic activity was demonstrated.

C. *In Vitro* Studies

In vitro *studies:* Table F summarizes relevant information from *in vitro* experiments with saw palmetto. Inhibition of androgen-dependent proliferation and cellular stimulation have been demonstrated for extracts of saw palmetto fruit.

In vitro inhibition of testosterone metabolism through inhibition of steroid 5-α-reductase and 3-α-hydroxysteroid dehydrogenase was demonstrated. Inhibition of androgen binding was demonstrated in some model systems.

Classical *in vitro* toxicity data available are minimal (Degenring et al., 2001; Ondrizek et al., 1999a, 1999b) and do not address antiandrogenic concerns in females.

D. Related Substances

Table G contains information relevant to antiandrogenic safety issues for substances related to saw palmetto. Information about substances that are functionally related because they inhibit steroid 5-α-reductase is included. In summary, several of the substances functionally related to saw palmetto extract are contraindicated for use in women because of potential deleterious effects on the external genitalia and internal reproductive organs of the male fetus.

III. OTHER RELEVANT INFORMATION

A. Sources

The saw palmetto is one of the "fan palms"; it is also called the American dwarf palm tree or cabbage palm. The plant is sometimes called sabal and the fruit is called sabal fructus. This can be confusing because the saw palmetto is not a member of the genus *Sabal*; it is a distinct plant that can be confused with the *Sabal palmetto*. Other names for saw palmetto include shrub palmetto, juzhong, and palmier nain. Botanical descriptions of saw palmetto can be found in the literature (Leung and Foster, 1996).

Saw palmetto is an evergreen shrub, usually 2 to 10 feet tall. It is indigenous to undeveloped areas of the southern costal regions of the United States, especially Florida and Georgia, and is also abundant in Cuba and the Bahamas. Most saw palmetto fruit used in dietary supplements is harvested in Florida. It grows rapidly in sandy soil (either acidic or alkaline) and forms prominent colonies in sandy dunes, hammocks, or costal prairies. In the Northern Hemisphere, the plant blooms from April to early June and the fruit ripens in September and October.

Analytical issues: Saw palmetto was defined in the U.S. Pharmacopeia (USP) formulary in the early 1990s, but was eventually dropped. The 2002 National Formulary describes saw palmetto and powdered saw palmetto as preparations of partially dried, ripe fruit (USP, 2002). The USP requirements are voluntary, but must be met for any product bearing the USP designation. The USP formulary contains general tests for quality assurance[3] and specific tests for saw palmetto or powdered saw palmetto[4] (USP, 2000). Because these tests are voluntary, consumers have little assurance of product quality; variability in products is high (Feifer et al., 2002).

B. Relevant Conditions of Use Suggested or Recommended in Labeling or in Other Marketing Material

Occasionally, saw palmetto is marketed to women for urinary function, milk production during lactation, and, rarely, breast enlargement.

---

[3]General USP tests for quality assurance are (i) foreign organic matter, (ii) loss on drying, (iii) total ash, (iv) acid-insoluble, (v) pesticide residues, (vi) heavy metals, and (vii) microbial limits.

[4]Specific USP tests for saw palmetto or powdered saw palmetto are (i) botanic characteristics, macroscopic and microscopic (not applicable for powdered saw palmetto), (ii) identification, (iii) volatile oil content, (iv) content of lipophilic extract, and (v) content of fatty acids. The latter test includes identification of 11 USP methyl fatty acid RS standards (C6:0 through C18:3).

C. Cautions About Use

***Cautions provided in labeling[5] or other marketing material*:** A review of saw palmetto product labels and Internet marketing materials indicated that many (but not all) provide cautions to consumers to seek advice from health care providers before using the products if they have had prostate disorders or hormone-dependent cancers or are taking prescription medication, are pregnant, or are nursing. Some products carry warnings to discontinue use two weeks prior to surgery.

D. Usage Patterns

Total usage patterns and usage by men have been studied, but very little information is available about usage by women.

Saw palmetto has been used extensively in Europe and Asia. European sales figures for 1997 were $4 billion (Levy, 1998). In the United States, sales data reported by the Natural Marketing Institute ranked saw palmetto as the thirteenth best selling dietary supplement (Marra, 2002); however, sales growth has decreased 11 percent since 2001 (Marra, 2002). Sales for the U.S. market for saw palmetto supplements have been reported as $18 million in 1997 (Levy, 1998), $140 million in 1999 (Anon, 2000b), and $640 million in 2000 (Anon, 2000a). In a survey that examined the prevalence of use of herbal products among 752 randomly selected adults in Minnesota, saw palmetto was reportedly used by 4.3 percent of 376 respondents within the past 12 months to treat or prevent enlarged prostate, and to a lesser extent to promote general health and well-being and stimulate the immune system (Harnack et al., 2001).

It is estimated that 50 percent of men over the age of 50 have some symptoms of BPH (Berry et al., 1984). The incidence of BPH is 80 percent in men over the age of 80 (Berry et al., 1984). Urinary symptoms due to BPH result in 300,000 prostatectomies in the United States each year (Pinn, 2001). In a survey of patients in a U.S. urology clinic, 20 percent were combining conventional and botanical therapies, and 15 percent were using botanical dietary supplements alone (Bales et al., 1999). Over 30 percent of men with prostate problems have ingested saw palmetto for some period of time (Anon, 2000a).

---

[5]As defined in the Federal Food, Drug, and Cometic Act (FDCA) as currently amended, "The term 'labeling' means all labels and other written, printed, or graphic matter (1) upon any article or any of its containers or wrappers, or (2) accompanying such article." The term "label" is not being used; label means "a display of written, printed, or graphic matter upon the immediate container of any article" (FDCA, 21U.S.C. § 201(k) and (m)).

E. Information on Regulation and Regulatory Actions

Foreign regulatory status: Saw palmetto is approved as a drug with prescription status in Austria, Italy, and Poland (Vallancien and Pariente, 2001). It is approved as a drug with over-the-counter drug (OTC) status for use in various urinary problems associated with BPH in Switzerland, Sweden, and Denmark. In Spain, standardized lipid/sterol extracts are approved as a drug with prescription status, and nonstandardized extracts are approved as dietary supplements. In France, saw palmetto has OTC status but is primarily prescribed by physicians. In Germany, the Commission E has evaluated saw palmetto as safe and effective for urination problems in mild to moderate BPH; extracts of saw palmetto fruit have OTC status but are primarily prescribed by physicians (Blumenthal, 1998). In Canada, saw palmetto is authorized for sale as a traditional herbal medicine with the indication of increasing the flow of urine.

F. Available Information on Physiological and Biochemical Aspects

Very little is known about the digestion, absorption, distribution, metabolism, and excretion of some components of saw palmetto fruit (i.e., phenolic components, phytosterols, flavonoids, and polyprenoids). Other components have been well characterized (i.e., sugars, fatty acids, and other hydrocarbons).

Distribution: In a study of rats given a radioactive *n*-hexane LESP, tissue concentrations of radioactive labeled isolates of lauric acid, oleic acid, and β-sitosterol were highest in abdominal fat tissue, prostate, and skin. Lower concentrations were distributed to the liver and urinary bladder (Chevalier et al., 1997). No other studies reporting on the distribution of components of saw palmetto fruit were identified. Saw palmetto components were not clearly identified in any reports found in the literature.

G. Supplementary Information

Rectal administration: Extract of saw palmetto fruit was administered rectally (De Bernardi di Valserra and Tripodi, 1994) to show that the bioavailability and pharmacokinetic profile was quite similar to oral administration. T_{max} occurred about 1 hour after administration and a component was still detectable in plasma after 8 hours.

Topical use: A lotion containing cystine and saw palmetto extract is of possible use in alopecia (Morganti et al., 1998).

IV. TABLES ON SAW PALMETTO[6]

Table A	Individual Components of Saw Palmetto Fruit
Table B	Saw Palmetto: Summary of Adverse Effects in Clinical Trials
Table C	Saw Palmetto: Summary of a Clinical Case Reports (no relevant data available)
Table D	Saw Palmetto: Summary of Adverse Event Reports (no relevant data available)
Table E	Saw Palmetto: Summary of Animal Studies
Table F	Saw Palmetto: Summary of *In Vitro* Studies
Table G	Saw Palmetto: Related Substances that Might Suggest Risk

V. SUMMARY AND CONCLUSIONS

A. Summary

Saw palmetto is being widely used by men for prostate-related conditions, most notably benign prostate hyperplasia. Descriptions of saw palmetto are appearing in pharmacology texts for use in cystitis and for its antiedematous and antiandrogenic properties (Gennaro, 2000). There is a concern that these antiandrogenic properties pose a risk to males *in utero* because of the potential for deleterious effects on male genitalia.

Several pieces of evidence integrated together demonstrate that while there have not been documented cases of saw palmetto-induced birth defects in male offspring of humans or animals, there is a risk associated with saw palmetto ingestion by women.

It is well understood that testosterone, an androgen, or male sex hormone, is required for developing and maintaining masculine sexual characteristics. Testosterone is converted to the most active androgen DHT by 5-α-reductase, which then exerts the androgen action via androgen receptors.

In vitro data consistently demonstrate that saw palmetto extracts inhibit the testosterone conversion to DHT, including by inhibiting the 5-α-reductase enzyme. They also inhibit binding of DHT to androgenic receptors. Both of these actions would inhibit the androgen pathway if they occurred *in vivo*.

Animal data indicate that orally consumed saw palmetto preparations are antiandrogenic *in vivo*. Several animal studies were completed with oral administration of saw palmetto extracts following androgen stimulation of prostate hyperplasia. Studies indicate that saw palmetto extract at 50 to

[6]Tables appear at the end of this appendix.

300 mg/kg/day inhibit the androgen-stimulated hyperplasia in what appears to be a dose-dependent manner within studies. The 50 mg/kg/day is higher than the ~5 mg/kg/day ingested by humans (assuming 320 mg/day of LESP and 70-kg weight), but not high enough to mitigate concern for such serious effects as teratogenicity.

Inhibitors of 5-α-reductase are known to cause adverse effects and are thus contraindicated in women who may become pregnant (Table G). They are classified as pregnancy category X, the category indicating the greatest concern for pregnant women. As described in Table G, the pregnancy category X of these drugs results from teratogenicity studies in animals. These studies have shown that male offspring of animals (including monkeys) that consumed 5-α-reductase inhibitors exhibit abnormal male genitalia development.

Finally, the presumed mechanism for effectiveness of saw palmetto in prostate disorders is inhibition of androgen-sensitive pathways. This is partly because the prostate problems being investigated are generally treated by steroid 5-α-reductase inhibitors (Thomson PDR, 2004). Along these lines, the effect of saw palmetto on androgen pathways has also specifically been examined in humans. In a clinical study of healthy young males, no change in serum DHT was observed from ingesting the extract of saw palmetto fruit (320 mg/d, two divided doses, for 1 week) (Strauch et al., 1994). However, it was shown that activity of 5-α-reductase was decreased in prostate tissue and the content of DHT was markedly decreased in prostate tissue (mainly in the periurethral zone) in patients with benign prostatic hyperplasia who had ingested extract of saw palmetto fruit for 3 months.

The historical use of saw palmetto does not mitigate any concern about safety for pregnant women for several reasons. Most obvious is that saw palmetto has been predominantly used by men, and there is no indication that it has been safely used by pregnant women.

B. Conclusions and Recommendations About the Safety of the Ingredient Based on the Strength of the Scientific Evidence

At the present time, the weight of scientific evidence suggests that consumption of saw palmetto poses a risk to unborn male fetuses. This overall public health concern is mitigated somewhat by the much lower popularity of saw palmetto with women, but as noted previously, saw palmetto use is not limited to men. In summary, unless information becomes available to suggest that the antiandrogenic activity in humans is not high enough to cause birth defects in male offspring, a concern exists.

VI. LITERATURE CITED

Anon. 2000a. Herbal Rx for prostate problems. *Consum Rep* 65(9):60–62.

Anon. 2000b. The mainstreaming of alternative medicine. *Consum Rep* 65(5):17–25.

Bales GT, Christiano AP, Kirsh EJ, Gerber GS. 1999. Phytotherapeutic agents in the treatment of lower urinary tract symptoms: A demographic analysis of awareness and use at the University of Chicago. *Urology* 54:86–89.

Barsanti JA, Finco DR, Mahaffey MM, Fayrer-Hosken RA, Crowell WA, Thompson FN Jr, Shotts EB. 2000. Effects of an extract of *Serenoa repens* on dogs with hyperplasia of the prostate gland. *Am J Vet Res* 61:880–885.

Bayne CW, Donnelly F, Ross M, Habib FK. 1999. Serenoa repens (Permixon®): A 5α-reductase types I and II inhibitor-new evidence in a co-culture model of BPH. *Prostate* 40:232–241.

Berry SJ, Coffey DS, Walsh PC, Ewing LL. 1984. The development of human benign prostatic hyperplasia with age. *J Urol* 132:474–479.

Blumenthal M, ed. 1998. *The Complete German Commission E Monographs: Therapeutic Guide to Herbal Medicines.* Austin, TX: American Botanical Council.

Bombardelli E, Morazzoni P. 1997. *Serenoa repens* (Bartram) J.K. Small. *Fitoterapia* 68:99–113.

Breu W, Hagenlocher M, Redl K, Tittel G, Stadler F, Wagner H. 1992. Anti-inflammatory activity of *Sabal* fruit extracts prepared with supercritical carbon dioxide. *In vitro* antagonists of cyclooxygenase and 5-lipoxygenase metabolism. *Arzneimittelforschung* 42:547–551.

California Department of Health Services. 2002. *State Health Director Warns Consumers about Prescription Drugs in Herbal Products.* Online. Available at http://www.applications.dhs.ca.gov/pressreleases/store/pressreleases/02-03.html. Accessed January 8, 2003.

Carilla E, Briley M, Fauran F, Sultan C, Duvilliers C. 1984. Binding of Permixon®, a new treatment for prostatic benign hyperplasia, to the cytosolic androgen receptor in the rat prostate. *J Steroid Biochem* 20:521–523.

Chevalier G, Benard P, Cousse H, Bengone T. 1997. Distribution study of radioactivity in rats after oral administration of the lipido/sterolic extract of *Serenoa repens* (Permixon®) supplemented with [1-14C]-lauric acid, [1-14C]-oleic acid or [4-14C]-beta-sitosterol. *Eur J Drug Metab Pharmacokinet* 22:73–83.

Cristoni A, Morazzoni P, Bombardelli E. 1997. Chemical and pharmacological study on hypercritical CO2 extracts of *Serenoa repens* fruits. *Fitoterapia* 68:355–358.

De Bernardi di Valserra M, Tripodi AS. 1994. Rectal bioavailability and pharmacokinetics in healthy volunteers of *Serenoa repens* new formulation. *Arch Med Interna* 46:77–86.

Degenring FH, Sokolowski A, Suter A, Weber M. 2001. *Salmonella typhimurium* reverse mutation assay with the *Serenoa repens* extract Prostasan®. Online. *The European Phytojournal* Vol. 2. Accessed December 12, 2002.

De Swaef SI, Vlietinck AJ. 1996. Simultaneous quantitation of lauric acid and ethyl laureate in *Sabal serrulata* by capillary gas chromatography and derivatisation with trimethyl sulphoniumhydroxide. *J Chromatogr A* 719:479–482.

De Swaef SI, Kleibohmer W, Vlietinck AJ. 1996. Supercritical fluid chromatography of free fatty acids and ethyl esters in ethanolic extracts of *Sabal serrulata. Phytochem Anal* 7:223–227.

Délos S, Iehlé C, Martin PM, Raynaud JP. 1994. Inhibition of the activity of "basic" 5α-reductase (type 1) detected in DU 145 cells and expressed in insect cells. *J Steroid Biochem Mol Biol* 48:347–352.

Délos S, Carsol JL, Ghazarossian E, Raynaud JP, Martin PM. 1995. Testosterone metabolism in primary cultures of human prostate epithelial cells and fibroblasts. *J Steroid Biochem Mol Biol* 55:375–383.

Düker EM, Kopanski L, Schweikert HU. 1989. Inhibition of 5α-reductase activity by extracts from *Sabal serrulata. Planta Med* 55(Supplement):587.

Elghamry MI, Hansel R. 1969. Activity and isolated phytoestrogen of shrub palmetto fruits (*Serenoa repens* Small), a new estrogenic plant. *Experientia* 25:828–829.

El-Sheikh MM, Dakkak MR, Saddique A. 1988. The effect of Permixon® on androgen receptors. *Acta Obstet Gynecol Scand* 67:397–399.

Fang S, Wang X, inventors. International Medical Research I, assignee. 1995. *Composition of Herbal Extracts.* U.S. Patent 5,417,979.

Feifer AH, Fleshner NE, Klotz L. 2002. Analytical accuracy and reliability of commonly used nutritional supplements in prostate disease. *J Urol* 168:150–154.

Gennaro AR, ed. 2000. *Remington: The Science and Practice of Pharmacy.* 20th ed. Baltimore, MD: Lippincott, Williams and Wilkins.

GlaxoSmithKline. 2001. *Approval Package. Duagen (Dutasteride) Soft gel Capsules. Pharmacology Review(s).* Online. Available at http://www.fda.gov/cder/foi/nda/2001/21319_Duagen.htm. Accessed January 8, 2003.

Griebel C, Bames E. 1916. Über eine zur aromatisierung des kognaks dienende palm-frucht. [German]. *Zeitschrift Für Untersuchung Der Nahrung-Und Genussmittel, Sowie Der Gegrauchsgegenstände* 31:282-290.

Harnack LJ, Rydell SA, Stang J. 2001. Prevalence of use of herbal products by adults in the Minneapolis/St Paul, Minn, metropolitan area. *Mayo Clin Proc* 76:688–694.

Harnischfeger G, Stolze H. 1989. Portrait of a medicinal plant *Serenoa repens.* Saw palmetto. *Zeitschrift Für Phytotherapie* 10:71–76.

Hatinguais P, Belle R, Basso Y, Ribet JP, Bauer M, et al. 1981. Composition of the hexane extract from *Serenoa repens* Bartram fruits. *Trav Soc Pharm Montp* 41:253–262.

Hiermann A. 1989. About contents of sabal fruits and their anti-inflammatory effect. *Arch Pharm* (Weinheim) 322:111–114.

Hiipakka RA, Zhang HZ, Dai W, Dai Q, Liao S. 2002. Structure-activity relationships for inhibition of human 5α-reductases by polyphenols. *Biochem Pharmacol* 63:1165–1176.

Iehlé C, Délos S, Guirou O, Tate R, Raynaud JP, Martin PM. 1995. Human prostatic steroid 5α-reductase isoforms. A comparative study of selective inhibitors. *J Steroid Biochem Mol Biol* 54:273–279.

Jommi G, Verotta L, Gariboldi P, Gabetta B. 1988. Constituents of the lipophilic extract of the fruits of *Serenoa repens* (Bart.) small. *Gazz Chim Ital* 118:823–826.

Kloss P. 1966. Steam vaporizable constituents of pressed juice of *Sabal serrulatum* (Roem et Schult). *Arzneimittelforschung* 16:95–96.

Kokkalou E, Souleles C. 1988. Flavonoid constituents of Pelargonium × asperum Enrh. ex Willd. Geraniaceae. *Plant Med Phytother* 22:247–253.

Leung AY, Foster S. 1996. Saw palmetto. *Encyclopedia of Common Natural Ingredients Used in Food, Drugs, and Cosmetics.* 2nd ed. New York: John Wiley & Sons. Pp. 467–469.

Levy MA, Brandt M, Sheedy KM, Dinh JT, Holt DA, Garrison LM, Bergsma DJ, Metcalf BW. 1994. Epristeride is a selective and specific uncompetitive inhibitor of human steroid 5α-reductase isoform 2. *J Steroid Biochem Mol Biol* 48:197–206.

Levy S. 1998. Can saw palmetto be used to treat benign prostatic hypertrophy? *Drug Top* 142:53.

Lowe FC. 2001. Phytotherapy in the management of benign prostatic hyperplasia. *Urology* 58:71–76.

Marra J. 2002. The state of dietary supplements. Even slight increases in growth are better than no growth at all. *Nutraceut World* 5:32, 36, 38, 40.

Medical Economics Co. 2003. *Physicians' Desk Reference*. 57th ed. Montvale, NJ: Medical Economics Co.

Medsafe (New Zealand Medicines and Medical Devices Safety Authority). 2001. *Proscar™ (Finasteride)*. Online. Available at http://www.medsafe.govt.nz/profs/Datasheet/p/proscartab.htm. Accessed November 22, 2002.

Morganti P, Fabrizi G, James B, Bruno C. 1998. Effect of gelatin-cystine and *Serenoa repens* extract on free radicals level and hair growth. *J Appl Cosmetol* 16:57–64.

Nemecz G. 1998. Saw palmetto. *US Pharmacist* 23:97–98, 100, 102.

Niederprüm HJ, Schweikert HU, Thüroff JW, Zänker KS. 1995. Inhibition of steroid 5α-reductase activity by aliphatic fatty acids. Candidates for chemoprevention of prostate cancer. *Ann NY Acad Sci* 768:227–230.

Ondrizek RR, Chan PJ, Patton WC, King A. 1999a. An alternative medicine study of herbal effects on the penetration of zona-free hamster oocytes and the integrity of sperm deoxyribonucleic acid. *Fertil Steril* 71:517–522.

Ondrizek RR, Chan PJ, Patton WC, King A. 1999b. Inhibition of human sperm motility by specific herbs used in alternative medicine. *J Assist Reprod Genet* 16:87–91.

Palacios P, Gutkind G, Rondina RV, de Torries R, Coussio JD. 1983. *Genus Baccharis. II.* Antimicrobial activity of *B. crispa* and *B. notosergila*. *Planta Med* 49(2):128.

Paubert-Braquet M, Cousse H, Raynaud JP, Mencia-Huerta JM, Braquet P. 1998. Effect of the lipidosterolic extract of *Serenoa repens* (Permixon®) and its major components on basic fibroblast growth factor-induced proliferation of cultures of human prostate biopsies. *Eur Urol* 33:340–347.

Peirce A. 1999. *The American Pharmaceutical Association Practical Guide to Natural Medicines*. New York: William Morrow and Company.

Pinn G. 2001. Herbal medicine in renal and genitourinary disease. *Aust Fam Physician* 30:974–977.

Plosker GL, Brogden RN. 1996. *Serenoa repens* (Permixon®). A review of its pharmacology and therapeutic efficacy in benign prostatic hyperplasia. *Drugs Aging* 9:379–395.

Ravenna L, Di Silverio F, Russo MA, Salvatori L, Morgante E, Morrone S, Cardillo MR, Russo A, Frati L, Gulino A, Petrangeli E. 1996. Effects of the lipidosterolic extract of *Serenoa repens* (Permixon®) on human prostatic cell lines. *Prostate* 29:219–230.

Rhodes L, Primka RL, Berman C, Vergult G, Gabriel M, Pierre-Malice M, Gibelin B. 1993. Comparison of finasteride (Proscar®), a 5alpha reductase inhibitor, and various commercial plant extracts in in vitro and in vivo 5alpha reductase inhibition. *Prostate* 22:43–51.

Schöpflin G, Rimpler H, Hänsel R. 1966. Beta sitosterol as an active principle of *Sabal* fruit. *Planta Med* 14:402–407.

Shimada H, Tyler VE, McLaughlin JL. 1997. Biologically active acylglycerides from the berries of saw-palmetto (*Sernoa repens*). *Journal of Natural Products* 60:417-418.

Stenger A, Tarayre JP, Carilla E, et al. 1982. Pharmacology and biochemistry of hexane extract of *Serenoa repens* (PA-109). *Gaz Med Fr* 89:2041–2048.

Strauch G, Perles P, Vergult G, Gabriel M, Gibelin B, Cummings S, Malbecq W, Malice MP. 1994. Comparison of finasteride (Proscar®) and *Serenoa repens* (Permixon®) in the inhibition of 5-α reductase in healthy male volunteers. *Eur Urol* 26:247–252.

Sultan C, Terraza A, Devillier C, Carilla E, Briley M, Loire C, Descomps B. 1984. Inhibition of androgen metabolism and binding by a lipidosterolic extract of "*Serenoa repens* B" in human foreskin fibroblasts. *J Steroid Biochem* 20:515–519.

Thomson PDR. 2004. *Physicans' Desk Reference*. 58th ed. Montvale, NJ: Thompson PDR.

Timmermans LMJ, Timmermans LGJ Jr. 1990. The efficacy of the extracts of *Echinacea* and *Sabal* in the treatment of female idiopathic hypotonic bladder. *Acta Urol Belg* 58(2):43-59.

Tzeng SH, Ko WC, Ko FN, Teng CM. 1991. Inhibition of platelet aggregation by some flavonoids. *Thromb Res* 64:91–100.

USP (United States Pharmacopeia). 2000. *Dietary Supplements. Botanical Monographs. Saw Palmetto.* Online. Available at http://www.usp.org/frameset.htm. Accessed May 24, 2002.

USP. 2002. *The United States Pharmacopeia. The National Formulary. USP 25-NF 20.* Rockville, MD: USP.

Vacherot F, Azzouz M, Gil-Diez-De-Medina S, Colombel M, De La Taille A, Lefrere Belda MA, Abbou CC, Raynaud JP, Chopin DK. 2000. Induction of apoptosis and inhibition of cell proliferation by the lipido-sterolic extract of *Serenoa repens* (LSESr, Permixon®) in benign prostatic hyperplasia. *Prostate* 45:259–266.

Vallancien G, Pariente P. 2001. Treatment of lower urinary tract symptoms suggestive of benign prostatic obstruction in real life practice in France. *Prostate Cancer Prostatic Dis* 4:124–131.

Van Coppenolle F, Le Bourhis X, Carpentier F, Delaby G, Cousse H, Raynaud JP, Dupouy JP, Prevarskaya N. 2000. Pharmacological effects of the lipidosterolic extract of *Serenoa repens* (Permixon®) on rat prostate hyperplasia induced by hyperprolactinemia: Comparison with finasteride. *Prostate* 43:49–58.

Wagner H, Flachsbarth H. 1981. A new antiphlogistic principle from *Sabal serrulata*, I. *Planta Med* 41(3):244-251.

Wagner H, Proksch A, Riess-Maurer I, Vollmar A, Odenthal S, Stuppner H, Jurcic K, Le Turdu M, Fang JN. 1985. Immunostimulating action of polysaccharides (heteroglycans) from higher plants. *Arzneimittelforschung* 35:1069–1075.

Wang C, Makela T, Hase T, Adlercreutz H, Kurzer MS. 1994. Lignans and flavonoids inhibit aromatase enzyme in human preadipocytes. *J Steroid Biochem Mol Biol* 50:205–212.

Weisser H, Tunn S, Behnke B, Krieg M. 1996. Effects of the *Sabal serrulata* extract IDS 89 and its subfractions on 5α-reductase activity in human benign prostatic hyperplasia. *Prostate* 28:300–306.

Wilt TJ, Ishani A, Stark G, MacDonald R, Lau J, Mulrow C. 1998. Saw palmetto extracts for treatment of benign prostatic hyperplasia: A systematic review. *J Am Med Assoc* 280:1604–1609.

TABLE A Individual Components of Saw Palmetto Fruit

Hexane-extractable components[a]

Fatty acids – Breu et al., 1992; Cristoni et al., 1997; De Swaef and Vlietinck, 1996; Hatinguais et al., 1981; Jommi et al., 1988; Kloss, 1966. No data suggestive of toxicity are available.

Valeric acid – C5:0; a possible constituent of fresh saw palmetto fruit (Kloss, 1966).

Caproic – C6:0; contributes to characteristic odor of fresh saw palmetto fruit.

Caprylic acid – C8:0; < 2% of total fatty acids; contributes to characteristic odor of fresh saw palmetto fruit.

Capric acid – C10:0; caprinic acid; < 2% of total fatty acids). *In vitro*: inhibited type 2 steroid 5-α-reductase in homogenates of human genital fibroblasts grown in culture (IC_{50} 1.0 mM) (Niederprüm et al., 1995).

Lauric acid – C12:0; 24% of total fatty acids.

Lauric acid – 0.5 mg/mL ethanol extract (De Swaef and Vlietinck, 1996). *In vitro*: lauric acid inhibited type 2 steroid 5-α-reductase in homogenates of human genital fibroblasts grown in culture (IC_{50} 0.2 mM). Inhibited type 1 steroid 5-α-reductase in homogenates of human prostate tissue (IC_{50} < 0.5 mM) (Niederprüm et al., 1995).

Ethyl laurate – 0.7 mg/mL ethanol extract (De Swaef and Vlietinck, 1996). *In vitro*: ethyl laurate or other esterified forms of lauric acid did not inhibit type 2 steroid 5-α-reductase.

Myristic acid – C14:0; 12% of total fatty acids. *In vitro*: inhibited type 2 steroid 5-α-reductase in homogenates of human genital fibroblasts grown in culture (IC_{40} 0.6 mM) (Niederprüm et al., 1995).

Palmitic acid – C16:0.

Palmitoleic acid – C16:1; 9% of total fatty acids.

Stearic acid – C18:0.

Oleic acid – C18:1; 33% of total fatty acids. *In vitro*: inhibited type 2 steroid 5-α-reductase in homogenates of human genital fibroblasts grown in culture (IC_{50} 0.4 mM) (Niederprüm et al., 1995).

Linoleic acid – C18:2; 4% of total fatty acids. *In vitro*: inhibited type 2 steroid 5-α-reductase in homogenates of human genital fibroblasts grown in culture (IC_{50} 0.08 mM) (Niederprüm et al., 1995).

Linolenic acid – C18:3. *In vitro*: inhibited type 2 steroid 5-α-reductase in homogenates of human genital fibroblasts grown in culture (IC_{50} 0.1 mM) (Niederprüm et al., 1995).

Arachidic acid – C20:0.

Most fatty acids are also present as ethyl esters. Some reviewers reported relatively small proportions as ethyl esters 1 (Nemecz, 1998); however, some investigators reported relatively large amounts (De Swaef and Vlietinck, 1996; De Swaef et al., 1996).

Phenolics – Some of these components have also been reported to be ethanol extractable. No data suggestive of toxicity are available.

Anthranilic acid – an aromatic amine (2-aminobenzoic acid)

Trans-ferulic acid – 3-(4-hydroxy-3-methoxyphenyl)-2-propenoic acid.

Syringaldehyde – 4-hydroxy-3,5-dimethoxy-benzaldehyde.

Vanillic acid – 4-hydroxy-3-methoxy-benzoic acid.

continued

TABLE A Continued

Phytosterols – Sterols may also be present as glycosides. No data suggestive of toxicity are available.
Campesterol – 0.07% of dry weight (Hatinguais et al., 1981).
Cycloartenol – Cristoni et al., 1997; Hatinguais et al., 1981; Jommi et al., 1988.
24-Methylene cycloartenol – Jommi et al., 1988.
Daucosterol – 0.0047% of dry weight (Hiermann, 1989; Schöpflin et al., 1966).
Lupen-3-one – Paubert-Braquet et al., 1998.
Lupeol – Jommi et al., 1988.
β-Sitosterol – 0.0033–0.22% of dry weight (Cristoni et al., 1997; Elghamry and Hansel, 1969; Hatinguais et al., 1981; Hiermann, 1989; Jommi et al., 1988; Schöpflin et al., 1966).
β-Sitosterol, lauroyl
β-Sitosterol, myristoyl
β-Sitosterol, palmitoyl
β-Sitosterol diglucoside
β-Sitosterol 6-O-caprinoyl-β-D-glucoside
β-Sitosterol 6-O-lauryl-β-D-glucoside
β-Sitosterol 6-O-myristyl-β-D-glucoside
Stigmasterol – Cristoni et al., 1997; Hatinguais et al., 1981; Jommi et al., 1988.

Other lipid components – No data suggestive of toxicity are available.
Carotenoids – Griebel and Bames, 1916.
Monoacylglycerols – 1-monolaurin, 1-monomyristin (Shimada et al., 1997).
Triacylglycerols – tridecanoic acid and others (Kloss, 1966).
Valerianic acid ethyl ester – Kloss, 1966.

Ethanol-extractable components

Fatty alcohols – Cristoni et al., 1997; Hatinguais et al., 1981. No data suggestive of toxicity are available.
Behenyl alcohol – C22; docosan-1-ol.
Tricosan-1-ol – C23.
Lignoceryl alcohol – C24; tetracosan-1-ol; 0.004% of dry weight.
Ceryl alcohol – C26; hexacosan-1-ol.
Octacosan-1-ol – C28; 0.46% of dry weight.
Melissyl alcohol – C30; triacontan-1-ol; 0.033% of dry weight.

Flavonoids – May be present as aglycones and/or glycosides. Glycosides are listed in this table indented below the relevant aglycone flavonoid. Flavonoids are widespread in the human diet and no toxicities have been associated with them.
Apigenin – 4′,5,7-trihydroxyflavone. *In vitro*: weak cytotoxicity (0.8 mgdisc) (Palacios et al., 1983).
Rhoifolin – apigenin 7-O-neohesperidoside (Hiermann, 1989).
Kaempferol – 3,4′,5,7-tetrahydroxy-flavone (Hiermann, 1989). *In vitro*: inhibitor of human prostate type 2 steroid 5-α-reductase (transfected as cDNA into rat 1A cells in culture; IC_{50} 12 μM) (Hiipakka et al., 2002). Inhibited platelet aggregation (Kokkalou and Souleles, 1988; Tzeng et al., 1991). Competitive inhibitor of aromatase in human preadipose cells in culture (Ki 27 μM) (Wang et al., 1994).

TABLE A Continued

Quercitrin – 3,3′,4′,5,7-pentahydroxyflavone (Hiermann, 1989). *In vitro*: inhibitor of human prostate type 1 steroid 5-α-reductase (transfected as cDNA into rat 1A cells in culture; IC_{50} 23 μM) (Hiipakka et al., 2002). Inhibited platelet aggregation and (Kokkalou and Souleles, 1988).
Isoquercitrin – quercetin-3-glucoside (Hiermann, 1989).
Rutin – quercitin-3-O-rutinoside (Hiermann, 1989).
Polyprenoids – No data suggestive of toxicity are available.
Farnesol – C15:3; 3 isoprenic units (Jommi et al., 1988). *In vitro*: farnesol or geraniol (30 ηg/mL) inhibited proliferation of human prostate cells in culture induced by basic fibroblast growth factor (BFGF) or epidermal growth factor (EGF) (Paubert-Braquet et al., 1998; data not shown). Geraniol is a precursor of farnesyl pyrophosphate and geranyl geraniol.
Phytol – C20:1; 4 isoprenic units (Jommi et al., 1988).
Geranyl geraniol – C20:4; 4 isoprenic units (Jommi et al., 1988).
Serenoa polyprenol 2 – C30; 0.0005% of dry weight (Jommi et al., 1988).
Serenoa polyprenol 3 – C35; 0.0035% of dry weight (Jommi et al., 1988).
Octamethyldotriacontaoctaenol – C40:8; 8 isoprenic units; 0.027% of dry weight (Jommi et al., 1988).
Nonamethylhexatriacontanonaenol – C45:9; 9 isoprenic units (Jommi et al., 1988).
Phenolic glycosides – No data suggestive of toxicity are available.
Populin – 2-(hydroxymethyl)phenyl-β-D-glucopyranoside 6-benzoate (Hiermann, 1989).
Water-soluble components
Saccharides – No data suggestive of toxicity are available.
Monosaccharides – Glucose, fructose, galactose, mannose, arabinose, fucose, rhamnose, glucuronic acid, uronic acid, xylose (Harnischfeger and Stolze, 1989; Jommi et al., 1988; Wagner and Flachsbarth, 1981).
Polysaccharides: galactoarabane.
High-molecular-weight polysaccharides: acidic high molecular weight polysaccharides (25–500 kDa with immunostimulating activity) (Wagner et al., 1985).

NOTE: IC_{50} = concentration at which response has decreased to 50 percent of the original response, cDNA = complementary to mRNA.

TABLE B Summary of Adverse Effects in Clinical Trials Using Saw Palmetto in Blended Preparations

Study Design	Subjects	Parameters Monitored	Supplement / Placebo / Reference	Adverse Effects and Related Findings
Clinical Trial Using Blended Preparations with Female Subjects 1 trial, 20 subjects ingested blended saw palmetto-containing preparations, 10 subjects in placebo group				
Timmermans and Timmermans, 1990 Randomized? Double-blind? Placebo-control	*Condition:* **Hypotonic bladder** [incontinence (18 subjects) and other conditions] *Age:* 25-76 y ***All subjects were female.***	*Parameters monitored:* Unknown	Saw palmetto group: *Number of subjects:* **20** (25–68 y, mean age of 45 y) *Type:* **Extract of saw palmetto fruit** plus extract of *Echinacea purpurea* in drops[a] *Amount:* **78-104 mg/day** (90-120 drops/day) *Route:* Oral *Frequency:* ~3 times/day (20–25 drops/dose) *Duration:* ~77 **days** (mean)	**Saw palmetto group:** **Adverse effects:** Unknown
			Placebo group: ***Number of subjects:*** **10 (29–76 y, mean age of 52 y)** *Form:* **Drops** *Duration:* **~52 days (mean)**	**Placebo group:** **Adverse effects:** Unknown

[a] Urgenin® (Madaus GmbH, Wien, Austria) contained an extract/tincture of saw palmetto fruit (78-104 mg/day) and an extract of rhizomes/roots of purple coneflower (*Echinacea purpurea*) (84-112 mg/day). This product was a liquid intended for use as drops (~25 drops) to be ingested in water before meals (or after meals in subjects with gastric disturbances). **Urgenin was used in the one clinical trial with female subjects summarized in this table.**

TABLE C Saw Palmetto: Summary of a Clinical Case Reports (no relevant data available)

No relevant clinical case reports

TABLE D Saw Palmetto: Summary of Adverse Event Reports (no relevant data available)

No relevant adverse event reports

TABLE E Saw Palmetto: Summary of Animal Studies

Study Design	Results and Conclusions
Studies with rats (oral administration)	
Male Wistars Extract of saw palmetto fruit (several hypercritical CO_2 extracts)	Rat model of prostate hyperplasia due to androgen stimulation: in castrated prepubescent rats, administration of testosterone (15 µg/d, subcutaneously, for 10 d) stimulated prostate hyperplasia Oral administration of an extract of saw palmetto fruit inhibited testosterone-induced increase in prostate weight by 38% (150 mg extract/d) or 76% (300 mg extract/d); two other extracts were less effective (Cristoni et al., 1997)
Male Wistars Extract of saw palmetto fruit (50 mg/kg body weight/d, oral gavage, for 90 d; control was 2.5% ethanol vehicle) Castrated on day 0, hormone implants (estradiol implanted on day 7; testosterone implanted on day 21)	Rat model of prostate hyperplasia due to androgen stimulation: in castrated rats, administration of estradiol plus testosterone (over 3 mo following castration) stimulated prostate hyperplasia (maximal effect at 30 d) Oral administration of extract of saw palmetto fruit (50 mg/kg body weight/d) inhibited hormone-induced increase in prostate weight (maximal effect at 60 d and 90 d for the dorsal and lateral regions of the rat prostate; maximal effect at 30 d and 60 d for ventral region) (Paubert-Braquet et al., 1998)
Males Extract of saw palmetto fruit	Rat model of prostate hyperplasia due to androgen stimulation: in castrated rats, administration of testosterone stimulated prostate hyperplasia Oral administration of an extract of saw palmetto fruit (200 mg/d, for 6 d) inhibited hormone-induced increase in prostate weight (Plosker and Brogden, 1996; Stenger et al., 1982)
Immature males Extract of saw palmetto fruit (180 or 1,800 mg/d, in methyl cellulose in water, by gavage, BID), finasteride (0.1 or 10 mg/d, oral, BID) or cottonseed oil (2 ml, 5% ethanol, by gavage, control) Castrated; treatment was started on the day following castration and continued for 7 d: testosterone propionate (10 µg/d, subcutaneously), dihydrotestosterone (DHT) propionate (20 µg/d, subcutaneously), or	Rat model of prostate hyperplasia due to androgen stimulation: in castrated rats, administration of testosterone or DHT stimulated prostate hyperplasia; coadministration of finasteride inhibited testosterone-stimulated prostate growth Coadministration of an extract of saw palmetto fruit did not inhibit testosterone-stimulated prostate growth Coadministration of finasteride or extracts of saw palmetto fruit did not inhibit DHT-stimulated prostate growth (Rhodes et al., 1993)

TABLE E Continued

Study Design	Results and Conclusions
cottonseed oil (0.2 mL/d, subcutaneously, control); prostate was removed and weighed	
Mature male Wistars Sulpiride (40 mg/kg/d, ip); extract of saw palmetto fruit (100, 320, or 640 mg/kg/d, in 2.5% ethanol, by gavage), finasteride (5 mg/kg/d, in 2.5% ethanol, by gavage), or vehicle (2.5% ethanol, by gavage); treatments conducted for 30 days Control, castrated, sham-castrated, castrated/testosterone-implanted (resulting in subnormal testosterone level), castrated/DHT-implanted; castrated/adrenalectomized rats also mentioned (data not shown)	Rat model of prostate hyperplasia due to androgen stimulation: in castrated rats, administration of testosterone or DHT stimulated prostate hyperplasia Administration of extract of saw palmetto fruit (at 100 or 320 mg/kg/d) did not alter weight of the lateral lobe of the prostate in castrated, castrated/testosterone-treated, or castrated/ DHT-treated rats; only at 640 mg/kg/d did the extract decrease (by 59%) the weight of the lateral lobe in castrated/ testosterone-treated rats For comparison, finasteride (5 mg/kg/d) decreased (by 67%) the weight of the lateral lobe in castrated/testosterone-implanted rats (but not in castrated/DHT-implanted rats) (Van Coppenolle et al., 2000)
Studies with mice (oral administration)	
Males Extract of saw palmetto fruit	Murine model of prostate hyperplasia due to androgen stimulation: in castrated mice administration of testosterone stimulated prostate hyperplasia Oral administration of an extract of saw palmetto fruit (300 mg/d, for 12 days) inhibited hormone-induced increase in prostate weight (Plosker and Brogden, 1996; Stenger et al., 1982)
Studies with dogs (oral administration)	
20 males with moderate-severe prostate enlargement, but without clinical signs of prostatic hyperplasia, > 4 yr, 25–30 kg body weight) Extract of saw palmetto fruit Group A: 8 dogs, 1,500 mg/d, TID, orally, five 100-mg capsules per treatment, ~10 mg/kg/d, for 91 days Group B: 6 dogs, 300 mg/d, TID, orally, one 100-mg capsule per treatment, ~10 mg/kg/d, for 91 days	Benign prostatic hypertrophy model in dogs (the only domestic animal that commonly develops prostatic hyperplasia in aging)

continued

TABLE E Continued

Study Design	Results and Conclusions
Group C: 6 dogs, vehicle alone Vehicle was a meatball of canned dog food	

NOTE: BID = twice per day (amount listed is the total amount administered per day), TID = three times per day (amount listed is the total amount administered per day). Other animal toxicity studies in rats, mice, and dogs have been reported in a review article (Bombardelli and Morazzoni, 1997); however, primary publications of these studies were not available.

TABLE F Saw Palmetto: Summary of *In Vitro* Studies

Substance	Study Design	Results and Conclusions
Alteration of cells		
Saw palmetto, extract of fruit (Permixon)	Cells in culture: PC3 cells cotransfected with androgen receptor (wild-type) and CAT reporter genes (under control of androgen response element)	Addition of extract (25–50 µg/mL) inhibited CAT transcription induced by androgen (methyltrienolone) stimulation. No effect was observed in the absence of androgen-stimulation or in mock-transfected cells (Ravenna et al., 1996).
Saw palmetto, extract of fruit (Permixon), 10 µg/mL for 24 hours	*In situ* studies in human prostate biopsy samples: Normal tissue donors: 10 donors; 9 were ages 20–29 y, 1 was age 51 y BPH biopsy tissue samples: 10 from subjects without medical treatment, ages 62–83 y; 10 from subjects ingesting extract of saw palmetto fruit for previous 3 mo, 320 mg/d, BID	Model of proliferation/ apoptotic balance in prostate tissue samples: in epithelial tissue from subjects with BPH who had ingested extract, apoptotic index was increased (as assessed by TUNEL) compared with samples from subjects with untreated BPH. A small increase in the apoptotic index was observed in stromal tissue. In epithelial and stromal tissue from subjects with BPH who had ingested extract, proliferative index was decreased (as assessed by a MIB-1 immunohistochemical stain for Ki-67 proliferation antigen) compared to samples from subjects with untreated BPH (Vacherot et al., 2000). (The proliferative index is increased in untreated BPH tissues as compared with normal tissues. Ingestion of extract returned the proliferative index to the level found in normal tissue.)

continued

TABLE F Continued

Substance	Study Design	Results and Conclusions
Inhibition of enzymes		
Saw palmetto, extract of fruit	5-α-reductase from human prostate (obtained from patients undergoing surgery for BPH)	Addition of any of 4 extracts inhibited 5-α-reductase. IC_{50} values: 5.6 μg/mL (Permixon), 7.0 μg/mL (Talso, presumed to be the same as Talso uno), 31 μg/mL (Strogen forte), 40 μg/mL (Prostagutt, presumed to be the same as Prostagutt uno) For comparison, IC_{50} for finasteride: 1 μg/mL (Rhodes et al., 1993).
Saw palmetto, extract of fruit (Permixon)	Cells in culture: human foreskin fibroblasts (from healthy infants or adults)	Addition of extract inhibited steroid 5-α-reductase (conversion of testosterone to DHT) and 3-α-hydroxysteroid dehydrogenase (conversion of DHT to androstanediol) in assays using intact cells. Addition of extract inhibited binding of [^{3}H]-DHT to androgen receptor(s) in cytosolic, nuclear, and whole cell fractions. Addition of extract inhibited binding of [^{3}H]-methyltrienolone (R1881) to cytosolic components of rat prostate (Sultan et al., 1984).
Extract of fruit (Permixon)	Cells in primary culture: Human prostate epithelial cells: from subjects with PBH (IC_{50} = 40 μg/mL); from subjects with prostate adenocarcinoma (IC_{50} = 90 μg/mL) Human prostate fibroblasts: from subjects with PBH (IC_{50} = 200 μg/mL); from subjects with prostate adenocarcinoma (IC_{50} = 70 μg/mL)	Addition of extract inhibited metabolism of [^{3}H]-testosterone (0.1 μM) to all metabolites (DHT, androst-4-ene-3,17-dione, 5-α-androstane-3,17-dione). By comparison, finasteride inhibited metabolism of [^{3}H]-testosterone (0.1 μM) to DHT and 5-α-androstane-3,17-dione (IC_{50} = 20–40 ηM for fibroblasts; IC_{50} = > 100 ηM for epithelial cells),

TABLE F Continued

Substance	Study Design	Results and Conclusions
		but not androst-4-ene-3,17-dione (Δ4-A) (Délos et al., 1995).
Extract of fruit (Permixon), 10 μg/mL	Cells in coculture: human prostate fibroblasts and epithelial cells	Addition of extract inhibited type I and type II steroid 5-α-reductase activity (Bayne et al., 1999).
Extract of fruit (Permixon)	Cells in culture: human prostatic carcinoma cell line (DU 145)	Addition of extract inhibited metabolism of [^{3}H]-testosterone (0.1 μM, 1–6 h) by intact cells in culture (Délos et al., 1994).
Extract of fruit (Permixon)	Human steroid 5-α-reductase, type 1 and 2 isoforms expressed in insect cells (fall armyworm, *Spodoptera frugiperda* Sf9) transfected with baculovirus DNA (*Autographa californica* nuclear polyhedrosis virus, AcNPV)	Addition of extract inhibited baculovirus DNA steroid 5-α-reductase activity in cell homogenates of transfected cells (using 5 mM NADPH; 1 μM [^{3}H]-testosterone for IC_{50} assays; 0.1–10 μM [^{3}H]-testosterone for K_i assays). Type 1 isoform: noncompetitive inhibition; IC_{50} = 4 μg/mL, K_i = 7–8 μg/mL (Délos et al., 1995; Iehlé et al., 1995). Type 2 isoform: uncompetitive inhibition; IC_{50} = 7 μg/mL, K_i = 5 μg/mL (Iehlé et al., 1995). For comparison, finasteride was found to be a competitive inhibitor of 5α-reductase type 1 (IC_{50} = 0.5 μM, K_i = 0.3 μM) and type 2 (IC_{50} = 11 ηM, K_i = 7 ηM).
		Addition of extract inhibited activity of partially purified, expressed type 1 steroid 5-α-reductase (liposome entrapped to preserve activity of this nuclear membrane-associated enzyme) (Iehlé et al., 1995).

continued

TABLE F Continued

Substance	Study Design	Results and Conclusions
Extract of fruit (Palmae, prepared by supercritical CO_2 extraction)	Homogenate of human prostatic tissue (obtained during suprapubic prostatectomy)	Addition of extract (0.5 mg/mL) inhibited steroid 5-α-reductase activity in prostate epithelium and stroma (Weisser et al., 1996)
Alcoholic extract of fruit (Remigeron, alcoholic extract)	Cells in culture: human genital skin fibroblasts	Addition of alcoholic extract inhibited steroid 5-α-reductase in homogenate of fibroblasts (IC_{50} 0.005% solution of the dried extract) and in intact fibroblasts (IC_{50} 0.01% solution of the dried extract). Binding to the androgen receptor could not be demonstrated (Düker et al., 1989).
Petroleum ether extract of fruit	Cells in culture: human genital skin fibroblasts	Addition of pet ether extract inhibited steroid 5-α-reductase of fibroblasts. The inhibitory activity was enriched in the pet ether extract vs. an alcoholic extract (Remigeron) (Düker et al., 1989).
Other		
Extract of fruit (Permixon), 10 μg/mL for 4 d	Cells in coculture: human prostate fibroblasts and epithelial cells	Addition of extract did not inhibit secretion of PSA (Bayne et al., 1999).
Extract of fruit (Permixon)	Cytosolic androgen (DHT) receptor binding assay in rat prostate	Addition of extract inhibited binding of [^{3}H]-methyltrienolone (R1881). IC_{50} was 0.4 μg/mL (Carilla et al., 1984).
Extract of fruit (Permixon)	Cytosolic androgen receptor (DHT) binding assay in human tissues: uterus (1 specimen, 42-year-old female); vaginal skin (2-, 30- and 33-year-old females) Abdominal wall (2-, 30-, and 32-year-old females) Foreskin (6, newborn males)	Addition of extract inhibited binding of radiolabeled DHT and testosterone (El-Sheikh et al., 1988).

TABLE F Continued

Substance	Study Design	Results and Conclusions
Extract of fruit	Rat prostate androgen (DHT) receptor binding assay	Binding of DHT was not inhibited by the extract (data not shown) (Rhodes et al., 1993).

NOTE: 3-α-hydroxysteroid dehydrogenase is also called 3-ketosteroid reductase. CAT = chloramphenicol acetyltransferase, BPH = benign prostatic hypertrophy, TUNEL = terminal deoxynucleotidyl transferase dUTP nick end labeling, BID = twice a day, MIB-1 = a monoclonal antibody used to detect Ki-67 antigen, Ki-67, a proliferation antigen, a cellular protein which is not present during G_0 phase of cell cycle, IC_{50} = concentration at which response has decreased 50 percent of the original response, DHT = dihydrotestosterone, PBH = prostate benign hyperplasia, PSA = prostate-specific antigen.

TABLE G Saw Palmetto: Related Substances That Might Suggest Risk

Related Substance	Safety Issues
Functionally related therapeutic substances[abc]	
Steroid 5-α-reductase inhibitors[d]	Pregnancy category X: Dutasteride is contraindicated for use in women (GlaxoSmithKline, 2001). Finasteride is contraindicated in pregnancy or in women who may become pregnant (Medical Economics Co., 2003) and is classified as not intended for use by women (Medsafe, 2001). Possible adverse effect: low plasma level of DHT caused by exposure of women to dutasteride may inhibit fetal development of male external genitalia and internal reproductive organs (GlaxoSmithKline, 2001). Animal studies Mice – the maximum tolerated dose of finasteride was 250 mg/kg/d. Rats, teratogenicity studies – finasteride was not teratogenic in rats (320 mg/kg/d, 24 mo). Rats, developmental studies – in pregnant rats treated with finasteride (0.1–100 μg/kg/d), male offspring developed hypospadias (penile defect, urethral opening is displaced to the under surface) in a dose-dependent manner (3.6% incidence at 0.1 μg/kg/d; 100% incidence at 100 μg/kg/d). In pregnant rats treated with finasteride (≥ 30 μg/kg/d), male offspring were observed to have smaller prostate, smaller seminal vesicles, delayed preputial/foreskin separation, and transient nipple development as compared to control animals. In pregnant rats treated with finasteride (≥ 3 μg/kg/d), male offspring displayed a decreased anogenital distance. The critical period is day 16 to day 17 during gestation (a total of 21 d in the rat) for male offspring exposed *in utero* to manifest the effects already described. No developmental effects were observed in female offspring exposed *in utero* to finasteride at any dose studied. Rabbits, developmental studies – no developmental defects were observed in rabbit pups exposed to finasteride (up to 100 mg/kg/d) *in utero* (days 6–18 of gestation). Monkeys, developmental studies – finasteride (0.8 μg/d, i.v.) was administered to pregnant rhesus monkeys (days 20–100 of gestation); no developmental abnormalities were observed in the male fetuses. In other studies, finasteride (2 mg/kg/d) administered orally to pregnant rhesus monkeys resulted in defects in the formation of the external genitalia of male fetuses; female fetuses were not affected.

TABLE G Continued

[a] To construct this table, substances were considered that are structurally, taxonomically, and functionally related to saw palmetto fruit, extracts saw palmetto fruit, or their constituents (see Table A). Only the substances considered to be relevant to the risk of saw palmetto as a dietary supplement are included in the table. "Functionally related" substances may exhibit an activity that saw palmetto exhibits, based on *in vitro* or other data; they are not listed here because they have a similar chemical composition

[b] Botanical ingredients in dietary supplements with uses similar to extracts of saw palmetto fruit were considered. No data suggestive of toxicity are available and thus these substances were omitted from this table. The following substances were considered: extract of African palm tree bark (*Pygeum africanum*); extract of bark or leaves of aspen trees (*Populi tremula*); goathead vine (*Tribulus terrestris*); pumpkin seed (*Cucurbita pepo*; whole seeds, coarsely ground seeds or extract of seeds); extract of rhizomes/root purple coneflower (*Echinacea purpurea*); extract of stinging nettle root (*Urtica dioica*) (**should be avoided by pregnant women**) (Peirce, 1999).

[c] SPES® (Botanic Labs, Brea CA), a blend of 15 botanical ingredients, was also considered but was not included in this table because it is not related to saw palmetto. Three of the ingredients of SPES are also in PC SPES® (a saw palmetto-containing blend of 8 botanicals); however, SPES does not contain saw palmetto. Additionally, SPES is used for cancer, not BPH. PC SPES is used in prostate cancer and BPH. The ingredients of PC SPES are described in a footnote to **Table B-2**. The ingredients of SPES are as follows: licorice (rhizome/root of *Glycyrrhiza glabra* Fisch/*Glycyrrhiza uralensis* Fisch, gan-zao), blushred rabdosia (leaf of *Rabdosia rubescens* Hara, dong-ling-cao), ginseng (root of *Panax pseudoginseng* Wall, jen-sheng), reishi mushroom (stem of *Ganoderma japonicum*, ling-zhi), desert ginseng (*Cistanche deserticola*, cheng-min chou), pear-leaf wintergreen (*Pyrola rotundifolia* L., lu-ti-cao), hairy agrimony (*Agrimonia pilosa* Lebed/*Agrimonia japonica*, xian-he-cao), yenhusuo/yan-hu-so (*Corydalis yanhusuo*/*Corydalis bulbosa*), higanbana/red spider lily (*Lycoris radiata*, shi-suan), mou-hui tou (*Patrinia heterophylla*), di-bu-long (*Stephania delavayi* Diels), runan/shan-wu-gui (*Stephania sinica* Diels, hua-jian-jiu-teng), golden cow in the soil/prickly-ash (*Zanthoxylum nitidum*, liang-mian-zhen), rokujo (*Cervus nippon* Temminck, lu-jung), and pollen (hua-feng) (Fang and Wang, 1995). SPES may also contain soy milk. During analysis of specific lots of SPES substantial amounts of a synthetic drug (alprazolam, Xanax®) were identified (California Department of Health Services, 2002). SPES is no longer available on the market in the United States.

[d] Steroid 5-α-reductase inhibitors include: **finasteride** (Proscar®, MK-906; competitive inhibitor, selective inhibitor of human type 2 steroid 5-α-reductase, 50-fold selectivity), **dutaseride** (Duagen, GI-198745; inhibitor of human type 1 and type 2 steroid 5-α-reductase), **epristeride** (SKF 105657, a 3-androstene-3-carboxylic acid; uncompetitive inhibitor; selective inhibitor of human type 2 steroid 5-α-reductase, 400-fold selectivity), **izonsteride** (LY320236, a benzoquinolinone; competitive inhibitor of human type 1 steroid 5-α-reductase; noncompetitive inhibitor of type 2 steroid 5-α-reductase), and **4MA** (N,N-diethyl-4-methyl-3-oxo-4-aza-5-α-androstane-17-β-carboxamide, a 3-oxo-4-aza steroid; potent inhibitor of type 1 and type 2 steroid 5-α-reductase; potent inhibitor of 3β-hydroxysteroid dehydrogenase). Type 2 steroid 5-α-reductase is the predominant activity in human prostate; rat prostate contains equal activity of type 1 and type 2 (Levy et al., 1994). DHT = dihydrotestosterone.

Appendix L

Acknowledgments

The Committee on Framework for Evaluating the Safety of Dietary Supplements and the Food and Nutrition Board and Board on Life Sciences staff are grateful for the time and effort of the many contributors who participated in the workshops and meetings leading up to this report. Through openly sharing their considerable expertise and perspectives, these individuals brought clarity and focus to the challenging task of developing a useable and science-based framework for evaluating the safety of dietary supplement ingredients.

The list below mentions those individuals with whom we worked closely, but many others also deserve mention. Those individuals, whose names we do not know, made important contributions to the report by offering suggestions and insight at the many professional meetings and workshops the committee members attended. A number of the organizations listed below provided nominations for committee membership. The committee members, as well as the project staff, thank the following named (as well as unnamed) individuals and organizations.

INDVIDUALS AND ORGANIZATIONS

F. Alan Andersen
Cosmetic Ingredient Review

Valdimir Anisimov
N.N. Petrov Research Institute Oncology

Dennis Awang
Mediplant

Adrianne Bendich
Council for Responsible Nutrition

Joseph Betz
American Herbal Products Association

Kristen Blanchard
Nutramax Laboratories, Inc.

Paul Bolar
Pharmavite LLC

Luke Bucci
Weider Nutrition International & Schiff Vitamins

Walter Chambliss
American Pharmaceutical Association

Keith Cheng
Pennsylvania State University

Edward Croom
Council for Responsible Nutrition

Steven Dentali
American Herbal Products Association

Annette Dickinson
Council for Responsible Nutrition

John Doull
Kansas University Medical Center

Debora Ferrier
Self-employed

Kenneth Fisher
Consultant

Albert Fleischner
Goen Technologies

David Graham
Food and Drug Administration

Marcia Greenblum
American Dietetic Association

Richard Hall
Flavor and Extract Manufacturers Association

John C. Hammell
International Advocates for Health Freedom

John Hathcock
Council for Responsible Nutrition

J.T. Heimbach
JHeimbach LLC

James Kababick
Flora Research

James Komorowski
Nutrition 21, Inc.

Claire Kruger
Environ International

Gilbert A. Leveille
Consultant

Jeffrey Lipsius
Threshold Enterprises

Peter Ludwell
The Law Loft

Richard Malter
Retired

Hulon McClain
Whitehall-Robins Healthcare

David Roll
United States Pharmacopeia

Alan Rulis
Food and Drug Administration

Louis Scarano
Environmental Protection Agency

David Schardt
Center for Science in the Public Interest

Bruce Silverglade
Center for Science in the Public Interest

R. William Soller
Consumer Healthcare Products Association

Christine Lewis Taylor
Food and Drug Administration

Thomas N. Tiedt
Med-Tox Group

Susan Trimbo
Nutricia

Roy Upton
American Herbal Pharmacopoeia

José Vergés
BIOIBÉRICA S.A.

John Vincent
University of Alabama

John Walker
Environmental Protection Agency

Sidney Wolfe
Public Citizen's Health Research Group

Snow Wynter
Dietary Supplement Quality

Anthony Young
American Herbal Products Association

Appendix M

Biographical Sketches of Committee Members

Barbara O. Schneeman, Ph.D. (*Chair*), currently serves as a professor of nutrition in the Department of Nutrition and in the Division of Clinical Nutrition and Metabolism, is Associate Vice Provost for University Outreach, and previously served as dean, College of Agricultural and Environmental Sciences at the University of California at Davis. Her professional activities include membership on the U.S. Department of Agriculture (USDA)/Department of Health and Human Services 1990 and 1995 Dietary Guidelines for Americans Advisory Committee, the Board of Trustees of the International Life Sciences Institute-North America, and the editorial boards of *Proceedings of the Society of Experimental Biology and Medicine*, Food and Nutrition Series of Academic Press, *Nutrition Reviews*, *Journal of Nutrition*, and *California Agriculture*. Professional honors include the Institute of Food Technologists' Samuel Cate Prescott award for research, the Commissioner's Special Citation, and the Harvey W. Wiley Medal from the Food and Drug Administration (FDA) in recognition of her contributions toward the advancement of scientific research. Dr. Schneeman has also been active in developing state and national nutrition policy as an appointed member of the California State Board of Food and Agriculture and USDA public advisory board. She is currently president of the Dannon Institute, is a member of the Board of Trustees of the International Life Sciences Institute, and has been elected a Fellow of the American Association for the Advancement of Science. She recently served as Assistant Administrator for Human Nutrition of the USDA Agricultural Research Service (on leave from U.C. Davis). Dr. Schneeman's research areas include fat absorption, complex carbohydrates, dietary fiber, and gastrointestinal function.

Daniel L. Azarnoff, M.D., is president of D.L. Azarnoff Associates, through which he does consulting with the pharmaceutical industry. He also serves as senior vice president of Clinical/Regulatory Affairs at Cellegy Pharmaceuticals, Inc. Dr. Azarnoff's expertise includes pharmaceutical industry administration, pharmacology, clinical pharmacology, and general internal medicine. His research interests include the drug approval process, including preclinical (pharmacology, toxicology, pharmaceutics) and clinical (therapeutic, bioequivalence trials), drugs to treat hyperlipoproteinemia, and transdermal drug delivery. Dr. Azarnoff earned his M.D. from the University of Kansas where he became KUMC Distinguished Professor of Medicine and Pharmacology and previously served as president of Research and Development for the Searle Pharmaceutical Company.

Cindy L. Christiansen, Ph.D., is director, Statistics Section, Center for Health Quality, Outcomes, and Economic Research, which is a Veterans Health Administration Center of Excellence, and is an associate professor of health services at Boston University School of Public Health. Dr. Christiansen, a fellow of the American Statistical Association, has served as chair of their Section on Health Policy Statistics, is an associate editor for the *American Statistician,* and a column editor for the publication *Chance*. She is one of the country's leading experts on hierarchical and predictive models and their use in health services research. Her research interests include the development and implementation of multilevel and prediction models for health service and medical applications, and her methodological work has focused on Poisson models and on models for grouped ordinal data.

Alice M. Clark, Ph.D., serves as vice chancellor for Research and Sponsored Programs at the University of Mississippi and is a Frederick A.P. Barnard Distinguished Professor, as well as a professor of pharmacognosy and research professor of the Research Institute of Pharmaceutical Sciences at the University. Prior to assuming her current position in July 2001, Dr. Clark was director of the National Center for Natural Products Research (NCNPR), which operates as a drug discovery and development program that works on acquisition, preparation, and *in vitro* evaluation of extracts of higher plants and marine organisms for beneficial activity. Dr. Clark's research interests are in evaluation of natural compounds for antibiotic and antifungal activity, as well as in the utilization of microorganisms as predictive models for drug metabolism and as synthetic adjuncts. She was part of an NCNPR group working on a Centers for Disease Control and Prevention-funded project to evaluate the potential for botanical dietary supplements to interact with pharmaceuticals, to review the scientific literature on specific botanicals, and to review consumer use of botanical dietary supplements. Dr. Clark also serves as associate editor for the *Journal of Natural Products*.

Norman R. Farnsworth, Ph.D., is a distinguished university professor, research professor of pharmacognosy, director of the Pharmacognosy Graduate Program, and the director of the Program for Collaborative Research in the Pharmaceutical Sciences at the University of Illinois at Chicago (UIC). Dr. Farnsworth also serves as Director of the UIC/National Institutes of Health (NIH) Dietary Supplements Research Center at UIC. He is credited with designing a worldwide computer database, NAPRALERT, that compiles scientific literature on the safety and efficacy of herbal medicines, plants, marine organisms, and fungi. Dr. Farnsworth is also director of the World Health Organization (WHO) Collaborating Center for Traditional Medicine; using the NAPRALERT database, he has lead WHO's publication of numerous monographs reviewing traditional medicinals. He is a member of Health Canada's Expert Advisory Committee on Natural Health Products and served on the U.S. Commission on Dietary Supplement Labels authorized by the Dietary Supplement Health and Education Act of 1994. Dr. Farnsworth serves on the Scientific Advisory Board of the Herb Research Foundation, the Board of Trustees of the American Botanical Council, and the editorial advisory board of several peer-reviewed journals and *Herbalgram.* He has authored a number of publications about botanicals, including *Botanical Dietary Supplements Quality, Safety, and Efficacy.* His research interests include analysis of chemical and biological data on natural products, and isolation, identification, and structure elucidation of biologically active plant constituents.

Ted Gansler, M.D., M.B.A., is director of Medical Information Strategy at the American Cancer Society (ACS) and editor of the ACS publication *CA: A Cancer Journal for Clinicians.* At ACS, Dr. Gansler is responsible for assuring the accuracy of printed and electronic information products for patients, the general public, and health professionals. He is a graduate of Duke University, University of Pittsburgh School of Medicine, and Georgia State University School of Business Administration, and he completed a pathology residency and cytopathology fellowship at the University of Pennsylvania. Until recently, Dr. Gansler practiced cytopathology and surgical pathology at Emory University, and is currently an adjunct associate professor of pathology at Emory.

James E. Gibson, Ph.D., is a research professor of pharmacology and toxicology with the Brody School of Medicine at East Carolina University. Prior to his current appointment, Dr. Gibson was with Dow Agro Sciences, a world leader in the development and manufacture of chemicals and biotechnology for agriculture; former positions include global director for Regulatory, Toxicology and Environmental Affairs for Dowlanco and director of Toxicology Affairs for the Dow Chemical Company. In addition to teaching and establishing a program in toxicology, Dr. Gibson is currently pursuing research in developing and evaluating innovative *in vitro* methods for the safety and exposure assessments of biotechnology products. He received the Alexander von Humboldt Senior U.S. Scientist Award and is a recipient of the Society of Toxicology Achievement Award.

Stephen A. Goldman, M.D., F.A.P.M, F.A.P.A., is the managing member of Stephen A. Goldman Consulting Services, LLC, an independent consultancy that specializes in all aspects of medical product safety. He has extensive experience in academic/clinical medicine, public health, federal medical product safety regulation, and the pharmaceutical industry, with fellowship training in both clinical pharmacology/regulatory drug evaluation sciences and consultation-liaison psychiatry. Dr. Goldman was formerly medical director of the FDA MedWatch postmarketing surveillance and medical product safety information program. Prior to his work at FDA, he was director, Pharmacoepidemiology, at Knoll Pharmaceutical Company (Abbott Laboratories). He has performed original lithium/neuroleptic neurotoxicity research utilizing the FDA Spontaneous Reporting System database, and published numerous articles on medical product safety, adverse event reporting, and clinical psychiatry. Among honors received at FDA were the Commissioner's Special Citation/Harvey W. Wiley Medal and the Office of the Commissioner's Commendable Service Award. He is a fellow of the Academy of Psychosomatic Medicine and distinguished fellow of the American Psychiatric Association and holds an academic appointment as adjunct assistant professor of psychiatry at the Uniformed Services University of the Health Sciences. Dr. Goldman is a recognized expert in assessment, communication, and management of risk associated with medical product use.

Philip S. Guzelian, M.D., serves as the director of Medical Toxicology and codirector of the Hepatobiliary Research Center at the University of Colorado Health Sciences Center. Dr. Guzelian earned his M.D. at the University of Wisconsin-Madison. His research interests include liver disease, hepatic drug metabolism and toxicity, medical toxicology, and cytochrome P450. His research objective is to understand how cells recognize the presence of foreign chemicals and activate host defenses. Dr. Guzelian has been elected to membership in the Association of American Physicians and the Academy of Toxicological Sciences. He has been a member of the NIH National Advisory Environmental Health Sciences Council, chairman of the Toxicology Advisory Committee of the Burroughs Wellcome Fund, and a member of the drug safety scientific advisory committee for Rhone-Poulenc Rorer Pharmaceuticals, the Board of Scientific Directors of the International Life Sciences Institute, and the Board of Scientific and Policy Advisors of the American Council of Science and Health. He is also an *ad hoc* member of the Environmental Protection Agency's (EPA) Office of Science Coordination and Policy Scientific Advisory Panel and has served on EPA's Science Review Board for the Food Quality Protection Act.

Elizabeth Jeffery, Ph.D., serves as professor of nutritional toxicology at the Department of Food Science and Human Nutrition, the Division of Nutritional Sciences and the Department of Pharmacology at the University of Illinois, Urbana-Champaign. She has a Ph.D. in biochemistry from the University of London (U.K.) and teaches and conducts research in the area of safety and efficacy of functional foods and dietary supplements. Dr. Jeffery investigates the potential for soy to affect bone health and for broccoli and other crucifers to prevent cancer. Dr. Jeffery is a past editor of the American Society for Pharmacology and Experimental Therapeutics *Drug Metabolism* Newsletter and past associate editor of *Toxicology and Applied Pharmacology*. She is presently chair of the Bioactive Components Research Interest Section of the American Society for Nutritional Sciences, chair of the Toxicology Division of the American Society for Pharmacology and Experimental Therapeutics, and secretary/treasurer of the Food Safety Specialty Section of the Society of Toxicology.

Loren D. Koller, D.V.M., Ph.D., is an independent consultant with over 30 years of experience as a researcher in the areas of pathology, toxicology, immunology, carcinogenesis, and nutrition. Dr. Koller's past employment has been with National Institute of Environmental Health Sciences, Oregon State University, and University of Idaho. He has published in numerous refereed journals in his areas of interest, and served on several editorial boards, grant review panels, and as a consultant to government, business, and private firms. Dr. Koller has been engaged in biomedical environmental research relating to health effects in humans most of his career, including while serving as a dean in the College of Veterinary Medicine at Oregon State University for 10 years. He has experience and knowledge in agriculture, biomedicine, and environmental health, with an appreciation and sensitivity of the issues involved in developing federal regulations. He has served on committees for the National Cancer Institute, Agency for Toxic Substance and Disease Registry, Centers for Disease Control and Prevention, and U.S. Army, and on the National Advisory Committee to Establish Acute Exposure Guidelines for Hazardous Substances. Dr. Koller is a fellow of the Academy of Toxicological Science. He has cotaught veterinary microscopic anatomy, pathology, advanced clinical and diagnostic toxicology, tumor pathology, principles of toxicology, environmental and comparative toxicology, and target organ toxicology.

Joseph Lau, M.D., is a professor of medicine at the Tufts University School of Medicine and professor of clinical research at the Sackler School of Graduate Biomedical Sciences at Tufts University. He is also director of the Boston branch of the U.S. Cochrane Center and director of one of the 13 Agency for Health Care Research and Quality designated Evidence-based Practice Centers, located at the Tufts-New England Medical Center in Boston. Dr. Lau also directs the evidence review team of the National

Kidney Foundation's clinical practice guidelines program. Dr. Lau is interested in methodological issues in meta-analysis and the translation of evidence into practice. He has published extensively on the methodologies and clinical applications of meta-analysis. He is a member of the editorial board of *Clinical Evidence* and has served on FDA advisory committees and on study sections for the Agency for Health Care Research and Quality. Dr. Lau received his M.D. from the Tufts University School of Medicine.

Russell J. Molyneux, Ph.D., is a research chemist and project leader with the Western Regional Research Center of USDA in Albany, CA. He received his Ph.D. in organic chemistry from the University of Nottingham, United Kingdom, and was a postdoctoral fellow at the University of Oregon. Dr. Molyneux's primary field of interest is natural products chemistry, especially isolation and identification of compounds responsible for toxicity of plants to mammals, insects, or other plants (allelopathy). His recent research has focused on fused bicyclic alkaloids of the pyrrolizidine, quinolizidine, indolizidine, and nortropane classes, in particular the isolation and detection of new structural types from novel sources. Dr. Molyneux's current research is concerned with polyhydroxylated alkaloids, phytochemical constituents of crop plants that confer resistance to colonization and contamination by toxin-producing fungi, and metabolites of fungi responsible for grapevine diseases. He served as associate editor of the journal *Phytochemical Analysis* and is currently associate editor of the *Journal of Agricultural and Food Chemistry,* an American Chemical Society publication.

Susan S. Percival, Ph.D., is a professor of food science and human nutrition at the University of Florida. Dr. Percival is a recipient of the Future Leaders Award from the International Life Sciences Institute Nutrition Foundation. Her research interests include nutrition and immunity; effects of botanicals, phytochemicals, and trace elements on immune function; antioxidant bioavailability and impact on immunity; efficacy of dietary supplements in humans; and mechanistic studies in animal and cell culture models. While much of her research has focused on the metabolism of copper and other trace elements, Dr. Percival's research currently focuses on health effects of different fruit phytochemicals, Echinacea, and components of green tea.

Cheryl L. Rock, Ph.D., R.D., is a professor in the Department of Family and Preventive Medicine and the Cancer Prevention and Control Program at the University of California, San Diego, School of Medicine. She received her doctoral degree in nutritional sciences from the University of California, Los Angeles, School of Public Health. Dr. Rock's primary research efforts are focused on the role of nutritional and dietary factors in the development and progression of cancer in women, particularly breast and cervical cancer, and her research efforts also address eating pathology and weight concerns in women. She is presently involved in randomized trials that are testing whether modifications in diet and level of physical activity can alter biological processes and progression of cancer. She currently serves on editorial boards for several peer-reviewed journals and has been an invited participant in several NIH review committees, workshops, and meetings.

Jerrold M. Ward, D.V.M., Ph.D., recently became chief, Infectious Disease Pathogenesis Section, National Institute of Allergy and Infectious Diseases, Bethesda, Maryland, under a contract to So Bran, Inc.; most recently he was chief of the Veterinary and Tumor Pathology Section, Center for Cancer Research, National Cancer Institute (NCI), Frederick, Maryland, during the period of report preparation. He was also formerly head, Tumor Pathology, National Toxicology Program (NTP), NCI, Bethesda. Dr. Ward is an expert in the field of veterinary and toxicologic pathology. He was involved with the early development of the NCI bioassay program, publication of the first 200 NCI and NTP carcinogenesis bioassay reports (blue books), and was later a member of the NTP Technical Reports Subcommittee of the NTP Board of Scientific Councilors. Dr. Ward received his D.V.M. from Cornell University and his Ph.D. in comparative pathology from the University of California, Davis, and is board-certified in veterinary pathology (Diplomate, ACVP). He has served on several editorial boards of pathology journals and as an advisor for safety evaluation of toxins, carcinogenesis, and pathology in several capacities. Dr. Ward has also contributed to writing the *Society for Toxicologic Pathology Guidelines for Toxicologic Pathology* and has over 350 publications. He is the recipient of the NIH Director's Award for the discovery of a new Helicobacter and the FDA Commissioner's Special Citation for contribution to the Interagency Working Group on Nitrite Research.

Index

A

B

D

E

F

G

H

I

N

National Center for Complementary and Alternative Medicine, 66-67

O

P

R

S

W

X